The Medical School App Guide - Worldwide 2012-2013

For students with an undergraduate degree

3rd Edition

Dibah Jiva, Nottingham Medical School, UK, 2012

Bijan Teja, Dartmouth Medical School, US, 2013

To request permission, email admin@themsag.com

ISBN: 978-0-9869269-0-7

Published by Dibah Jiva and Bijan Teja

■ *About the authors*

D ibah Jiva is a fourth year medical student in the Graduate Entry Medicine program at the University of Nottingham (UK), who has been helping students gain admission to medical school for the past four years. She graduated with an honors degree in Nutrition from McGill University (Canada).

Her current projects and work alongside medical school include the Nutrition Center (www.TheIsmaili.org/nutrition) and a collection of 4 medical school application guides known as the MSAGs. The Nutrition Centre is a guide to traditional foods of African, Central Asian, South Asian, and Middle Eastern origin. She previously worked in clinical research and has given talks on healthy eating.

Bijan Teja is a fourth year medical student and second year business student in the MD/MBA program at Dartmouth College, one of the Ivy League universities in the US. He graduated with great distinction from Mcgill University in 2007 with a BSc. in physics, and since graduating has personally helped many students with their medical school applications, essays, and interviews.

Alongside his medical education, he co-writes and co-publishes four guides to medical school application. He previously worked in cancer research at the Tom Baker Cancer Center in Calgary, volunteered with cancer patients and conducted smoking cessation counseling for the community in New Hampshire (US). At business school he has developed business strategies for a struggling non-profit agency dedicated to keeping the elderly in their homes, and has worked with ophthalmologists at the university's medical center to help them improve cataract care processes. Bijan is currently taking a year off before his final year of the dual degree program to work in Tajikistan with the Aga Khan Development Network.

Between the two authors, they have gained admission to medical school in Canada, the United States and the United Kingdom. They have personally helped applicants successfully gain admission in the Canada, the United States, the United Kingdom, Ireland and the Caribbean.

■ *Preface*

We have create a unique guidebook that is now the most comprehensive resource available on the market on applying to medical school abroad. This guide is written for students who are currently completing an undergraduate degree or who have completed an undergraduate degree and are considering applying to medical school. It covers everything you need to know to apply to medical programs offered in English in the following countries:

1. Canada
2. United Kingdom
3. United States
4. Australia
5. Caribbean
6. Croatia
7. Czech Republic
8. Hungary
9. Ireland
10. Poland
11. Romania
12. Slovak Republic
13. Ukraine

Among these 13 countries, we have covered 115 programs open to students who have completed an undergraduate degree worldwide. This is the only guide on the market that gives such global information on medical school application for prospective students, all in one book.

This guide aims to be a user-friendly and up to date resource to prepare for medical school applications and increase your chance of admission. It is full of essential information to help you secure your place at the medical school of your choice.

It includes **for each** of the **115 programs in English** in the 13 countries (for the US and Caribbean, it is for a selection of programs):

• Admissions policies

- Selection formulas
- Entrance statistics
- Course requirements
- Degree requirements
- Entrance exam requirements
- Interview structure and content information
- Tips from the medical school admissions offices
- Tuition fees
- Contact details

The guidebook has been written in partnership with the medical schools, getting all the information from them directly mostly by phone, but also by email and personal visits. Alongside the complete information available for each medical program, other sections are packed with expert advice, insider's tips and very useful summary tables so you can refer to everything you need at a glance.

The sections with **expert advice, insider's tips** and very useful **summary tables** are:

✦ Entrance statistics section
- Statistics are presented for each medical program.
- Find out how many students apply and how many get admitted.
- Competitiveness is a key factor in deciding where to apply.

✦Returning to practice at home section
- If you choose to study medicine abroad, one of the key factors in choosing your medical school is the ease with which you can come back to practice at home.
- 3 sections dedicated to explaining the procedures involved in coming back to practice medicine in Canada, the UK and the US.
- Information on exams to write and level of competitiveness to help you make an informed decision.

✦ What are your chances section for Canada and the UK
- These are 2 unique sections, not available in any other guidebook or online.
- Find out which medical schools may consider your profile more favorably
  - If you do not have a 2:1 (have a 2:2 or a third)
  - If you have a low MCAT score
  - If you do not have healthcare experience

- If you have a low or high GAMSAT score
- If you have a low or high UKCAT score
- If you have a bad year in your GPA
- Etc.
- Medical school admissions is so competitive that it is essential to know where you have the greatest chances, as well as where you do not based on your profile.

◆ Personal statement section
- We explain using quotes from medical schools, what the admissions committees are looking for in your personal statement and essays.
- Also find expert help on how to plan, structure and write your personal statements, with tips on style, content and professionalism.
- Find examples of successful personal statements and essays from graduate applicants covering different profiles and anecdotes such as healthcare work experience, teaching experience, non-scientific background, research experience, explaining low grades, why medicine, etc.
- All personal statement extracts come with critiques that highlight particular strengths and weaknesses of the extract to help you evaluate your own drafts.

◆ Medical school interview section
- Unique summary table of the interview structures at each medical school
- Expert advice on how to structure answers for different types of questions:
  - Questions asking for examples / anecdotes
  - "Dealing with" or "handling difficult situations" questions
  - Expression an opinion, point of view, ethical questions
- Most common interview questions explored in detail with a structure and method to help you prepare a personal answer to all questions.
- A variety of medical ethics and scenario questions presented and explained.

For completeness the guidebook also includes **all other essential information** you may need to apply to medical school:

◆ University rankings
- Global university rankings and medical school specific rankings from different sources for all countries.
◆ International applicants

- Information on admissions policies as well as entrance statistics for international students in the different countries.
✦ Reference letters
  - Expert advice on who to ask and how to ask in order to obtain the best reference letters for your application.
✦ GAMSAT, UKCAT, BMAT, MCAT
  - Everything about the tests, timings, structure, marking system, content.
  - Scoring and your chances at medical schools explained. Each university uses scores very differently and this is an essential factor in deciding where to apply.
  - Full guide on all the resources available to you in order to prepare including books, practice tests, personal tutors, courses and interactive resources.
✦ Cost of applying to and studying medicine
  - Information on costs of applying and studying medicine, as well as information on loans and bursaries to help finance your medical education in different countries.

We have spent over 2000 hours compiling this information over three years and updating it each year. It should save you time, provide you with information that is not easily found elsewhere on all your options and most importantly, help you get into medical school successfully.

Dibah Jiva and Bijan Teja

■ *Acknowledgements*

We would also like to thank the following friends and colleagues for their various contributions to this guide:

Rahima Alani, SABA School of Medicine 2012
Shahid Ali, Dartmouth Medical School/Harvard School of Public Health 2013
Aja Bjerke, Dartmouth Medical School 2011
Laura Brown, Dartmouth Medical School 2012
Adam Kassam, Dartmouth Medical School/Columbia School of Public Health 2013
Suzanne Kellman, Dartmouth Medical School 2010
Farhan Merali, Harvard Medical School 2012
James Peers, University of Nottingham 2012
Omar Samji JD, Associate Attorney, Gibson Dunn
Alia Teja, Royal College of Surgeons in Ireland 2011
Joseph Westaby, University of Nottingham 2012
Ben Young, Dartmouth Medical School 2011

In order to write this book, we have needed help from many people and institutions. We are particularly grateful to the staff who work in the medical school admissions offices. They spent a considerable amount of time responding to our questions by email and on the phone, providing us with the material to write this guide.

We would also like to thank Jamil, Shabrina, Aziz, Fuibah, Jabin and our parents for their love, help and support.

Application process summaries & general information

Where to apply

Whether you have excellent grades or have not achieved the grades you hoped to achieve in your undergraduate degree, "where to apply" is one of the most important and challenging question to answer. In this section we hope to give you a concise summary of the competitiveness and important application considerations when applying to medical schools in the countries covered in this guide. For each country below, you will find information on:

1. Number of medical programs in English
2. General admissions statistics
3. Competitiveness - GPA and academic requirements
4. Pre-requisites, entrance exams and other entrance requirements
5. Application process summaries

You will find more details on class structures, detailed statistics and detailed admissions requirements in the country specific sections on the following pages:

Students from the US, Canada, the UK and elsewhere may choose to study medicine abroad such as in Australia, the Caribbean, Ireland or Eastern Europe. Medical schools in these countries are usually easier to gain admission to with lower GPA and lower MCAT or GAMSAT score requirements. Some schools in countries like the Czech Republic and Australia also allow students to enter a 4 year program without a completed undergraduate degree (as several schools in Canada do), allowing some students to finish their medical training earlier than they would have had they waited to apply in their home country. If for some personal reasons, you were not able to complete your undergraduate degree, these medical schools can be a good option. For some countries such as Australia, Romania and the Caribbean, the application deadlines are usually later than the final decision dates for Canadian, UK and US schools, allowing students to apply after they have heard back from schools in their home country.

There are many advantages to applying to medical schools abroad and these are detailed in the country specific introductions below. However, downsides also need to be considered. When returning to your home country to practice, you might be at a disadvantage when competing for residency/training posts compared to local medical graduates. Match rates tend to be higher for US students who graduated from US schools than US students who studied abroad (see page 108 for more details). However, in the US for example, USMLE scores carry a lot of weight in the residency match and thus you can make up for this by doing well in your USMLE examination. There are other minor disadvantages you might want to consider such as the more limited number of hospitals available during your rotation years at some programs such as those at some Caribbean schools. This being said, the most significant thing you want to be careful about is the accreditation of the medical school you are choosing, to make sure you can work where you plan to once you graduate. Even if a school is WHO (World Health Organization) listed, medical graduates from certain medical schools may not be allowed to practice in their country/state of choice. Refer to the "returning home to practice" section on page 93 for information on returning to practice in your home country after graduation from an international medical school.

Canada

There are 17 medical schools in Canada, 13 of which offer their medical program in English, 3 of which offer their medical program in French and 1 that offers 2 medical programs, one in English and one in French. In this guide, we cover application to the 14 English taught medical programs in Canada (but not the French medical programs). Most medical programs in

Canada are 4 years in length except the two 3-year programs offered at the University of Calgary and at McMaster University [3, 4].

In 2009, there were 10,457 Canadian applicants. Approximately 2,815 Canadian applicants received at least one offer of admission (approximately 2535 enrolled, 30 deferred and 250 declined). This means that approximately 27% of Canadian applicants were offered admission that year. In 2009, there were also 189 applicants from the US, of whom 14 were granted at least one offer of admission, for an admission rate of 7.4%. Finally, 299 students from other foreign countries applied, of which 34 were accepted to at least one school, for an admission rate of 11.4% [5]. (see page 122 for more details on international application in Canada).

In general, Canadian medical schools place more weight on grades and test scores in their admissions processes than medical schools in the US. The average GPA in 2010 for entering students at Canadian medical schools ranges between roughly 3.66 to 3.88, and the average MCAT scores range from roughly 28 to 33, but note that schools vary significantly in their GPA calculation methods (see page 110 for more details).

Although every school accepts some out-of-province students, almost all schools favor in-province applicants. The two schools in Canada that do not favor in-province students are the University of Toronto and Queen's University [6, 7]. See page 122 for the number of out-of-province and international students accepted at each school.

Many schools require applicants to complete prerequisite courses and/or a certain number of credits before applying, but unlike some European medical schools, there are no universities in Canada that require applicants to have an undergraduate degree in a scientific discipline to be eligible. All undergraduate majors are accepted equally as long as the prerequisite and minimum credit requirements are met, and the courses taken show academic endeavor. The five medical programs in Canada that do NOT require any prerequisite courses are those offered at McMaster university, the University of Calgary, the Northern Ontario School of Medicine, the University of Western Ontario and Dalhousie Medical School. The University of Saskatchewan does not require prerequisite courses for certain applicants.

Outside Ontario, prospective students apply directly to the medical school through their website. In Ontario (6 universities), the application process is centralized through the Ontario Medical School Application Service (OMSAS, available at www.ouac.on.ca/omsas). Most applications close between September and November.

Many medical schools in Canada do not require students to hold an undergraduate degree to enter their program and allow students who are in their second or third year of their undergraduate studies to apply for admission. See page 121 for more information on this.

Regarding standardized examinations, most schools require the MCAT except the University of Ottawa [8], the Northern Ontario School of Medicine [9], and the 3 programs in Quebec taught in French [10-12]. At McGill University, CEGEP students are exempt from taking the MCAT, and submission of MCAT scores is optional for students applying with degrees from Canadian universities. The University of Saskatchewan does not require the MCAT for in-province applicants under certain conditions [13].

In addition to grades and MCAT scores, the application consists of reference letters, personal statements, essays and/or activity lists. The specific requirements for each medical school are outlined in the school specific sections (page 147) and in table format on page 140. All medical schools in Canada interview students before offering a place. Most Canadian schools now use MMI format interviews (see page 447 for information on interviews).

Application statistics and selection ratios for each school are listed in the school specific sections on page 110 and in table format on page 116. Web links to the schools' statistics are also provided on page 114.

United Kingdom

If you are a student with an undergraduate degree, a healthcare professional or any other professional who wants to study medicine, you may have the option to apply to any of the 53 available programs in the UK. These programs can take 4, 5 or 6 years to complete. Out of the 53 medical programs, 16 are 4 year programs, 27 are 5 year programs and 10 are 6 year programs. In general, 6 year programs tend to be for applicants who do not have a scientific background and 4 year programs tend to be the most competitive programs to gain admission to. However, this is not true for every medical school. The admissions policies and academic requirements for each school can be found in the school specific sections on page 190.

In 2010 there were 7,947 places to study medicine in the UK for 20,938 applicants, meaning that approximately 40% of students were offered a place in at least one program.

Most 4 year programs are open only to 'home applicants', which include UK and European Union applicants; however, a few of them, such as the programs at the University of Warwick and Imperial College London, also have some places reserved for non-E.U applicants. Most 5 year and 6 year programs are open to international applicants, although the number of allocated spaces is limited by a governmental quota. Refer to page 206 for information on international entrance statistics and number of places.

Medical Schools in the UK are generally more forgiving than Canadian medical schools toward students with lower performance in their undergraduate degree, with most schools requiring an upper second class honours degree (equivalent to a GPA of approximately 3.4 - 3.6, or lower in some cases). Some programs such as the University of Nottingham require a lower second class honours degree, and Peninsula Medical School requires a third class honours degree (see "what are your chances with a 2:2 in your undergraduate degree" on page 210 for more details).

About 50% of 4 year programs in the UK consider applications from students who completed their first degree in a scientific discipline. The other half considers any undergraduate degree, including arts, social sciences or humanities. Most of the 5 year programs accept all undergraduate degree. There are a few exceptions to this such as the University of Dundee who consider applications to their 5 year program only from students with an undergraduate degree in a scientific discipline. All 6 year programs open to graduate applicants allow students to apply with degrees from non-scientific disciplines. Each school's policy regarding which undergraduate degrees are accepted is outlined in the section "undergraduate science degree vs. non-science degree" on page 203.

The application process for most programs is centralized through UCAS and is exclusively online (www.ucas.co.uk). The application opens the week of June 15th. Applicants can only apply to 4 medical programs at a time. Making a well informed decision in choosing which schools to apply to significantly increases the chances of admission.

Note that the only program that does not use the UCAS application form is the University of Liverpool Foundation for Health Studies program (6 years). See the school specific section on page 265 for more details.

Some schools like Cambridge and Oxford ask applicants to submit an additional personal statement and ask for additional reference letters. Alongside the UCAS application, most, but not all schools, require applicants to write either the GAMSAT, BMAT or UKCAT. The GAMSAT is offered once a year in the UK and is also offered in Australia, New Zealand, London, Singapore and Washington, USA. As the exam is not offered year round, applicants should make sure not to miss the deadline for registration for their application year. Once the

UCAS applications are submitted and the schools receive the applicants' GAMSAT, BMAT or UKCAT scores, applicants may be notified of an unsuccessful application or be invited for an interview. One exception is the University of Southampton, where graduate applicants to the 5-year program are normally not interviewed (only international graduates are interviewed).

For details on the interview structures of each school and advice on how to prepare for interviews, please refer to page 447. After the interview stage, applicants either receive a refusal, a notification that they are on the waiting list, a conditional offer or an unconditional offer.

United States

There are currently 133 medical schools in the United States offering 4 year programs in medicine. In 2010, there were 580,304 applications from 42,742 applicants. Out of the 42,742 applicants, 18,665 matriculated to a medical school. Overall, approximately 47% of US students applying to medical school in the US are accepted each year [14]. Acceptance percentages for international applicants tend to be slightly lower.

Most programs are open to out-of-state and international applicants, but the number of international applicants accepted at each medical school varies widely. Approximately 17% of US schools are relatively open to international applicants and accept 5 or more international students each year, while roughly 40% accept no international students at all (see page 301 for more details on foreign application in the US).

The US medical schools vary substantially in the weight they place on grades and test scores in their admission process, as well as their ratios of number of applicants to number of students accepted. There are some very competitive schools in the US that accept as few as 3-4% of applicants such as Harvard University and Yale university, but also many well established schools in the US that have higher acceptance percentages than Canadian and UK schools.

As is the case in Canada, medical schools in the US usually require applicants to complete prerequisite courses before applying, but unlike European medical schools, there is no preference given to students with scientific degrees. All undergraduate majors are accepted equally provided the prerequisite requirements are met, and the applicant has shown academic endeavor in their studies. A study at Harvard Medical School found that students are successful in medical school regardless of their undergraduate major, as long as they have adequate preparation in sciences.

Unlike Canada and the UK, most US medical schools use a rolling admissions process. This means that at schools where this is the case, students are only accepted until the class is full, causing students who apply early to have a very significant advantage over those who apply later.

There are four steps in the US medical school application process.

Step 1: The first step is completing the primary application (AMCAS application), which is sent to nearly all schools. It includes a 5300 character personal statement and 15 activity/award descriptions. Only 9 schools are not using the AMCAS application in 2011. These are the seven schools using the Texas Medical and Dental School Application Service (TMDSAS), the University of Missouri-Kansas City, and the University of North Dakota. The updated list of medical schools using the AMCAS application for entry in 2011 is available one the AAMC website: https://www.aamc.org/students/applying/amcas/participating_schools/

Step 2: You will then complete a secondary application for each school, which usually involves school specific essays, reference letters and a secondary application fee. Some schools screen applicants before inviting them to complete a secondary application while others allow all students to complete it.

Step 3: Many schools then use certain unspoken MCAT and GPA cutoffs to screen applicants (this is done either after step 1 or 2). If the baseline academic cutoffs are met, the applicant's essays, references etc. are read by a subcommittee and if the subcommittee agrees that holistically, you are a good candidate, they request that you be granted an interview. Interviews usually take place on campus but you can occasionally request to interview with alumni close to your home or your university.

Step 4: Admissions decision - once interviewed, your application file and interview scores are sent to a committee where the admissions decision is made.

Students can apply to as many schools as they like. We recommend applying to many schools as this significantly increases your chances of admission. The average student applying in the United States applies to 13.6 medical schools [14].

Australia

There are 12 graduate entry programs in Australia offered by 11 universities. Nine medical programs accept international applicants offering a total of approximately 400 places in 2012 for international applicants. The University of Queensland and the University of Melbourne accept the greatest number of international applicants.

All graduate entry programs in Australia require applicants to have completed or be in the final year of a bachelor's degree. No preference is given to any particular major in the undergraduate degree, but note that the University of Melbourne has prerequisite courses that must have been completed.

All applicants for Commonwealth Supported Places and other domestic places at graduate-entry schools (i.e. citizens/permanent residents of Australia and citizens of New Zealand) must have a current GAMSAT (Graduate Australian Medical School Admission Test) score. Scores from either the current or previous year can be used for the application. This means if one applied in 2012, he or she can use test scores from 2011 or 2012.

The GAMSAT Consortium is introducing an on-line application and matching system for applicants to Australian graduate-entry medical schools. This is a new centralized system that all graduate entry programs participate in except the program at the University of Sydney. GEMSAS will increase the number of preferences available for applicants to medical schools and provide an equitable and transparent allocation process. Details on the GEMSAS application can be found on page 326. The fact that the University of Sydney does not participate means that you can apply through GEMSAS and get a medical school interview this way, but can also have a second chance at interview by applying to the University of Sydney separately.

Please note that at the time of publication of this guidebook, GEMSAS is not yet certain if they will manage international student applications through GEMSAS in 2012, but this issue is currently being discussed with the universities. If this new system is approved, international applicants will have the choice of applying directly to the universities or applying to them through GEMSAS. If they apply through GEMSAS, they will be offered up to six preferences said the GEMSAS office. However, the ACER applicant guidebook states that international applicants will be offered up to 2 places only. Please monitor the ACER and GEMSAS websites where information will be posted later this year revealing whether or not international applicants will be eligible to apply through GEMSAS.

All applications from local students will be handled by GEMSAS.

Although most Australian Universities have a mandatory interview, which can sometimes be done by phone for international students, the University of Queensland no longer interviews applicants for their graduate entry program. The GPA, GAMSAT and MCAT minimum requirements in Australia tend to be slightly lower than those in North America and the UK; the minimum GPA is usually 5.0 out of 7.0 (roughly 2.67 out of 4.0 or a lower second class honours). In general, the minimum requirement for the MCAT is 8/8/8/M, but for some universities, applicants need to score significantly higher to be competitive. Some schools set more competitive cutoffs based on competition, and many weigh the most recent years of study at university more heavily than the first years. Specific GPA and GAMSAT/MCAT score requirements for each medical school are listed in the school specific sections on page 331.

Applications to Australian medical schools open in early May. Offers of admission are made between late October and mid-December. Australian schools begin classes in February. Since the application deadline for Australian schools is around the end of June, as an international applicant, you can wait to hear from Canadian, US and/or UK schools and then apply to Australian schools to start the following February if you wish.

Caribbean

As of June, 2010, we have identified 30 medical schools operating in the Caribbean teaching medical programs in English. There may be more than 30 schools, as new schools are created frequently and although there are lists of schools on different websites, we did not find any of the lists to be 100% accurate. The medical schools listed in this guidebook are medical schools that we verified exist and operate. Also note that we did not include medical schools that teach in Spanish and medical schools in Cuba. A paper on the performance of Caribbean medical school graduates on the USMLE tests published by FAIMER in the Journal 'Academic Medicine' in 2011 found that as of June 2010, there were 56 schools in the Caribbean, including Cuban medical schools and schools without English programs. In the past 10 years, 5 schools have closed. 22 schools have been educating students for 10 years or less, and 90% of the students in Caribbean schools are taught at medical schools where English is the language of instruction [15]. Note that of the approximately 10,400 international medical graduates certified to practice in the US in 2009, approximately 25% (2,600) graduated from the Caribbean. Around 2000 Canadian students are estimated to be currently studying in the Caribbean.

It is notable that although a few medical schools close down every couple of years, approximately 10 new medical schools are in development and this shows a trend towards more places to study medicine in the Caribbean in the years to come.

Although most 4 year Caribbean medical programs require applicants to have completed an undergraduate degree at an accredited university before starting the medical program, some medical schools allow applicants to enter after completing 90 credits. It is good to note that even with travel and insurance costs, schools in the Caribbean are usually less expensive than US medical schools.

Students usually submit applications directly to the medical schools and complete an interview by phone or at a site near them with a university representative. Application requirements include reference letters, 1 or 2 essays, and an application form with work, academic and personal information. Just like most US schools, most Caribbean schools use rolling admission which means that a student increases his or her chances of acceptance by submitting their application form early.

One major difference compared with the application process for North American and E.U medical schools is that there are 3 applications periods in the year for most Caribbean schools, so you can apply and matriculate at 3 different times in the year. At some schools, it can be advantageous to apply for the January and May start dates as the September start date tends to receive more applications per place. Details on the application periods are given in the school specific sections on page 355. The average GPA of entering students at Caribbean medical schools is roughly 3.2 to 3.4 out of 4.0, with scores ranging from 2.7 to 4.0 at some schools, but also lower GPAs at other schools. The average MCAT scores for enrolling medical students is usually around 26, with most competitive applicants generally scoring above 20.

Croatia

There are currently 2 medical schools in Croatia offering programs in English: the University of Split, which offers one 6 year program, and the University of Zagreb, which offers a 4 year program and a 6 year program. Students with premedical university courses or students who wish to combine the first two years can finish the 6 year program in 5 years at the University of Zagreb. Both programs are open to students from all nationalities.

The application form at the University of Zagreb includes basic information such as educational background and passport information. Students also submit a copy of their CV. Students who have not completed secondary school (high school) physics, chemistry and biology usually need to write an entrance examination covering these subjects. Sample examinations and a list of topics are available from the university's website. For US applicants, the ACT and/or SAT I and SAT II exams may be acceptable in place of the university's entrance exam. The University of Split gives advantages to students who have taken the MCAT or the SAT, and also requires a CV. In addition, students write a statement about their reasons for wanting to study medicine in English in Split.

In the 2010-2011 application cycle, the deadline for application was July 1st and late applications could sometimes be accepted until mid-September. The deadlines for next year's entry have not been released at the date of publication of this guidebook.

Czech Republic

There are seven 6 year medical programs offered in English in the Czech Republic at the five Charles University Faculties, Masaryk University and Palacky University. At Masaryk University, students can receive credit for the first two years of the program if their premedical courses cover the same material as the first two years of the program (anatomy, physiology, etc.). All programs are open to all nationalities.

A few universities like Charles University Faculty of Medicine in Hradec Králové and Palacky University ask for reference letters and a copy of the applicant's CV, but most universities like Masaryk University base their admissions decision primarily on an entrance examination. The entrance examinations, when required, are usually offered both at the university and in other countries (UK, USA, Taiwan, Norway and other countries depending on the university) where the university has official representatives. A few medical schools like Charles University Second Faculty of Medicine and Palacky University allow students who have taken the MCAT or SATs to be exempted from writing their entrance examination. Strong grades can also allow students to gain exemption from the entrance examinations at some universities like Palacky University and Charles University in Hradec Králové.

All universities except for Charles University, Faculty of Medicine in Pilsen and Masaryk University require an interview at least for some applicants. At some medical schools like Charles University Faculty of Medicine in Hradec Králové, the interviews are very short and are used to assess English language proficiency and basic motivation for a career in medicine. At other medical schools, the interview is performed by a board of admissions and may evaluate students' motivation, problem solving skills and communication skills in more depth. See the school specific sections on page 369 for more details on the requirements and admissions details of each medical school.

Application deadlines are usually in May-June, and the entrance exams normally take place between May and September. Resources for the exams including sample questions and a list of topics covered are available on most universities' websites.

Competitiveness for places ranges between the schools but in general, the medical schools have 2 applicants for each place on average. Keep in mind of course that not all applicants accept an admission offer, and the rate of acceptance is thus higher than 50%.

Charles University Second Faculty of Medicine has commented on application agencies, who help students with the application process for additional fees:

"Some agencies provide a reliable service (we have had decent experience with Academic Agency, www.academicstudy.eu). However, there are also other recruitment agencies that might help the applicants with only part of the required paperwork or just charge a ridiculous amount of money virtually for nothing." [16]

Hungary

Hungary is a European Union member country situated in the middle of Europe with borders to Austria, Slovakia, the Ukraine, Romania, Croatia and Slovenia. There are four 6 year English taught medical programs in Hungary offered by the University of Pécs, Semmelweis University, the University of Debrecen and the University of Szeged. At the University of Pécs and the University of Szeged, students can receive credit for having taken premedical courses if they covered similar material to the courses taught in the programs (anatomy, physiology etc). All three programs are open to students of all nationalities. Most students apply to the universities through university representatives in their country or region.

All four medical programs require an entrance examination for admission, however, note that at the University of Pécs, the University of Debrecen and the University of Szeged, students with undergraduate degrees or strong grades may be granted exemption (see the school specific sections on page 378 for more details). Otherwise, the exams can be scheduled with the university's representatives in the applicant's country (or in the closest country with a university representative).

Details on the examinations including topics covered and practice questions are available from the schools' websites. The schools' application processes include basic information, and students generally need to submit a copy of their CV and 1 or 2 reference letters as well. Most applicants are interviewed as part of the admissions process, and the interviews generally cover chemistry or biology, as well as communication skills and the applicant's motivation. More details about each medical school are available from the school specific sections.

The application deadlines are between April and June, and the examinations can be scheduled around those times with the universities or the university representatives. Late applications can sometimes be accepted.

The programs tend to accept quite a few English speaking students each year, and actively recruit students from around the world. At the University of Pécs and Semmelweis University, there are approximately 3 applicants for each position offered. Remember, of course, that some applicants get into more than one school and thus the universities accept more students than the number of places available.

For Canadian students, one website outlining the application requirements for each school is available from Julia Barta (international representative): www.getglobaleducation.com/application.html Some other international representatives also have their own websites, including www.studymedicineineurope.com/about.html for US students.

Ireland

There are 6 medical schools in Ireland offering a total of 12 medical programs that are either 4, 5 or 6 years in length. This guide covers the application process for E.U and non-E.U undergraduate students and professionals. It does not discuss the application process for students finishing secondary school (high school). Of the 12 medical programs offered, four are 4-year graduate entry programs (GEPs), five are 5-year medical programs and three are 6-year medical programs.

In Ireland, E.U students are usually admitted based on achieving an upper second class honours degree and their performance on the GAMSAT exam for the 4 year programs, or based on their secondary school examination results and the HPAT-Ireland exam for the 5 and 6 year programs. Most non-E.U students including North Americans apply through an agency in their country. Competition for places varies significantly, but some schools like RCSI have average MCAT scores as high as Canadian and US schools (29 in recent years at RCSI) and GAMSAT cutoffs higher than most UK schools (63 in 2010 at RCSI), while other programs may be less competitive.

There is a different application process for E.U students, North American students and other students. E.U students apply through the Central Application Office (CAO) of Ireland (www.cao.ie) and Canadian and US students apply through the Atlantic Bridge Program (www.atlanticbridge.com), an organization established to coordinate admission of North American students applying to Irish medical schools. There are also other international agencies that coordinate admissions for students from Singapore, Malaysia and other non-E.U countries that will not be explored in this book.

Students are **not** required to be Canadian or US citizens to apply through the Atlantic Bridge Program [17]. However, they are required to have completed a significant portion of their education in North America [18]. If you are unsure of your eligibility, you can contact the Atlantic Bridge Program at +1 (949) 723-6318.

The CAO application deadline is usually around the beginning of February, and the Atlantic Bridge deadline is November 15th. Non-E.U, non-North American students may have different deadlines depending on their agency.

The detailed application process and requirements for E.U and non-E.U applicants to all medical programs in Ireland is provided on page 384.

Poland

There are 11 schools in Poland offering a total of 17 medical programs in English to which graduate applicants are eligible to apply. Seven are 4 year programs and ten are 6 year programs. Within those programs, one 4 year program is only open to North American students, and one six year program is only open to students from Norway, Sweden and Denmark. More details are available in the school specific sections on page 407.

Most of the 4 year programs require applicants to write the MCAT, but non-North American students are sometimes exempt, or may write a different exam through a recruitment agency.

The Jagellonian University Medical College requires applicants to write either the MCAT or the GAMSAT.

Some 6 year programs require applicants to write a university admissions exam, usually in biology and chemistry only. Many programs also require an interview, which may focus on biology and chemistry or other topics related to the applicant's experience and motivation.

Application deadlines for the Polish medical programs are usually between May and August. Many schools ask students to submit their applications through recruiting agencies abroad such as the Hope Medical Institute in North America and M+D Europe.

Most students in the 4 year programs tend to be from North America, while most students in the 6 year programs come from Europe and Asia. Most programs receive between 2 and 3 applications per place available. More details are available in the school specific sections on page 407.

Romania

There are seven 6 year medical programs in Romania offered in English. To gain admission, E.U students need to have their credentials accepted by the National Center for Recognition and Equivalence of Diplomas (referred to as CNRED in Romanian), and non-E.U applicants need to get permission to study from the Romanian Ministry of Education, Research and Innovation. Many schools including Iuliu Hatieganu University and Gr. T. Popa University do not have an entrance examination for international applicants, but some like Carol Davila University have an examination that tests English language skills, while others like Victor Babes University require an exam that tests biology and chemistry. Universities requiring an entrance examination post details on their website including sample questions and topics covered.

To apply, students usually submit their documents (transcripts, application form, CV, etc.) to the schools' international offices, who then forward them to the appropriate institution (CNRED, the Romanian Ministry, etc.). Students are then sent a letter of acceptance from the institutions.

Some schools have examination fees (application deadlines are usually between July and October, but note that applicants sometimes have to start the application process several weeks before the deadline to have their acceptance letter issued before the final deadline).

As is the case in Poland, several schools have over 100 international students studying medicine in English, coming from several countries including countries in Europe, North America, Asia and Africa. See the school specific sections on page 422 for more details.

Slovak Republic

There are three 6 year programs taught in English in the Slovak Republic at the two Comenius University in Bratislava Faculties as well as Pavol Jozef Šafárik University. Students submit an application form with a CV to all three programs, and must also write a multiple choice entrance exam at all three schools to gain admission. None of the three schools require an interview. Some students apply directly to the schools, while others may apply to a university representative in their country if one exists.

The entrance examinations are the most important part of the application process in the Slovak Republic. The schools provide materials for their entrance examinations on their websites. Comenius University in Bratislava, Faculty of Medicine in Bratislava also offers a 1000 practice question review booklet for their entrance exam.

The universities generally have their entrance exams between June and August or September every year, and registration deadlines for the examinations can be as early as mid-May.

The schools have between approximately 50 and 100 places available for international students each year, with many students from Europe, as well as students from other parts of the world including some from North America.

Ukraine

There are currently eleven 6 year programs taught in English in the Ukraine. At Kharkov State Medical University, students have been eligible to receive credit for the first year of the program based on undergraduate courses they took previously.

To apply, students usually send their application directly to the university, alongside their secondary school certificate, and the medical school then sends them an invitation letter to study in the Ukraine (after the student's file is approved by the Ministry of Education in the Ukraine). Applicants need to bring this letter along with supporting documentation (photographs, medical test results, and other documents specified by the universities) to the nearest Ukrainian embassy where they are then issued a visa to study in the Ukraine. Some schools may interview students before enrollment, usually to ensure that they are proficient in

English. There are usually no admissions exams required. Some universities like Lugansk State Medical University have international recruitment agencies through which students submit their applications.

Applications deadlines vary significantly, and at some schools like Bukovinian School of Medicine and Ternopil State Medical University, students can gain admission as late as mid-November, two months after the course has started. Note that it takes 10 - 30 days for the Ministry of Foreign Affairs in the Ukraine to process the documentation, and may take longer with bank transfers, university processing and mailing.

The English program class sizes tend to be smaller in the Ukraine compared to other countries, with most schools offering between roughly 20 to 80 places each year. Some schools like M. Gorky Donetsk National Medical University divide students into groups of 8 or 9 for their classes, as is done at several other Eastern European schools.

The MCAT

General information

The MCAT is an American test that is accepted in most countries except the UK. It is required for application in the US, and most Canadian schools require the MCAT as well (see page 110 for more details on how the MCAT is used in Canada). Schools in Australia, the Caribbean, Ireland, Poland and some other Eastern European schools will also consider the MCAT.

The MCAT is a time constrained, computer-based exam. Unlike some other computer-based exams, the MCAT is not an adaptive test (an adaptive test is one where the next questions are chosen based on how well the test writer performed on the previous ones). For the MCAT, the questions are fixed before you start, which means you can review and change answers on the current section, just like on a paper exam. There is no penalty for wrong answers.

There are four parts in the exam: Physical Sciences, Verbal Reasoning, Written Sample and Biological Sciences.

Physical Sciences: 52 multiple-choice questions in 70 minutes on first year university physics and first year university chemistry. Calculators are not allowed. Note that there is no calculus required for this section. Test writers will need to be able to do multiplication, long division and estimation of log conversion (like $\log(107) \approx 2$) by hand to answer questions. Techniques on how to do this quickly are taught in courses and in MCAT preparation books.

Verbal Reasoning: 40 multiple choice questions in 60 minutes. Usually, students will read a passage and answer 4 to 10 questions on it before moving on to the next passage. This is not the same as reading comprehension. The questions ask students to draw inferences and understand the author's intentions. For example, they may ask "how would it change the author's argument if this fact turned out to be false?" or "why did the author choose to bring up this fact?" Although this is not based on content, practice goes a long way.

Writing Sample: There are two writing samples, each 30 minutes long. Students will get a statement like "The object of education should be to teach skills, not values" or "The nature of democracy requires that its citizens be dependent upon one another", which have been used in previous exams and are posted on the AAMC website along with many other examples. Test takers are then given three specific tasks for each statement. These tasks are explained on the AAMC website: www.aamc.org/students/mcat/preparing/writingsampleitems.htm. The following three tasks are assigned for the first example above.

1. Explain what you think the statement means
2. Describe a specific situation in which the object of education might be teaching values rather than skills.
3. Discuss what you think determines when the object of education is to teach skills and when it is to teach values.

The first task is the same for each question. It requires students to interpret and define the words in the statement – for example, you could define education as being education in a classroom, or you could say education is any occasion where one person teaches something to another, or any other reasonable definition you choose. This will set the stage for the rest of your essay. The next two tasks are phrased differently for each question, but ask for basically the same things each time. The second task is to find an example of when the statement is false, and the third is to find a way to determine when the statement will be true and when it will be false. Preparation courses and books have advice and instructions on how to structure your essay, as well as examples of essays that scored very well.

Biological Sciences: 52 multiple choice questions in 70 minutes on first year university biology and first year university organic chemistry.

Uses, scoring and your chances

The three multiple-choice sections are graded on a bell-curve and given a score from 1 to 15. A score of 8 roughly corresponds to the mean (50th percentile), with every ~2.5 points representing a standard deviation. For the exam overall, the mean is roughly 25 and the standard deviation 6.4. These are estimates and vary slightly each year. Below is a table from the AAMC website showing what each score means in terms of percentile.

Hypothetical Examinee Score Distribution

Scaled Score	% Achieving Scaled Score	Range of Percentile Ranks		
15	1.1	98.8	–	99.9
14	2.7	97	–	98.7
13	3.6	93	–	96
12	4.5	88	–	92
11	8.6	79	–	87
10	11.3	68	–	78
9	12.7	55	–	67
8	15.0	40	–	54
7	12.1	29	–	39
6	9.5	20	–	28
5	7.4	12	–	19
4	4.5	7	–	11
3	3.1	4	–	6
2	2.7	1.3	–	3
1	1.2	0	–	1.2

Scaled Score Mean – 8.0
Standard Deviation – 2.5

Figure 1. Approximate relationship between section scores and percentiles
More detailed tables are available from https://www.aamc.org/students/applying/mcat/admissionsadvisors/mcat_stats/

The writing section is given an alphabetical grade between J (lowest) and T (highest). Each essay is graded twice – once by a computer program and once by a person. If the grades are significantly different, a second person marks the essay and determine the final score for that essay.

For Canadian and US schools, applicants may write the MCAT once, twice, three times or even more sometimes trying to obtain the highest possible scores. As the MCAT is a key element of an application, it is essential to understand how an MCAT score can help or hurt one's application to medical schools. In Canada, applicants with very low MCAT scores are not affected at all when applying to the medical schools that do not use the MCAT. The universities in this category are the Northern Ontario School of Medicine, the University of Ottawa and the 3 French medical programs in Quebec. Also note that at McGill University, MCAT score submission is optional for Canadian students under certain conditions, and at the University of Saskatchewan, in-province applicants do not need to submit MCAT scores if their pre-requisite courses meet certain grade requirements, but out of province students must submit MCAT scores.

At the University of Toronto, once an applicant meets the minimum expected score requirements of 9 in each multiple choice section and N on the writing sample, a higher

MCAT score does not increase the chances of admission (note that those who fall slightly below these requirements may be granted admission if the rest of their application is very strong). This also means that if an applicant has not excelled in their MCAT but meets these cutoffs, they will not be disadvantaged at the University of Toronto compared to applicants with very high MCAT scores.

It is also important to consider that when the MCAT has been written more than once, policies differ as to which scores are used by the admissions offices. Some universities like the University of Toronto consider only the latest MCAT score, while other universities like the University of British Columbia consider the best MCAT score. Also, some universities will recalculate the MCAT score based on their formula which may be beneficial to some applicants. One example is the University of Manitoba, where applicants are given an operative MCAT score equal to: 0.3(Verbal Reasoning) + 0.2(Physical Science) + 0.3(Biological Science) + 0.2(Written Sample).

The exact MCAT policies, cutoffs and entering class averages are available for each medical school in Canada under "MCAT" in the school specific sections.

In the US, the MCAT is usually used as an initial screening tool alongside the GPA before a full file review, or as part of a global assessment before students are invited for interview. More statistics and information on MCAT scores in the US is available in the country's section on page 296.

At the American University of the Caribbean, the average MCAT score for entry in 2009 was 25. At Ross University in the Caribbean, although there is no minimum MCAT requirement, the average MCAT scores of matriculants was 27, and most students accepted in recent years had scores above 17. More details on the admissions processes at Caribbean medical schools are available in the school specific sections on page 355.

At the Royal College of Surgeons in Ireland, the MCAT average for admission was 29 in 2009, and scores were considered as part of the full application including reference letters, academics, personal statement and an interview. At Jagiellonian University Medical College in Poland, a minimum MCAT score of 21 was required for applicants to be considered for admission.

Many other schools in Eastern Europe and in Australia use the MCAT scores as part of their assessment as well. Most Australian schools require a minimum of 8/8/8/M to apply.

Cost of the MCAT

The cost of the exam is USD235 in the US and Canada. There is an additional USD70 fee in most other countries where the exam is offered . Fee assistance is available for eligible test-takers who are US citizens, permanent residents or refugees. The program reduces the fee from USD235 to USD85.

Resources for the MCAT

There are plenty of resources to help students prepare for the MCAT. Amongst them, you can find live courses, software programs, question banks, private tutors, books and study guides. In this section, we will review some of the resources most commonly used by students to prepare for and excel on the MCAT exam.

Courses

Large scale studies have looked at whether students who enroll in test preparation courses perform better on the MCAT. One study in particular looked at students who took the exam in 1980 (excluding those students who had written the MCAT previously), and found that those who took a course scored about 0.13 points higher on the reading section (lowest difference) and 0.43 points higher in physics section (highest difference), and had a 5% greater likelihood of getting into medical school [19]. Although this study is over 25 years old and there are many other factors influencing how well applicants do on the test, the study shows that there is a small statistical difference between students who take an MCAT preparation course and those who do not. Overall, MCAT courses help with the following:

•Learning and reviewing the content of the test
•Learning to apply the content to specific types of questions
•Keeping to a study timeline
•Obtaining answers to students' specific questions
•Practicing full length exams under exam conditions, which helps build the endurance needed for the 5.5 hour exam.
•Getting comments and help with writing samples
•Meeting with mentors one on one to get help with any trouble areas.

There are several MCAT courses available in Canada.

Agency	Description	Rough cost (USD)
Kaplan private tutoring	15 - 35 hours over 1-9 months. Students make a schedule with their tutor after taking a diagnostic test. The tutors are normally students who scored "above the 95th percentile on each section of the test". Students who sign up for tutoring can also attend any classroom or online lectures, and get access to all the course materials, including the 11,000 questions and the 8 AAMC exams. Writing samples can be corrected by the tutor.	35 hours: Approximately $5000 25 hours: Approximately $3900 15 hours: Approximately $2800
Oxford Seminars private tutoring	Tutors are available in Toronto, York, Kingston, Calgary, Burnaby and Vancouver, but tutors may be available in other cities upon request. Tutors are generally people who have done well on the exam.	If the student has taken the classroom course, the cost is approximately $50 per hour. If not, the cost is approximately $100 per hour with a minimum of 3 hours.
Princeton Review private tutoring	48 hours or more over approximately 4 months. Students can select their tutor's experience: Private, Master or Premier tutor. Students get access to 9 Princeton Review practice exams, the 8 AAMC exams and other questions and course materials available from the online student center. The course also comes with LiveGrader credits, which allow students to submit writing samples from all their practice tests for grading and feedback. Access to online or classroom courses is <u>NOT</u> included.	Approximately $15,600 for 48 hours with a premier tutor, or $3,650 for 10 hours in a single subject with a premier tutor. Approximately $11,280 for 48 hours with a master tutor, or $2,650 for 10 hours in a single subject with a master tutor. Approximately $7,680 for 48 hours with a standard level private tutor, or approximately $1,800 for 10 hours in a single subject with a standard level private tutor. Available tutor qualification levels and experience differ from city to city. Prices also vary between Canada and the USA
Princeton Review online private tutoring	Students set their own schedule with their tutor. They get access to LiveOnline credits for their practice exams (see private tutoring), as well as the same materials as those in the Princeton Review private tutoring course.	See Princeton Review private tutoring. Prices are usually approximately the same
Princeton Review small group tutoring	Group tutoring with one instructor for 2 to 4 students. Students can select their own group or can have the company find them a group. Same additional materials as private tutoring.	Approximately $2999 per student for 48 hours

Table 1. Individual and small group private tutoring for MCAT preparation
Information obtained from the company websites and by speaking to company representatives.

Course	Description	Rough cost (USD)
Dr. Ferdinand MCAT 1 week camp	Held in Montreal, QC and Las Vegas, NV. Approximately 50 hours of teaching and 50 hours of supplemental DVD video. Also includes one on one sessions and mock exams.	Approximately $1500 for the course only. Approximately $2400 with books and DVDs
Dr. Ferdinand Live Prep weekend course	Held in Toronto, ON twice a year over 2 days. Includes MCAT book and flashcards	Approximately $495
Kaplan classroom course	54 hours of classroom instruction and 32 hours of testing during 24 individual sessions. A total of roughly 11,000 questions are available to the student. The course can be done over 1 - 12 months. Written samples are corrected by local instructors. In some cities there is an instructor dedicated to teaching and correcting writing samples.	Approximately $2000
Kaplan summer intensive course	Held in Boston, MA and San Diego, CA. 320 hours total over the course of 6 weeks. Includes one-on-one tutoring and small group workshops, as well as 5 full-length practice MCATs under simulated testing conditions.	Approximately $7,500 without housing Approximately $11,100 with housing
Oxford Seminars	22 hour courses available in most provinces over 3 days. 40 hour courses over 5 days available across Canada and New York. Taught by students who scored in the top 2% on the exam. Course materials and practice exams are included (3 for 22 hour course, 4 for 40 hour course). No simulated exam is given.	Approximately $495 for 22 hour seminars. Approx. $745 for 40 hour seminars.
Prep 101 courses	Full course includes 54 hours of classroom instruction and 54 hours of in-class testing. Students also get access to the 8 AAMC practice exams. Offered in most provinces. 28 essays are also graded with feedback.	Approximately $1,595 for full course
Princeton Review classroom course	105 hours of classroom instruction over 42 individual sessions. Students also get access to LiveGrader, which allows them to submit their writing sample essays for grading and feedback. Usually done over 2 months, but different schedules available, particularly in larger cities.	Approximately $2000
Princeton Review summer intensive course	Six week program held in San Diego, CA and Austin, TX. 370 hours of instruction over the course of 6 weeks, as well as admission and application workshops.	Approximately $8000 without housing Approximately $11,000 with housing

Renert classroom course	Available in Calgary, AB. Includes approximately 35 1.5 hour lessons, access to 9000 practice questions and the 8 AAMC full length practice exams.	Approximately $1,300

Table 2. Classroom and summer intensive MCAT courses
Information obtained from the company websites and by speaking to company representatives.

Course	Description	Rough cost (USD)
Dr. Ferdinand MCAT home study course	20 hour video lecture series. Also includes books and 3 online practice exams.	Approximately $399
Dr. Ferdinand MCAT platinum study course	60 hours of live online MCAT review lectures and 16 hours of DVD science review. 8 writing sample essays corrected with feedback. 10 full-length MCAT practice exams	Approximately $1200
Kaplan MCAT online course	54 hours of lectures,, can be completed over 1 - 12 months. Sessions are pre-recorded. Writing sample grading and feedback is normally not included. Questions are answered by email. Comes with 11,000 practice questions, 8 AAMC exams and other course materials.	Approximately $2,000
Princeton Review MCAT LiveOnline course	105 hours of live online instruction. Access to 4 LiveGrader credits, which allow the student to submit writing samples for grading and feedback. Also get online coaching and email support. Comes with 11 Princeton Review practice exams, the 8 AAMC exams and other questions and course materials.	Approximately $1800

Table 3: Online MCAT preparation courses
Information obtained from the company websites and by speaking to company representatives.

Several courses including those from Kaplan and Princeton Review often offer a discount of a few hundred dollars if you enroll early (usually before April or May).

Books

Kaplan and Princeton Review have their own set of books available in stores and from their website. Many of them are also included in their MCAT courses. The ExamKracker books tends to be less detail oriented but in the view of some students, more clear and to the point. Some books available include:

Book	Description	Rough cost (USD)
Examkrackers MCAT Complete Study Package	1088 pages, 5 volume set of ExamKracker manuals. One full length practice exam and approximately 30 half hour mini-exams.	Approximately $110
Kaplan MCAT 45	324 pages, targeted at the more difficult questions and topics on the test.	Approximately $20
Kaplan MCAT in a Box	Approximately 700 flashcards covering biology, physics and chemistry terms, definitions and concepts.	Approximately $32
Kaplan MCAT Premier	1080 pages, comes with online resources, quizzes, short videos and 4 full-length practice tests	Approximately $65
Princeton Review, Cracking the MCAT	1080 pages. Covers all topics on the MCAT with practice passages and a tear-out reference guide. Also includes access to 4 full-length practice exams.	Approximately $62
Princeton Review, MCAT Workout	368 pages. Practice chapters on each section of the MCAT, as well as 2 full-length online tests	Approximately $15
The Gold Standard MCAT	1000 pages. Covers all components of the exam. Includes 3 online practice exams.	Approximately $60
The Official Guide to the MCAT Exam	400 pages. Includes passages and questions from previous MCAT exams with explanations. Also a lot of data including the percentages of applicants admitted to medical school with different MCAT and GPA scores (also available in the MSAR book).	Approximately $30

Table 4. List of some books to prepare for the MCAT

Although these are some of the more popular MCAT books, there are several other complete and subject specific books available.

Practice and mock tests

Practicing full length sections and full length exams is the best way to get used to the timing of the MCAT and the style of questions. Full length exams and question banks are usually included with review courses and tutoring programs, but are are also sold separately by some companies. Some of these separately sold question sets are listed below:

Name	Description	Rough cost (USD)
AAMC practice examinations	Full length practice exams sold individually. 8 available in total.	First exam free + approximately $35 for each additional exam
Dr. Ferdinand practice examinations	10 full length online examinations.	Approximately $150 for all tests, or $25 for each individual test. 1 free test is also available online.
Kaplan free full-length practice test	1 practice test, no writing sample. Includes assessment of strengths and weaknesses, and also includes answers and explanations.	Free
Kaplan Qbank	1000 questions with explanations	Approximately $200
Princeton Review free full-length practice test	1 practice test. Includes report of strengths and weaknesses, and also includes 1 LiveGrader Credit, which allows students to submit a writing sample for grading and feedback.	Free

Table 5. List of some online practice materials to prepare for the MCAT

There are also several practice question books and paper examinations available, most of them written before the MCAT was changed to a computer based exam in 2007. A list of previous writing sample topics is available from the AAMC at: www.aamc.org/students/mcat/preparing/ writingsampleitems.htm. Note that writing sample grading and feedback is not included with most of the question banks and practice examinations.

It can be beneficial to do as many of the tests as possible under real, time constrained test conditions, preferably with a few sections in a row. This can help build stamina for the test day.

When should you write the MCAT?

The course requirements for the MCAT are first year university physics, chemistry, biology and organic chemistry. There are some subtopics on the MCAT that are sometimes not covered in first year university courses (such as thermal expansion of metals or buoyancy), but these topics will be covered in the MCAT books and prep courses.

Some students finish the physics, chemistry and biology courses during their first two terms of university, take two 3-4 week intensive organic chemistry courses during the first two months of their first-year summer, then study for the MCAT the last two months of the summer and write the test. The advantage is that students using this approach study for and write the MCAT with all the material fresh in their minds. Consider, however, that although most Canadian schools accept MCAT scores from the past 5 years, the University of Manitoba and several US schools including the Yale University and Rosalind Franklin, Chicago Medical School only accept MCAT scores from the past 3 years. At the University of Manitoba, MCAT scores written before April 2008 are not acceptable for entry in 2012. At Stanford University, MCAT scores earlier than August 2008 are not acceptable for entry in 2012.

Thus, students writing the MCAT their first-year summer and graduating in four years will, at many US schools and at the University of Manitoba, only be allowed to use their MCAT scores until their last year of college (for matriculation the year after graduation). If unsuccessful, they would have to rewrite the MCAT to reapply to these schools the following year.

If you wish to write your MCAT during your first year summer and need to complete organic chemistry, some universities like the University of Alberta offer an intensive 6 week organic chemistry course (first three weeks for Organic Chemistry I and the last 3 for Organic Chemistry II) starting early May. With some companies like Kaplan and Princeton Review that are available in many cities or allow courses to be taken online, you can begin the MCAT course in the city in which you are taking the organic chemistry course, and finish it in another city. Alternatively, you can take the MCAT course at an accelerated pace after finishing organic chemistry or another spring/summer course.

The MCAT is offered several times each month and can be taken three times in one calendar year. It takes approximately one month to receive your tentative scores. Most North American universities require the MCAT to be written by August or September of the application year. Note that if the exam does not go well on the last possible test date, it will not be possible to submit another set of scores with your application. When possible, it is a good idea to write the test with enough time left so you can rewrite it if necessary.

The GAMSAT

Medical schools using the GAMSAT

The following programs require the GAMSAT to be eligible in the 2012-2013 application cycle.

1. Keele University (4 year)
2. University of Nottingham (4 year)
3. Peninsula Medical School (5 year)
4. St George's, University of London (4 year)
5. Swansea University (4 year)

Note that the University of Newcastle's 4 year program considers the GAMSAT scores in addition to UKCAT scores if the applicant believes this will strengthen their application. Also, students without a science degree or science A-levels can apply for the 5 year program at Keele University by scoring well on the GAMSAT (in addition to writing the UKCAT, which all applicants to the 5 year program must write).

The GAMSAT structure and timing

The GAMSAT is designed to test applicants' aptitude for critical thinking, written communication and scientific problem solving. Writing the GAMSAT exam requires knowledge of biology (1st year university), chemistry (1st year university), physics (A level) and English (general proficiency).

The GAMSAT exam consists of 3 sections:

I. Reasoning in humanities and social sciences (75 multiple choice questions in 100 minutes)
II. Written communication (2 essays of 30 minutes each)
III. Reasoning in biological and physical sciences (110 multiple choice questions in 170 minutes: 40% biology, 40% chemistry, 20% physics)

The GAMSAT scoring and your chances

Your score is calculated based on performance in all 3 sections with double weighting given to section III. Some medical schools also set minimum cutoffs for the individual sections. For example, at the University of Nottingham, applicants needed to achieve a minimum score of 55 in section 2, 55 in either section 1 or section 3 and at least 50 in the remaining section, in addition to meeting the overall GAMSAT cutoff.

A percentile scoring sheet is also included with each year's GAMSAT score report. In 2009, a score of 51 corresponded to the 25th percentile, 55.5 to the 50th percentile, 60 to the 75th percentile and 66 to the 90th percentile.

At St. George's, University of London Medical School, the University of Nottingham and Peninsula Medical School, those who meet the minimum academic criteria and meet the GAMSAT cutoff each year are routinely granted interviews.

Keele University uses the GAMSAT in conjunction with the full UCAS application to determine if applicants will be invited for interview, and Swansea University only takes the GAMSAT into account after the interview.

For universities setting a GAMSAT cutoff for interview, the cutoffs generally range from 58 (roughly 65th percentile) to 65 (roughly 88th percentile) depending on the competition that year and the university. Peninsula Medical School tends to have higher GAMSAT cutoffs (62 - 64 in recent years) because they do not set a minimum requirement for achievement in the undergraduate degree. This can be a good university to apply to for some students who have achieved lower than a 2:2 in their fist degree but have done well on the GAMSAT.

Other universities like the University of Nottingham and St. George's tend to have slightly lower cutoffs (usually low 60s or occasionally high 50s), but they also require applicants to have achieved a minimum of a lower second (2:2) in their undergraduate degree. Applicants are also often expected to achieve minimum scores of 50 or 55 in individual GAMSAT sections.

Cost of exam taking and preparation

In 2011, the cost of the exam is £195 to write, with an additional cost of £50 for late registration. Preparing for the exam can also be costly. Courses can cost between approximately £100 to £650 or more, and books can cost between £40 to £400 (books are normally included in the courses, but applicants sometimes buy additional books and practice materials). See the next section for the costs of some of the courses, books and practice material available.

Some students also find it helpful to have a one on one tutor for specific subjects. This can range in price from approximately £15 to £60 per hour depending on the tutor's qualifications and experience.

Resources for the GAMSAT

Courses, home study packages and private tutoring

Courses and private tutoring can help with several aspects of GAMSAT preparation:
•Learning and reviewing the content of the test
•Learning to apply the content to specific types of questions
•Keeping to a study timeline
•Obtaining answers to students' specific questions
•Practicing full length exams under exam conditions
•Getting comments and help with the writing section
•Getting additional help with any trouble areas quickly and easily

There are several GAMSAT courses, home study packages and private tutoring options in the UK. A few of them are listed in the table below:

Name	Description	Rough cost
Dr. O'Neill's GAMSAT courses	Although the courses are offered in Australia, some UK and correspondence packages are available.	Home study science review course: Approximately £195 (up from £130 last year) Home study MCQ practice course: Approximately £195 (up from £130 last year) Writing Better Essays Complete Course and 6 writing samples corrected: Approximately £165 (or 12 for £265)
Dr. Prep GAMSAT courses	One and three day courses in 2011 held in London covering different aspects of the exam. Mock exams are included in the course.	Three day course: £399 GAMSAT Reasoning and Written Communication (1 day course): £170
Gradmed GAMSAT full course and mock test	20 day weekend course covering all sections of the test, held at Imperial College in London. The course usually runs from June through September. Applicants can sign up for individual subjects in the course or for the full course. They can also sign up for a mock exam. Books and materials are not included, but a list of books relevant to the course is given to the student beforehand. The course will also been offered in Dublin between January and March.	Full 20 day course (excluding mock exam): Approximately £3180 All three science modules: Approximately £2450 One science module: Approximately £675-980 Written and verbal reasoning sections: Approximately £535 Maths for sciences module: £195 Mock test: £99
Gradmed GAMSAT intensive weekend course	Weekend intensive courses offered over 3 weekends covering all sections of the test. The course is held at Imperial College in London.	Approximately £1080
Medprep international home study GAMSAT courses	3 packages available, including as much as 1200 practice questions, 1100 pages of notes, 3 full length exams, 8 essays corrected with feedback and 30 hours of online audiovisual lectures.	Between £278 and £649 including shipping.
PrepGenie comprehensive GAMSAT course	Online course with tutorials in each subject, 5 full-length tests, approximately 4000 additional questions, and 20 essays with feedback.	Full course: Approximately £380 Individual modules in Humanities, Chemistry, Biology or Physics: Approximately £175 each

Table 6. Classroom and home-study GAMSAT preparation courses.
Information obtained from the company websites and by speaking to company representatives.

To our knowledge, there are no organizations in the UK that provide private tutoring specifically for the GAMSAT, however, there are private tutors available through organizations like 'tutors 4 me' who specify that they can tutor for the GAMSAT. On www.tutors4me.co.uk, tutors charge approximately £30 to £40 per hour. Some tutors also advertise on websites such as www.newmediamedicine.com. For applicants looking for tutoring in a specific subject, they can also find private tutoring through organizations like www.sciencetutors.co.uk or sometimes through organizations offering tutoring for the BMAT and the UKCAT, as the BMAT has a writing section that is similar in some ways to the GAMSAT writing section, and the UKCAT has a verbal reasoning section similar to the humanities and social sciences section on the GAMSAT.

Books

There are very few books written specifically for the GAMSAT. For this reason, some students find that books for the UKCAT (verbal reasoning), BMAT (written communication) or MCAT (a US based exam with similar biology, chemistry, physics, humanities, social sciences and written communication sections) are useful in preparing for the GAMSAT. Some find them to be even more useful than the books written specifically for the GAMSAT, while others prefer GAMSAT specific materials. Those that use the MCAT books for preparing for the GAMSAT science section often find it more time-efficient to use the more succinct, to the point guides such as the ExamKrackers series, rather than the more detailed books such as the Kaplan books.

Some of the books available for the GAMSAT are listed below:

Name	Description	Rough cost
ExamKrackers MCAT inorganic chemistry	Reviews all first year university inorganic chemistry tested on the MCAT (similar to the GAMSAT). Includes 7 thirty minute mock exams and 85 additional questions. 211 pages	Approximately £17
ExamKrackers MCAT organic chemistry	Reviews all first year university organic chemistry tested on the MCAT (similar to the GAMSAT). Includes 4 thirty minute mock exams and 60 additional questions. 154 pages	Approximately £14
Examkrackers MCAT Physics	Reviews all first year university physics tested on the MCAT (similar to the GAMSAT). Includes 8 thirty minute mock exams and 120 additional questions. 257 pages	Approximately £18

GAMSAT Guru books	10 books written on specific subjects, or specific sections of the test.	All books sold together for approximately £360
Griffiths GAMSAT review ebook	Ebook covering strategies for each section of the GAMSAT including some practice questions. 171 pages.	£34.95

Table 7. Preparation books for the GAMSAT

Some books specifically for the GAMSAT are available through the full courses listed above.

Practice questions and mock exams

There are several practice books available, including official practice materials from the GAMSAT test writers (the Australian Council for Educational Research). Most applicants planning to write the GAMSAT will purchase at least the official practice materials, as these materials are among the resources available that give the best sense of what the real exam is like.

Name	Description	Rough cost
Gradmed mini-mock exam	10 unit mini-exams with answers and explanations taking approximately 1 hour and 15 minutes to complete	Free
MedPrep international	2 full-length tests online and one sent by mail. Also 4 essays marked with feedback. Note that feedback often takes a week on average, or up to 20 days in periods of high demand.	30 day access: £149 60 day access: £169 90 day access: £189
Official GAMSAT practice materials	3 books available, including a full GAMSAT practice test and 2 practice question books.	GAMSAT Practice Test: £26 GAMSAT Practice Questions: £16 GAMSAT Sample Questions: £16
Ozimed GAMSAT tests	10 full length GAMSAT tests. Answers are included, but solutions to problems are not included.	5 tests: £119 10 tests: £203
PrepGenie GAMSAT tests	Comprehensive and section specific practice tests	Comprehensive tests (5 full length tests and 40 section tests with explanations): £271 Full length test papers (5 full length tests with explanations): £88 Section specific test papers (10 test papers per package, 40 questions per test): £63 per package

Table 8. List of GAMSAT practice tests and question books

When to write the GAMSAT?

The 2011 GAMSAT will be held Friday, September 16th, 2011 in the UK. Registrations open on June 3rd and close on August 12th, 2011. More information on the GAMSAT is available on the official website at www.gamsatuk.org. The GAMSAT is also offered in Ireland and Australia, usually in March each year. Applicants can write the exam in different countries each year without penalty. There is no maximum number of times an applicant can write the test. Since the exam is valid for 2 years, some applicants write it 2 years before applying so that if they do not obtain a good score, they can rewrite it again the next year to obtain a higher score.

The UKCAT

Medical schools using the UKCAT

The UKCAT is used in most programs in the UK. Below is the list of medical schools open to graduate applicants that use the UKCAT:

1. University of Aberdeen (5 year)
2. Barts and the London School of Medicine (4 and 5 year)
3. Brighton and Sussex Medical School (5 year)
4. Cardiff University (5 and 6 year)
5. University of Dundee (5 and 6 year)
6. University of East Anglia (5 year)
7. University of Edinburgh (5 year)
8. University of Glasgow (5 year)
9. Hull York Medical School (5 year)
10. Imperial College London (4 year)
11. Keele University (5 and 6 year)
12. King's College London (4 and 5 year)
13. University of Leeds (5 year)
14. University of Leicester (4 and 5 year)
15. University of Manchester (5 and 6 year)
16. University of Newcastle/University of Durham (4 and 5 year)
17. University of Nottingham (5 year)
18. Queen's University Belfast (5 year)
19. St. George's, University of London (5 year)
20. University of Oxford (4 year)
21. University of Sheffield (5 and 6 year)
22. University of Southampton (4 and 5 year)
23. University of St Andrews (6 year)
24. University of St. Andrews, North American Program (6 year)
25. University of Warwick (4 year)

The UKCAT structure and timing

The UKCAT is designed to be a test of aptitude rather than a test of academic achievement, however, preparation can substantially improve an applicant's score. The test assesses a wide range of mental abilities and behavioral attributes identified by medical and dental schools as important. The exam is only valid for one application cycle, thus students need to write it the year they are applying. In 2011, the exam can be taken between July 5th and October 7th. Students receive their results at the test center immediately after completing their test.

The UKCAT consists of four subtests:

1. **Verbal reasoning**: Assesses candidates' ability to think logically about written information and to arrive at a reasoned conclusion.

2. **Quantitative reasoning**: Assesses candidates' ability to solve numerical problems.

3. **Abstract reasoning**: Assesses candidates' ability to infer relationships from information by convergent and divergent thinking.

4. **Decision analysis**: Assesses candidates' ability to deal with various forms of information, to infer relationships, to make informed judgements, and to decide on an appropriate response, in situations of complexity and ambiguity.

The full test lasts just over 1 and a half hours. Students with special needs may be eligible to receive more time on the test. Each of the subtests is in a multiple-choice format and is separately timed.

The UKCAT scoring and your chances

The first four sections are marked based on the number of correct responses. No marks are deducted for incorrect answers. Each of the first four subsections is scored on a scale of 300 to 900. The nation average on the full test is usually around 2400-2500 [6].

The section on behavioral traits is no longer included, and thus the brief summary on the applicants personality will of course no longer appear.

There is wide variation in the way UKCAT scores are used in medical school admissions processes, ranging from setting absolute cutoffs for automatic interview as is done at Barts and The London School of Medicine, to having the UKCAT count for roughly 10% of the overall admission score once a base cutoff is achieved, as is done at the University of St. Andrews.

Some medical schools like Hull-York Medial School generally expect applicants to be within the top 25% on the UKCAT exam to be granted an interview. Others such as the University of Glasgow state that those below the national average (usually around 2400-2500) are unlikely to be invited for interview. Many medical schools have no cutoff for interview and applicants can conceivably make up for any deficit in the UKCAT score provided the rest of their application is exceptionally strong.

If the UKCAT does not go well for an applicant, they should consider which university will place less emphasis on this and will still give them a good chance of obtaining an interview. If an applicant does very well on the UKCAT, it opens several doors in terms of automatic or near automatic interviews at certain UK universities. Details on how each program uses the UKCAT are available in the "School by School" section.

Exemptions from the exam

Students who received their education in certain countries may not need to write the UKCAT. A list countries where the exam is required is available from the UKCAT website at:
http://www.ukcat.ac.uk/pages/details.aspx?page=whereICanTakeTest

Those who have received their secondary school education outside of the listed countries should complete the form available from the website below and submit it to the UKCAT administration:
http://www.ukcat.ac.uk/pages/details.aspx?page=whoMustTakeTest

They may be granted an exemption number allowing them to apply without writing the test, which will be forwarded to the appropriate medical schools. Note that applicants must submit the form before September 23rd, 2011.

It is somewhat difficult to tell how not writing the UKCAT will affect an applicant's chances of admission. Medical schools generally say "it will not affect their chances", but it is unclear how the applicant's pre-interview scoring might change. For some students with the means to fly to another country and write the exam, it may be more useful to discuss with the admissions office how their chances might improve if they write the UKCAT and do well in deciding whether or not to make the investment.

Cost of exam taking and preparation

The exam costs £65 to £80 for EU applicants depending on when the exam is taken, and £100 for non-E.U applicants. EU candidates may be eligible to receive a bursary for the full cost of the test if they meet one of the requirements listed at: http://www.ukcat.ac.uk/pages/details.aspx?page=Bursaries

Preparing for the exam can cost between roughly £40 to £260 for home and classroom course preparation, as well as roughly £10 to £100 for books and practice questions. Private tutoring usually costs between around £27 to £100 per hour depending on the materials included and the qualifications and experience of the tutor.

Resources for the UKCAT

Courses and home study packages

Most classroom courses are held over a weekend or a single full day. These courses do not have time to teach all of the test material, but can give applicants a sense of the overall content of the exam and provide some studying and test taking techniques. Study materials and some practice questions are also included in the price for several of the courses.

Name	Description	Rough cost
Develop Medica e-learning materials	Includes materials on each section of the UKCAT, practice questions and one full length mock exam.	Approximately £40
Develop Medica UKCAT review workshop	1 day small group workshop. Includes 7 hours of classroom teaching. The course is held several times a year in Central London and Nottingham.	Approximately £180

Duff Miller 1 day UKCAT course	Covers approach to abstract reasoning and decision analysis. Students will practice questions in the afternoon. Course held in London on September 10th, 2011.	Approximately £250
Get Into Medical School UKCAT classroom course	One day UKCAT course held a few times a year at Exeter College in Oxford. Includes tuition on all parts of the test with mock questions.	Approximately £149
Kaplan 2 day Live Online UKCAT course	Includes all materials from the Kaplan UKCAT classroom course.	Approximately £259 to £299 depending on the time of year the course is taken
Kaplan 2 day UKCAT classroom course	2 full-day classroom courses offered throughout the UK between June and early October. The course is also offered in Ireland. Courses include a full length test and teaching on each section of the exam. The course comes with at total of 5 full length exams and a UKCAT strategy book.	Approximately £259 to £299 depending on the time of year the course is taken
Medipathways UKCAT classroom course	A one day course held in London, includes two practice tests	Approximately £150
PreUKCAT course	One day UKCAT course held in London a few times in September. Course covers all every section of the exam with a 30 minute mini-mock exam.	Approximately £99
Testprep 2 day UKCAT course	Several weekend courses offered in London between July and September covering all aspects of the exam.	Approximately £225

Table 9. Classroom and home-study UKCAT preparation courses
Information obtained from the company websites and by speaking to company representatives.

Private tutoring

There are several private tutoring companies available, some of whom offer specific tutoring packages for the UKCAT. A few of the private tutoring companies also offer a mock exam before the start of tutoring to gauge what areas students may want to focus on. See the table below for a few companies that offer private UKCAT tutoring:

Name	Description	Rough cost
1-2-1 UKCAT tutoring through develop medica	Students take a full length mock exam (included in price) and meet with a tutor at the center in nottingham for a two hour tutoring session. Their UKCAT guide, which covers each section of the test, is also included, as well as one additional practice test.	Approximately £249
Kaplan online private tutoring	Packages start at ten hours of private online tutoring. Students take a diagnostic test and then create a study plan. A UKCAT strategy book and five full length practice tests are included.	Approximately £1250 for ten hours
Kaplan private tutoring in London	Packages start at ten hours of tutoring and include the UKCAT strategy book and five full length practice tests.	Approximately £1250 for ten hours
ScienceTutors.co.uk	One to one tutoring available in several locations throughout the UK. Some tutors in this organization offer tutoring for the UKCAT.	Approximately £27 per hour
Tutors 4 me	One to one tutoring available in a few locations in the UK	Price varies by personal tutor. Approximately £30 to £40 per hour.

Table 10. UKCAT private tutoring agencies

Books

There are several books available to help prepare for the UKCAT, most of which focus mainly on practice questions. Some books are listed in the table below:

Name	Description	Rough cost
BMAT and UKCAT uncovered	Book includes tips, strategies and practice questions and explanations for all sections of the UKCAT and BMAT exams. 344 pages.	Approximately £15
Elite Students Series: How to master the UKCAT	Book includes exam techniques section and over 750 practice questions with explanations covering all sections of the test. 320 pages.	Approximately £9
Get into medical school - 600 UKCAT practice questions	Book includes exam techniques and 600 questions with explanations covering all sections of the test. 420 pages.	Approximately £12

How to pass the UKCAT	Book includes exam techniques and over over 600 practice questions with explanations. 320 pages.	Approximately £10
Passing the UKCAT and BMAT, 2011 edition	Covers medical school application tips and each section of the UKCAT and BMAT with practice questions and explanations. 288 pages.	Approximately £14
Succeeding in the 2010 UK Clinical Aptitude Test	Book includes tips on each section of the exam as well as practice questions and explanations. Approximately 250 pages.	Approximately £11

Table 11. List of UKCAT preparation books

Practice questions and mock exams

There are several practice books available, including official practice materials from the UKCAT test writers.

Name	Description	Rough cost
123Doc online Qbank	Online question bank. 1-3 month subscriptions available	1 month: £30 2 months: £40 3 months: £50
AceMedicine UKCAT question bank	Online question bank, roughly 1,800 questions, available in 6 and 12 month subscriptions	6 months: £47 12 months: £57
onExamination online practice questions from BMJ (British Medical Journal) learning	Online question bank available for 1-3 month subscriptions	1 month: £26 2 months: £36 3 months: £41
Practice tests, questions and answers for the UKCAT	Written by the same authors as "Passing the UKCAT and BMAT, 2011 edition", includes 2 exams and additional sections for a total of 500 questions with explanations. 256 pages.	Approximately £13
UKCAT consortium practice materials	3 practice tests (not all full-length) available from the UKCAT Consortium	Free
UKCAT practice online	Online question bank with roughly 2,400 questions and explanations. Access available for several months (usually until November of the testing year)	2272 questions: £45 Individual subtest questions (50 to 882 questions per package): £7 to £18

Table 12. List of UKCAT question banks and question books

The BMAT

Medical schools using the BMAT

There are a few programs in the UK open to graduate applicants that use the BMAT.

1. Cambridge University (6 year program, but completed in 5 years by graduates)
2. Imperial College London (6 year)
3. University of Oxford (6 year program, but completed in 5 years by graduates)
4. University College London (6 year program, but completed in 5 years by graduates)

The BMAT structure and timing

The BMAT is designed to be a test of aptitude rather than basic knowledge, however, preparation can substantially improve an applicant's score, just as it can for the UKCAT. The test is written by candidates wishing to study medicine, pharmacology, biomedical science, physiological sciences and veterinary medicine. The exam is only valid for one application cycle, thus students need to write it the year they are applying. For the next application cycle, the exam will take place on November 2nd, 2011.

The BMAT consists of 3 subtests:

1. **Aptitude and skills**: Assesses candidates' ability to analyze data, solve problems, understand arguments and infer information.
2. **Scientific knowledge and application**: Assesses candidates' ability to apply knowledge in science and math. Background knowledge includes science and math courses up to key stage 4 of the national curriculum.
3. **Writing task**: Assesses candidates' ability to develop ideas, organize them and communicate them in writing concisely and effectively. Students write 1 essay from a choice of 4 questions.

The first section lasts 60 minutes and the next two sections last 30 minutes each, for a total of 2 hours. Students with special needs may be eligible to receive more time on the test.

The BMAT scoring and your chances

Each question in the first two sections is given a score of 1 to 9, 9 being the best achievable score. Average scores tend to be around 5.0, correlating to roughly half the questions answered correctly. Scores of 6.0 are considered very good, and scores above 7.0 are obtained by less than 4% of students. The essay section is marked by two assessors and given a total score between 0 and 15, with 7.5 being an average grade, and scores above 13.5 being attained by less than 4% of students. A score of 15 is given to applicants with excellent use of English, clear construction, and strong arguments. More details are available from: http://www.admissionstests.cambridgeassessment.org.uk/adt/bmat/about under "Explanation of Results 2010".

Each medical program listed above uses the BMAT differently in their admissions process. At University College London, those who score significantly below average on the BMAT are unlikely to be admitted. In addition, high scores do give applicants an advantage over those with average or slightly above average scores.

At the University of Oxford, the BMAT and GCSE scores are the main two factors that determine whether an applicant is given an interview. The university weighs each section of the BMAT separately. Last year section 1 was weighted at 40%, section 2 at 40% and section 3 at 20%. Note that for section 3, the "Quality of Content" score is given double the weight of the "Quality of English" score. The average BMAT scores for all applicants using this weighting was 55%, and the average weighted BMAT score for students receiving an interview was 66%.

At Cambridge University, the BMAT is considered among other factors before the interview, however, approximately 90% of students who apply are invited for interview. After the interview, every part of the application, including the BMAT, is considered in selecting applicants for admission.

At Imperial College London, applicants must perform well in all three sections of the BMAT in order to have their full application reviewed.

Cost of exam taking and preparation

The exam usually costs around £42 for UK applicants and £72 for international applicants applying prior to the late fee date, although fees may change slightly from year to year. The

normal registration period for 2011 ends on September 30th, 2011. EU candidates may be eligible to receive a bursary for the full cost of the test if they meet one of the requirements listed at:
http://www.admissionstests.cambridgeassessment.org.uk/adt/bmat/faqs#q6

Preparing for the exam can cost between roughly £180 to £420 for home and classroom course preparation, as well as roughly £10 to £100 for books and practice questions. Private tutoring usually costs between around £27 to £125 per hour depending on the materials included and the qualifications and experience of the tutor.

Resources for the BMAT

Courses

There are several courses available for BMAT preparation, most of which last 1 to 2 full days. Some courses like the Kaplan course include materials and mock exams. Some of the courses available are listed below:

Name	Description	Rough cost
Develop Medica 1 day BMAT course	A few one day sessions held in London each year with a maximum of approximately 16 students at each session. Includes a full length practice test.	Approximately £180
Duff Miller 2 day BMAT course	Weekend course held in London on the 24th and 25th of October, 2011.	Approximately £420
Get Into Medical School BMAT classroom course	One day BMAT course held a few times a year at Exeter College in Oxford. Includes tuition on all parts of the test with a full-length mock exam.	Approximately £175
Kaplan 2 day BMAT classroom course	2 full-day classroom courses offered throughout the UK. Includes BMAT strategy book and five full length practice tests.	Approximately £259 to £299 depending on the time of year the course is taken

Table 13. Classroom BMAT preparation courses

Note that some courses such as the Kaplan course offer small discounts for those who take the course before September 1st. This may work better or worse for some students depending on the study schedule they are planning.

Private tutoring

There are several private tutoring agencies available to help prepare for the BMAT. Some companies offer tutors specifically for the BMAT, while other general tutoring companies sometimes have tutors who specialize in a few subjects including the BMAT. Some companies offering BMAT private tutoring are listed in the table below.

Name	Description	Rough cost
Kaplan private tutoring	Packages start at ten hours of tutoring and include the BMAT strategy book and five full length practice tests.	Approximately £1250 for five hours
ScienceTutors.co.uk	One to one BMAT tutoring available in several locations throughout the UK.	£27 per hour
Tutors 4 me	One to one BMAT tutoring available in a few locations in the UK	Approximately £40 per hour

Table 14. BMAT private tutoring agencies

Books

There are several BMAT specific books available including a book from some of the BMAT test writers. Some of these books are listed in the table below. Note that the last 7 books in the table are listed on the official BMAT website: www.admissionstests.cambridgeassessment.org.uk/adt/bmat. These books cover the first section of the test on critical thinking. We encourage test writers to look at other websites such as www.newmediamedicine.com or www.amazon.co.uk with feedback on the books before purchasing them.

Name	Description	Rough cost
BMAT and UKCAT uncovered	Book includes tips, strategies and practice questions with explanations for all sections of the UKCAT and BMAT exams. 344 pages.	Approximately £15
Elite Student Series: How to Master the BMAT	Includes sections covering math, physics, chemistry and biology, as well as a writing section. Also includes review questions. 208 pages.	Approximately £9
Kaplan BMAT	Includes test strategies, complete review of all sections of the exam, practice questions and a full length practice test. 288 pages.	Approximately £20

Passing the UKCAT and BMAT, 2011 edition	Covers medical school application tips and each section of the UKCAT and BMAT with practice questions and explanations. 288 pages.	Approximately £14
Preparing for the BMAT: The Official Guide	Written by the BMAT test writers, includes approaches to questions and practice examples. 112 pages.	Approximately £12
Succeeding in the Bio Medical Admissions Test	Includes approaches to each section of the BMAT with practice questions and a mock exam. Approximately 210 pages.	Approximately £11
Critical Reasoning: A Practical Introduction	Covers the process of critical thinking with examples. 224 pages	Approximately £13
Critical Thinking for Students	Covers the process of critical thinking, particularly focused for students taking the critical thinking AS level course. 120 pages.	Approximately £9
Critical Thinking: A Concise Guide	Covers the process of critical thinking with examples. Companion website included with case studies and sample questions. 294 pages.	Approximately £12
Critical Thinking: An Introduction	Covers critical thinking, argument analysis, decision making and application to different subjects. 228 pages.	Approximately £9
The Logic of Real Arguments	Covers techniques to analyze logical arguments with examples. 236 pages	Approximately £13
Thinking from A to Z	A book covering arguing and critical thinking with examples. Focuses more on the types of arguments people make and the philosophy of argument. 176 pages.	Approximately £8
Thinking Skills	Covers critical thinking and problem solving skills with examples. 280 pages	Approximately £15

Table 15. List of BMAT preparation books

Practice questions and mock exams

One of the main resources for practice tests is the official BMAT website, which has several practice sections and full length exams with explanations available:
www.admissionstests.cambridgeassessment.org.uk/adt/bmat/Test+Preparation
To our knowledge, there are very few books available that provide only questions (one practice exam is available from www.drprep.net), however, several of the books listed in the previous section include practice questions and mock exams.

Extracurricular activities and volunteer work

General information

Although individual schools place different weight on your extracurricular activities, nearly all admissions committees will look at your activities outside of school as part of your application. This is particularly true at the more competitive programs. For more information on extracurricular requirements in Canada, see page 139; for the UK, see page 220.

Alongside the nature of your extracurricular commitments, many admissions advisors are also careful to look at the longevity of your commitments. It may not reflect well if a candidate never stays with a volunteer commitment or leadership position for more than a month or two. Your essays and interviews will require you to draw on what you learned from your volunteer, leadership, research and/or extracurricular activities. Your answers regarding these experiences will carry greater weight if you stayed with the commitments for a longer time. Holding strong leadership roles and taking initiative will also help in the application. It says a lot about someone when they head a project or organization, or take initiative and start something successful in their community. If you have a chance during your summers or during the year, getting research experience will go a long way in your application. Any research articles you can publish in academic journals will carry significant weight as well.

Regardless of the type of work, volunteer work also says a lot about an applicant. There are many selfish reasons to become a doctor: the salary, job security, and prestige, just to name a few. When reviewing your application, the admissions committee is trying to gauge how much of your motivation comes from your desire to serve others, and your volunteer work will speak louder than your words in many cases.

Whatever areas you like getting involved in, know that your pursuits in these areas will strengthen your application. Get a good mix of medically related and non-medically related work, and when appropriate, keep your commitments for a good length of time.

Clinical experience

Out of all the activities you may get involved in, clinical experience or work in a caring role is considered especially important by many admissions offices. Strong clinical experience shows that you have made efforts to find out what medicine really entails. It also gives you the chance to find out if you enjoy the medical environment and working with sick people. In Canada, although clinical experience is not cited as one of the admissions requirements by any Canadian medical schools, it is nearly impossible to get in without any clinical experience. An application with no medically related work at all is usually considered quite poor. Here is what Dalhousie Medical School says:

"The Admissions Committee considers it important that you have some medically related experience. This can be volunteer work or paid work depending on your circumstances. Applications from individuals who do not have such experience are rarely acceptable to the committee."

Some medical schools in the UK recognize that it may be easier for some applicants to gain medically related work experience than others, but it is more difficult to gain admission without any clinical experience at most schools. An application with no evidence of effort to find out what a career in medicine entails is often considered less favorable in the UK as well. Here is what Queen's University Belfast says:

"candidates are expected to state explicitly that Medicine is their career choice. There should be evidence of commitment and motivation in the personal statement; this is usually shown by 'workshadowing' in Medicine, attending medical careers conferences or undertaking voluntary work in a care setting."

1. For volunteer work, a great place to start is at your city hospitals. Most have a volunteer team and are constantly recruiting. Although many of them will first offer you an administrative position filing documents or working in a store, it is a good idea to insist to take positions where you get more patient contact, like working with geriatric patients, with sick kids or in palliative care. The more patient contact you have, the better you will know if you really enjoy this side of medicine, and these experiences will help you in many ways as a physician besides strengthening your application.

2. Another way to get hands on experience easily is to shadow a physician. You may know some doctors that you can ask, but if you do not, another option is to ask your family doctor if he or she can arrange for you to sit in with one of his or her colleagues.

3. You can also work in call centers for people in distress or in facilities for senior people or mentally challenged children and adults. If you approach a center by going there directly instead of just calling, it shows interest and dedication and they are more likely to welcome you. If they do not usually have volunteers working there, you can offer some ideas of how you may be useful by reading to patients, or playing a game with them or simply talking to them. You can offer to come and help serve the food or organize afternoon entertainment for the patients/residents. If you are a professional piano player, then why not come and play for the patients? What is important is that you have opportunities to interact directly with the patients and the healthcare team to understand the good aspects, but also the problems that they face.

4. You can call organizations in your community that deal with chronically ill patients such diabetics, patients with cystic fibrosis, spinal cords accident victims, AIDS patients, etc. These organizations are usually well organized and have extensive experience dealing with patients with chronic conditions.

If you can only do one extracurricular activity, try to make sure it is healthcare related. You will be able to talk about it in your personal statement, you essays and your interviews. You may also obtain reference letters from supervisors involved in your project.

Research experience

Research will always be a favorable feature in your application as it shows curiosity outside the classroom, commitment to hard work and interest in scientific matters. Furthermore, many of the admissions advisors are research faculty at the medical school, and value students who show promise in this area. It is also important to apply for funding. In Canada, scholarships for undergraduate research are available from the Natural Sciences and Engineering Research Council of Canada (NSERC), local foundations like the Alberta Heritage Foundation for Medical Research (AHFMR), and many others. Similarly, in the UK, scholarships for undergraduate research are available from the Biotechnology and Biological Sciences Research Council (BBSRC), the Medical Research Council (MRC), independent foundations like the Bupa Foundation, and many others. Wherever you hope to complete your research, it will likely be worth your while to consider applying for funding.

There are many great research opportunities through universities, research centers and through doctors or researchers you may know.

1. One way to find professors is to go on the schools' websites and look up faculty in the department you want to work in. You can email some professors to see if they are interested.

2. You can often enroll in a course at your university for credits that allows you to work with a faculty member on his or her research.

3. You can apply for sponsored summer research programs. Note that these programs often require previous experience as well as very competitive grades. The positive side is that being accepted to one of these prestigious summer programs will help in your medical school application.

4. If a student is unable to gain acceptance to a research position, they may be able to apply for a position in a lab as an assistant and through time and initiative, work their way up to doing research. It shows commitment and you will still be able to learn and make contacts even if it may not lead to a publication fast.

International experience

International work is very valuable in setting students apart, although volunteer work and work in a caring role might be considered more important. Medical schools also like to see applicants that demonstrate social understanding, appreciation of diversity and leadership. International experience may be the best way for some to demonstrate all of these.

1. There are several government and non-governmental organization (NGO) opportunities in HIV education and prevention, medicine and dentistry, research, economic development, women's health, etc. Programs like unite for sight or habitat for humanity offer great opportunities to go abroad. Both programs take students from around the world. There are also organizations like VSO in the UK, CIDA in Canada and others that take students from specific countries.

2. There are also companies like Projects Abroad or the Institute for Field Research Expeditions Abroad (IFRE) that you can pay to place you in a volunteer position as an English teacher, a medical assistant or at an orphanage caring for children. However, these companies tend to

get mixed reviews, and in many cases most of the money you pay stays in Europe or North America. If there is a country that attracts you particularly, it may be best to look for a local NGO in that country rather than a European or North American company that you have to pay.

3. Some students work at refugee camps or in disaster relief.

4. If you are looking for a summer experience, another option is to contact hospitals, clinics, senior's homes or women's shelters abroad directly. Rural ones are more likely to need your assistance and will often be willing to help you find accommodation. This is probably the cheapest way for an applicant to find an opportunity to volunteer abroad but it does have its security and safety risks as you will not be part of a group or an organization. A similar but maybe slightly safer way if to contact foreign doctors when they come for seminars or presentations in your home country. They might be able to help you arrange a volunteer position in the hospital or clinic they work in in their country.

Three websites that may be a good place to start are listed below:

1. www.gatesfoundation.org/jobs/pages/volunteering.aspx
   Links to several volunteering websites organized by category.
2. www.abroadreviews.com
   Reviews from volunteers after their experiences with different organizations. If you are thinking of volunteering, this may be a good place to start narrowing your decision. If the organization you want is not listed here or if you want more reviews, there are a few online forums like the one in the link below that may have some relevant posts. And of course searching google will usually bring up reviews as well.
3. boards.bootsnall.com under "living abroad"
   Online discussion boards, several of which are about volunteering abroad.

Other extracurricular experience

Teaching

Teaching is an experience that is common to many applicants. This can be private tutoring, teaching music, teaching abroad or many others. Although it is not medically related, it is a very valuable experience. It helps develop a skill that is essential in medicine: the ability to break down complex principles and convey them in a simple, easily understood and well-organized manner. This is helpful during your training when you have to present patient histories to your senior colleagues and is also very important when you have to explain to patients their disease process in a way they can understand. Communication skills are highly valued by admissions committees.

Sports, music, other

Some admissions committee members are careful to see that applicants lead a balanced lifestyle, as this shows them that they are more likely not to "burn-out" in medical school. Intramural or community league sports teams, music classes, a cappella groups, religious groups, etc. can be a great way to add balance to your application. Some applicants, particularly those playing sports or playing music at a higher level, may choose to discuss in their personal statement how their commitments helped them learn leadership skills, reliability, teamwork, or other qualities relevant to medicine.

What other students have done

We have asked second and third year medical students what extracurricular activities they had done before being accepted to medical school. Here are some answers:

Student 1: I volunteered at a therapeutic riding program where mentally and physically handicapped individuals would have the opportunity to ride horses, I also coached youth teams through 4-H, and of course the standard volunteering at a free clinic for migrant workers.

Student 2: I volunteered to help organize the Chicago (or any other) marathon. I also volunteered with the National Ski Patrol (alpine or Nordic).

Student 3: I volunteered with Aids Action, Big Brother/Big Sister and Habitat for Humanity.

Student 4: I volunteered as a third rider on an ambulance in Boston for two years, worked 4 PM to 12 PM shift. I also worked as a disaster services worker for the American Red Cross. I only went locally to fires, floods (and water-main breaks), but it was definitely worth doing (up in the middle of the night, having to practice being calm and nice to people who are totally wigging out). The Red Cross has a wide variety of volunteer work you can do, not all blood drives and the like.

Student 5: I was an English teacher and taught English in Toyama, Japan for one year. I also worked with the AmeriCorps National Civilian Community Corps where i volunteered for 10 months with 10 other 18-24 year olds.

Student 6: I worked as an outpatient clinical assistant in a busy clinic where I took blood, sorted notes, coordinated clinics, chaperoned doctors, etc. lots of relevant clinical experience. Developed great interpersonal skills. I qualified as a phlebotomist with a certificate, manual handling, etc. I worked in liver laboratories and worked at a family doctor's clinic as a receptionist. I also got relevant work experience at two other hospitals shadowing consultations, watching endoscopies and going on ward rounds.

Student 7: I worked as a chemical engineer manager for a pharmaceutical company for 10 years. While there, I did volunteer work in the hazmat team (a team that wears oxygen suits and is called when there are chemical leaks). I have also been teaching Sunday school and was part of a service that visited terminally ill patients.

Personal statement and essays

General requirements

Applicants are often required to write at least one essay or personal statement discussing why they want to become a doctor or why they believe they will make a good doctor. This is the essay required by the AMCAS application, the UCAS application and applications to other schools in several other countries.

In addition to this essay, some schools, particularly those in North America require additional essays. Here are a few examples of what the schools ask for:

"The HST Division represents a unique environment that draws on the combined resources of Harvard University and MIT to provide a distinct preclinical education tailored to preparing students for a career as a physician-scientist, with an emphasis on quantitative and analytic approaches to areas of critical importance to medicine. Please explain your interest in HST, including how your prior experiences, including research, have prepared you for this challenging opportunity." [Approximately 1 page, Harvard HST program, 2011]

"Describe a significant experience that you consider a success in your life. Reflect on the factors that led to this success." [Approximately 150-200 words, McMsater University, 2010]

"What makes you special, someone who will add to the Mount Sinai community." [250 words, Mount Sinai, 2008]

"Tell us about a difficult or challenging situation that you have encountered and how you dealt with it. Identify both the coping skills that you called upon to resolve the dilemma, and the support person(s) from whom you sought advice." [2400 characters, University of Chicago, 2008]

"Please use this space to write an essay in which you discuss your interest in the Yale University School of Medicine." [500 words, Yale University, 2010]

For details on specific essay requirements at schools in Canada, see page 140. For more information on the UCAS application essay in the UK, see page 221. For more details on admissions essays in the US, see page 307. Additional details on each school's requirements are also listed in the school specific sections.

What and how to write, and what not to write...

Opening lines

"Your opening line must be a kicker. I often would tune out with the more common opening statements, making a huge difference on the applicant's entire essay assessment." (admissions advisor). This is not an autobiography; it is an argumentative piece of writing, so be convincing and do not start with "I was born in London, England..." A better way to start the personal statement is with a compelling personal story or a poignant quote related to what you will be discussing. The University of Oxford advises that: "You will not be alone in trying to open your statement with an attention grabbing intro. If you try this, make sure it helps tutors to learn something about what motivates and enthuses you".

Example of a good opening line
Tears rolled down her cheeks as she walked away from the clinic with her tiny, underweight baby in her arms. She was a young mother, and despite how much I wished I could help her, I had to refuse her of her baby's monthly pack of vitamins because our supply had run out.

Elaborating on meaningful experiences

Particularly for those who have gained a substantial array of experiences, it is often much more engaging and effective to pick some of the most profound experiences and expand on these areas, rather than listing every award, accomplishment and position held. This is especially true when there is a place to list your activities in the application, as there is in the AMCAS and OMSAS applications. "The other annoying thing that many applicants do is reiterate their CV/activities. Don't follow your entire activity list; pick a few interesting experiences and expand on them" (admissions advisor discussing application in the US and Canada). In many ways, your essay is your chance to show that you are more than the sum of your test scores, academic transcript and extracurricular or volunteer accomplishments. While these components of the application are substantial, your essays and personal statements allow you to bring your experiences alive and feature how those experiences have developed your desire and ability to succeed as a physician.

Although there is no separate space in the UCAS application to list activities, applicants still need to be careful not to make their essay a list of accomplishments without discussing their meaningful experiences. Some applicants in the UK ask their referees to mention some elements that were important but that they did not have room for in their personal statements. Here is what the University of Oxford says about elaborating on meaningful experiences: "Do not simply recount everything you have ever undertaken. If you have undertaken extracurricular activities, or hold positions of responsibility at school, tell us why you sought these, and why they are important to you. You will not impress us by simply recounting that you took up a placement in Thailand, but we might be more appreciative if you tell us what you personally learnt from the experience, about your interaction with local people, and about shadowing the medical team working within your village."

Not sounding arrogant

It is a good idea to avoid blank statements such as "I am a very compassionate person" or "I can communicate very effectively." Anybody can say these things. A better approach is to describe your experiences and highlight what you learned from them. To give you some examples of what makes a successful essay or activity description, compare the first applicant to the second one below.

Description of 'Volunteering at the foothills hospital'

Weaker applicant: During my first year at the foothills hospital, I volunteered for four hours per week at the gift shop. I then began working with the "Art-a-la-carte" program. My work consisted of bringing a cart filled with paintings to patients every week and asking them if they wanted to borrow one. While working with the patients, I noticed that I was a very compassionate person and was really good at making patients feel better. I also got a truly amazing sense of satisfaction from helping the people on the wards. It was an incredible experience that I will never forget.

Stronger applicant: During my time with Art a la Carte, I "carted" various paintings around to patients. They could borrow as many of them as they wanted, and I would talk to them as I helped put their new paintings on their walls. My favorite moments were when a patient would find a painting that reminded them of their personal life. Whether it was of a skyscape or a Spaniel, it always held a story, and I loved to see the emotion in their eyes as they fondly remembered their past. Occasionally, I would meet a patient who did not want a painting, but wanted someone to visit with them. I remember one elderly lady who invited me in and asked me to sit next to the window with her. Despite the limited view, she appreciated what she had. We sat together admiring the sunshine in the parking lot below. I began to see that we are more than organs, skin and bones, and that healing can be an emotional process as much as it is a physical one.

Comments

The second essay is certainly not perfect and can be much improved - but it is here to convey a few key concepts. The second essay is stronger because it conveys emotion more creatively. What people do not enjoy reading are statements such as, "It was an incredible experience I will never forget" or "I will give 110% if I am accepted", which are used in the majority of personal statements. Limit hyperbole. It dilutes the meaning of your sentences. Anyone can say that they are compassionate. Rather than coming flat out and just saying it, convey your strengths by talking about what you learned from your experiences, much the way the second applicant did. The last line is a good example. Instead of just saying "I am a compassionate person who will be nice to patients", the second applicant comes at it from a fresh angle and uses a lesson he learned to convey something about himself.

Using diversity to your advantage

"Your essays have to be unique and interesting. Focus on your diversity... Mention it somewhere, bring it up on the side or directly; it will work towards your benefit [...] International work goes a long way as well" (US admissions advisor). Most admissions advisors aim to get a high level of diversity in their class, in terms of experience, cultural backgrounds, academic backgrounds, etc. Some universities even ask directly about how you will contribute to their class diversity in their interviews. The things that make you a unique applicant and allow you to contribute a unique dimension to the classroom will be powerful in your application in most cases.

Example of an extract highlighting diversity and discussing a meaningful experience

My experience living and working with people from different cultures has taught me several lessons, given me important perspective and helped me to understand that appreciating diversity is a state of mind, a function of seeing and learning from the best in others. At the age of fifteen I began volunteering as an English tutor for Afghan immigrants, and since then have befriended many Afghan members of my community. Their outlook on life has been shaped by their upbringing in a war-torn country, and they have helped me to gain new perspective on the value of education and the power of perseverance through difficult times. The relationships we forged have helped me internalize the importance of connecting with people of different cultures when working together. These individuals have lived without safety or freedom for most of their lives, and the courage and faith that they exemplify has taught me about the extraordinary obstacles that the human spirit can conquer.

Example 2 of an extract highlighting diversity
My own cultural background has shaped my appreciation for diversity as well. My ancestry stems from India, through East Africa, to Canada where my family now lives. My family has instilled in me an appreciation for the quality of life that we enjoy, and they have taught me the importance of helping those less fortunate. I have put these principles into action through my volunteer work at home and abroad. In Africa I learned the importance of empowering local communities and keeping an open mind to overcome language, age and cultural barriers. In Tibet and Nepal I learned a great deal about seeing and appreciating the best in others, as these cultures exemplify many humanitarian principles not always as evident in more materialistic societies. My experiences have enhanced my desire to continue working closely with people of different backgrounds and learning from their diversity, and have prepared me to excel in the increasingly diverse field of medical science.

Why not become a physiotherapist?

While dedicating your life to helping others is a very commendable reason to become a doctor, it begs the question – "Why not become a physiotherapist or a nurse?" Maybe you want to pursue medicine because it would allow you to combine analytical thinking or problem solving with an opportunity to work closely with families and patients. Maybe you want to take a leadership role in the health field and apply a broad range of knowledge in your work, maybe you are thinking about it from a global perspective. Whatever your reasons are, make sure that they do not beg the above questions. Your reasons may also be strengthened by including examples of efforts you have made to explore your desire to become a physician and/or evidence of preparation to excel as a physician (working in a hospital for example).

Description of 'interest in the healing profession"
My interest in the healing profession began in freshman year of high school when I began volunteering at Toronto's Sunnybrook Veterans Hospital at the age of 14. At first, I helped

to safely transport patients. Over time, I shouldered more responsibility and my experiences became more meaningful as I built personal rapport with veterans by listening attentively to their stories. My concern for patients and their care was noticed in my senior year by Dr. Pierre Francois, a cardiac surgeon. After speaking with him about my interest in medicine he invited me to observe a bypass operation. I still remember the buzz I felt from seeing this medical miracle.

At Sunnybrook, I gained insight into challenges facing geriatric medicine, especially the need for constant attention and support for elderly patients. What struck me was how isolated and depressed our veterans felt. I worried for them and for others, like my grandfather, who do not have access to the same care. I felt a certain calling to become a doctor.

Comments

The applicant does a good job of not only highlighting the efforts he has made to learn about a career in medicine, but also his curiosity to learn more about his patients' stories and the work of the surgeon. Curiosity is an important attribute which admissions advisors often look for. The language is simple and easy to read, while emotions are still conveyed powerfully, such as when the applicant discusses the "medical miracle." Another very good aspect of this extract is that the applicant not only describes what he or she experienced, but makes the paragraph stronger by reflecting on it: "I worried for them and for others, like my grandfather, who do not have access to the same care." Ability to reflect on situations is required throughout a medical course/medical career and will be seen as very positive by admissions committee.

Explaining any weaknesses in your application

If you have had a difficult semester or a poor grade in a course, the personal statement may be a good place to explain it. If there is a good reason, bring it in. If you have taken higher level courses in the same subjects and done well in them, it is a good idea to talk about how you overcame those difficulties and excelled in the higher level classes. You should be careful in the way you bring out a weakness as you do not want to emphasize any weakness to the admissions committee. However, if there is a true weakness in your application, the committee will eventually see it and the personal statement may be your only chance to provide a context in which to view the issue. The University of Oxford says the following about the personal statement: "Please do not be shy in declaring any mitigating circumstances. These may help us to put your achievements or personality within a finer context. We actively look for reasons why you may have under-performed in examinations, or performed well against the odds".

Description of a low GPA

I realize that a 2:2 (2.7/4.0) in my undergraduate may count against me but my motivation has changed considerably since undergraduate years. I have attempted to compensate by taking an MSc course in the pathology of viruses and by working full time within the healthcare system where I have gained a real appreciation of the commitment needed as a doctor.

Comments

One positive element in this extract is the way the applicant gives a context in which to consider his 2:2. For him, this involved gaining experience in healthcare and an advanced degree. Ways to improve this extract could include mentioning an award for academic excellence during the MSc, or including high grades during the MSc if appropriate. Another way to improve this may be to discuss the trend of the applicant's grades if they showed a steady increase from first year to fourth year and also give some explanation as to why the applicant only achieved a 2:2 in his undergraduate degree.

Making the personal statement personal

An essay that presents a list of extracurricular activities is likely not to be personal enough, as is an essay that is excessively creative with philosophical and theological explorations. As mentioned above, this is your chance to bring your application to life with your personality and your life experience. A good way to ensure your essay is personal enough is to ensure that each sentence written, or at least most of them, could not have been written by most other applicants. Once you have gone through the exercise of checking this, ask someone very close to you to read the essay and ask them if it really portrays who you are. You may think that the admissions committees do not know you and will not be able to tell, but the truth is, the more personal your essay is, the more unique it will be, and the more likely you will stand out from the pool of applicants and be selected for an interview.

Example of an essay that sounds personal: "What has been your most humbling experience"

When I was in high school, I strived to outdo others and to be the best. I took pride in my work, yet I felt unfulfilled. I had adopted the mantra of "be the best you can be" and I applied it to an extreme. In my mind, if I wasn't everything, I was nothing. However, as I worked harder and harder toward achieving this goal, I found myself feeling increasingly unfulfilled. A strange thing happened to me when I came to university. I discovered that I was not the best mathematician in the world, nor the best one at Stanford. Many people I met were unquestionably bright, and there was a wealth of talent that was truly unique and that out shot my own. I knew that I would maybe never reach the top. Although this thought was dreadful to me, I decided that whatever happened, I would work hard. I began placing a high value not only on my marks but on cultivating humility and the knowledge that I gained from it. The eyes with which I used to judge the world became the eyes with which I would observe and understand it. It was liberating not to pass judgment on it but to just take it in. I believe that humility is essential to seeing and learning from the best in others. As challenges in the future become more complex, I hope to be able to learn from the experiences and skills of my peers and mentors to continue to improve my abilities. The scientific knowledge that I will gain through seeking help when needed will enhance my ability to provide the very best medical treatment.

Comments

This essay is undeniably personal. The applicant takes us through a very meaningful experience in his life, outlining his thoughts, feelings, and the lessons he learned during this time. It is written in a candid manner, using frank and undisguised words such as "In my mind, if I wasn't everything, I was nothing" or "I discovered that I was not the best mathematician in the world". Because this essay is so personal, it is different from anything the admission advisor might have read that day and it is thus more likely to grab his or her attention and interest. The words "although this was dreadful to me" and "it was liberating" help us feel and relate to the same revelation the applicant had. Another good aspect of this extract is that the applicant clearly describe the evolution of his thought process and does not let the reader guess. Even if you write an essay well, it will not leave a good impression if the reader does not understand what your point is. In this extract, the sentence "The eyes with which I used to judge the world became the eyes with which I would observe and understand it" present the personal growth of the applicant in a strikingly concise manner. Finally, in the conclusion, the applicant links his story with the practice of the medical profession and presents one more reason why he or she will be a good doctor. This is a powerful and sensible ending.

On the downside, this essay can be risky as it presents a negative aspect of the applicant: his lack of humility initially. Discussing pride in any form could make an admissions advisor nervous to take a chance. If something like this is done on an application, it is important to include how the negative aspect presented may have improved or changed. Note that the applicant who wrote this essay was granted an interview.

Example 2 of an extract that sounds personal

Tears rolled down her cheeks as she walked away from the clinic with her tiny, underweight baby in her arms. She was a young mother, and despite how much I wished I could help her, I had to refuse her of her baby's monthly pack of vitamins because our supply had run out. I was in Píntag, a rural community in Ecuador, volunteering at a medical clinic and living with a host-family. It was one of my first experiences in the medical field, as well as one of the most meaningful. I had decided to embark on this three-month adventure after volunteering at a hospital in Richmond Hill, Ontario and realizing that I was ready to explore the career of a physician in a more hands-on manner. From the first day at the Subcentro de salud, I was shocked by the lack of doctors, equipment and other resources, including medication. I worked closely with the doctors and was given the opportunity to prepare charts, perform vaccinations, and assist in emergencies. From interacting with patients, hearing their stories, and working with the physicians, I realized that good doctors must go beyond treating the disease; they must have the ability to overcome barriers and make connections with the patients. At the Subcentro, I saw, with my own eyes, that a physician's work can determine one's fate: life from death, and happiness from sorrow.

Comments

This introduction captures the reader's interest and mind from the very first line. The wording is simple but powerful and expresses the social conscience of the applicant towards the less fortunate in the world. The applicant seems caring, compassionate, energetic and committed. International experience in the healthcare field shows real effort from the applicant to find out about medical practice and interact with patients. This makes the applicant a very competitive candidate for interview. Note that this extract is written in a very personal way "I saw, with my own eyes [...]", "hearing their stories", etc. This makes the story powerful and memorable.

Proofreading

Although you will not be disadvantaged for not being a professional writer, admissions committees do expect to read an essay that is free of spelling mistakes and uses correct grammar. They also expect applicants to have put considerable work into their personal statements and essays, and thus expect your writing to reflect strong communication skills. Remember that communication skills are very important in the training and practice of medicine and it is thus logical that admissions committees are looking for evidence of strong communication skills in the application.

Weaker applicant: I had wanted to be a physician since the age of eight. When I found out that my friend's mother had been diagnosed with a neurodegenerative disease, I had asked my parents how I could help her. When they told me she needed the help of a doctor, I immediately changed my career of choice from bus driver to brain surgeon.

Stronger applicant: At the age of eight, when I found out that my friend's mother was suffering from a neurodegenerative disease and was in need of a doctor, I changed my career of choice from bus driver to brain surgeon.

The stronger applicant says the same thing but cuts out a third of the text. This makes it easier on the admissions officer who may be tired after reading several applications that day, and allows the applicant to say more in the short word-limit given.

Weaker applicant 2: Although my ancestry stems from India, my parents grew up in East Africa before moving to Canada and raising me.

Stronger applicant 2: My ancestry stems from India, through Africa, to Canada where my family now lives.

Again, the second sentence conveys the same idea much more quickly, and is easier to read as a result.

To strengthen your personal statement, it is a good idea to get regular feedback from others on your essays plans and drafts, particularly from those in medical school or in the medical profession. It will take several drafts before coming to a strong final version.

Additional extracts and personal statements

Extract of a personal statement - hospital volunteering and research

[...] In secondary school and first year university I became a regular volunteer on the palliative care ward. I regard this time as being formative for the solidification of my drive to go into medicine. I started by doing simple tasks – bringing artwork, showing movies – and over time grew close to many of the patients. A very peculiar air pervades the palliative care ward – this is the last stop on many of the patients' paths. I was surprised to find the flourishing of hope even there and even more so to discover its' necessity. I recall wholeheartedly wishing to give support to my patients. It was not long before I started working in a cancer research lab. As a researcher I was determined, meticulous and vigilant. I knew that I needed this 'technical' ability to help people, my good will and support would only go so far. Great physicians empower people by weaving science and compassion, and I look forward to the challenges that lie ahead in practicing this noble art.

Comments

Instead of discussing the amount of hours spent or different positions held in different hospitals, the author discusses a lesson he learned from his work: "I was surprised to find the flourishing of hope even there and even more so to discover its' necessity". This reflection conveys that the applicant was actively learning and engaging on the job, is able to reflect on his experiences and is better prepared for a career in medicine as a result. This helps make the essay personal.

Perhaps one of the most powerful elements in this extract is the way the applicant shows maturity and reasoning in his choices "I knew that I needed this 'technical' ability to help people, my good will and support would only go so far'. A lot of applicant only describe their experiences, which may be appropriate. In this extract, explaining why the applicant made certain choices (in this case to start doing research) tells the admissions committee a lot about his active search for the right career, maturity and sense of initiative.

Finally, the author's reasons for wanting to become a physician are less likely to beg the question "why not become a physiotherapist, or a researcher, or something else". Few other careers "weave science and compassion" the way medicine does.

Extract of a personal statement - clinical research

[...] I am currently conducting a clinical research project. Our objective is to assess the benefits of a new medical device in treating rheumatic diseases. The first aspect of my work was to set up a protocol for the adequate analysis of the efficiency of the device. During one of the patient interviews I conducted, I was deeply touched by the euphoria of a middle aged woman. As she was telling me about difficult times when walking was a challenge, she got up and started flexing her knees up and down. I am not sure if she was convincing herself or me that she could finally walk normally, but what was certain was her gratitude towards her physician. Moments such as this one remind me of the human level involved in the practice of medicine, and strengthen my motivation to excel as a doctor whose work goes beyond the physical treatment of patients.

Comments

One good aspect of this extract is that the applicant does not waste words describing the role of the team but instead focuses on what he or she did. This is good because the admissions committees are interested in the work that you did, not the work that your team and colleagues did. The other important point in this extract is that the applicant links their experience to something that they learned that will have an impact on their career as a doctor: the understanding of "the human level involved in the practice of medicine" and that the "work goes beyond the physical treatment of patients."

Description of 'Volunteering in village orphanage'

I went to Africa to teach English, but found an opportunity to do much more. Whether we were playing sports or chasing the chicken we needed to catch for dinner, the connection I developed with the boys at the orphanage was truly special and culminated in our bonding together as a group to achieve a common goal. The dirt road the orphans played soccer on was covered in manure, and they badly wanted to do something about it; my goal was to show them that they could.

The next day, I brought five grass slashing knives to the orphanage, which lay adjacent to an unkept grassland. The boys' eyes lit up; we were going to build a soccer field! I taught them how to use an axe and set up a rotation so that everyone was involved. My role was to do as much as I could while still leaving it as their project; this was as much about building their confidence as it was a soccer field. After several days and many blisters, the field was ready, complete with wooden goal posts and stones for spectators to sit on.

Comments

The author shows a connection with the kids: "whether we were playing sports or chasing the chicken we needed to catch for dinner" by describing his experience. This is more effective than simply saying "the connection I developed with the boys was truly special", since anyone could have made this statement. The applicant also demonstrates in his story a sense of initiative, awareness of social disparity and genuine care. This is done in a simple and easy to read style of writing.

Extract of Personal Statement - 'Physician shadowing & Kenya project'

During winter and summer breaks away from Cornell, I shadowed Dr. John Laprey in the operating room and orthopedic clinic at Toronto's St. Michael's Hospital. I experienced some harsh realities of this profession in Toronto, including long patient wait-times and inadequate funding. Despite these challenges, it was Dr. Laprey's focus on patient care that made a profound impact on me. It had to do with HOW he practiced medicine. This was most evident during the miraculous recovery of a 22-year old trauma patient who was transformed from being paraplegic to having a full range of motion in 10 weeks. Despite his tireless efforts, Dr. Laprey modestly attributed the recovery to the patient and the resiliency of the human body. Dr. Laprey inspired me by being an empathetic listener and by being humble, caring and kind. There was no doubt that patients were at the core of his practice of medicine.

Working with four students under Joshua Hanson, Professor Emeritus of Nutrition at Cornell, I helped design an HIV/AIDS nutrition program for rural African communities. This culminated in a trip to Kenya during the '06/'07 winter break. Working in collaboration with ICODEI, a local NGO, we modified and implemented the program to suit local needs. This experience showed me that public health education programs which are culturally sensitive and delivered in a creative way can be effective. I also appreciated that not all medical interventions require millions of dollars or MRI machines. I was most impressed and motivated by the Kenyans' degree of commitment, despite their poverty, in learning how to prevent and better cope with illness.

Comments

The applicant goes well beyond a simple description of his experiences, highlighting important learnings from each activity that demonstrate his maturity. His description of the impressed and motivated group of Kenyan locals gives us a sense that his project was successful and meaningful to them. This essay could be improved by discussing more what his role was in the team of four students, or something interesting about their approach to the project which may have taught him something, possibly important to his career in medicine. He also provides good insight into why Dr. Laprey is an excellent role model for him, but applicants should be careful not to use this technique in too many paragraphs, as some applicants spend too much time discussing their role models rather than themselves.

Extract of Personal Statement - 'nutrition project in Tajikistan'

This past summer I dedicated myself to providing disaster-relief in Gorno-Badakshan, Tajikistan through Focus Humanitarian Assistance. As I immersed myself in the Pamiri culture and learned about everyday struggles, my concept of social justice evolved. In a country where the majority lived in extreme poverty, I felt empowered as I saw a simple two-hour training session on proper dieting help local Tajikis survive the harsh and debilitating winters. Although my work did not directly address the curative needs of the population, many disparities concerning healthcare constantly disturbed me. For example, upon realizing that no locals wore prescription lenses, I inquired about the reasons behind this oddity. As I heard each local proudly respond that they did not need corrective glasses, I wondered whether their pride was linked to their unfamiliarity with the concept of perfect vision and the lack of ophthalmological care in the region. After having such inspiring experiences, I have refined my goals as an aspiring physician: to utilize my medical training to empower other health professionals in these communities to address the urgent healthcare issues common to such underrepresented areas.

Comments

The story about his conversation with the elders is very effectively written. It is engaging for the reader and highlights something he learned about rural health challenges in a memorable way. His reflections throughout the description of events demonstrates his maturity "I wondered whether their pride was linked to their unfamiliarity with the concept of perfect vision and the lack of ophthalmological care in the region." The strongest aspect of this extract is the ability of the applicant to reflect on his experiences and convey that in an engaging manner. Possibly, there is not enough there about what the applicant did himself in Gorno-Badakshan and the admissions committees are always interested in what you did, rather than what your project or team did.

Extract of personal statement - academic achievement

Advancing directly from high school graduate to second year university student was a serious test of my independent learning abilities. Determined to keep pace with my classmates who until then had been one year my senior, I opted to take Calculus 2 and Calculus 3 in parallel. The undergraduate advisor for the Department of Chemistry gave me permission as well as exemption from two prerequisite courses. Without a basic understanding of the material from Calculus 2, I could not complete my assignments for Calculus 3. I resolved to teach myself Calculus 2 in the span of one month. I developed my own rigorous work schedule and self-imposed deadlines for the completion of various chapters. Heeding the advice of some of my mentors, I prioritized my tasks and kept focused to work efficiently. I directed my own progress, setting ambitious goals and working hard to reach them. That year I earned the highest grades in all my classes and proved to myself that self directed learning is one of my greatest strengths. This ability has been further developed through my three summers of research in Multiple Sclerosis at the National Institute of Health, where I was given the opportunity to study recent publications and to set up my own experiments. I have expanded my ability to understand concepts not presented in any textbook, to digest and synthesize the material published on a given topic in order to subsequently employ that knowledge in the design of new research experiments.

These experiences have greatly enhanced my capacity for self directed study, both inside and outside of the classroom. I am ready, motivated and driven to learn, and I believe that I am prepared to face the challenge of succeeding at the Schulich School of Medicine

Comments

The applicant gives context to the admissions committee for reading and understanding his transcripts. Moreover, rather than listing many occasions where he or she has been able to demonstrate self-directed learning, the applicant chooses to focus on one example and explores it in depth. The applicant first sets the stage of the problem faced providing clear reasoning of his or her actions "Without a basic understanding of the material from Calculus 2, I could not complete my assignments for Calculus 3", then explains his or her method of tackling the issue: "I developed my own rigorous work schedule and self-imposed deadlines for the completion of various chapters." In addition, the applicant shows maturity of thought by respecting advice of experienced senior mentors: "Heeding the advice of some of my mentors, I prioritized my tasks and kept focused to work efficiently."

Another strong element of this essay worth mentioning is the fact that the applicant applied self-directed learning to learning outside the classroom: "...have expanded my ability to understand concepts not presented in any textbook, to digest and synthesize the material published on a given topic in order to subsequently employ that knowledge in the design of new research experiments." This is particularly valuable in a medical school application since a lot of the clinical skills that medical students need to learn cannot simply be read in a textbook. Rather, they need to be practiced and applied.

Extract of a personal statement - anecdote from a hospital experience

[...] I first experienced this type of learning during my volunteer work on the palliative care ward. I had expected that patients would be depressed, but gradually I understood that their feelings were much more complex.

One of my fondest memories is of a man named Ken Smith (name changed) whom I met during my regular visits on the ward. Ken, a martial arts expert diagnosed with cancer, challenged me to a little demonstration. With a few quick movements, he surprised me by getting my hand in a vice grip and immobilizing my whole body. Later, when I reflected upon the incident, I understood that it was not just an expression of strength, but that Ken was trying to regain a sense of dignity. For many patients, the worst thing about cancer is not the end itself, but the demeaning way in which the illness runs its course. Ken taught me the importance of helping patients maintain their dignity, self worth and sense of self.

My experience on the palliative care ward has helped me to internalize important aspects of providing patient care. I have had a chance to develop an understanding of the emotions that patients and their loved ones experience during difficult times, and I believe that as a physician, understanding these complexities will better enable me to form trusting relationships and serve people in need of medical assistance.

Comments

This extract revolves around a patient-applicant interaction that occurred on the palliative care ward. The sole fact that the patient was able to "challenge [the applicant] to a little demonstration" shows that the applicant was able to get close to patients and befriend them. In many ways, presenting this story shows the ability of the applicant to interact with patients much more effectively that saying: "I befriended many patients on the palliative ward."

The other strong point of this extract is that the applicant not only showed that he had good interactions with patients but was also able to draw lessons from these interactions: "I had expected that patients would be depressed, but gradually I understood that their feelings were much more complex", "I have had a chance to develop an understanding of the emotions that patients and their loved ones experience during difficult times."

Obtaining the best reference letters

T he reference letter requirements can differ significantly between schools and countries. For example, most universities in the US and Canada ask for 2-3 letters of reference, while in the UK and at several schools in Eastern Europe, one reference letter is often all that is required. For details on the reference letter requirements in Canada, see page 142; in the UK, see page 223, in the US, see page 310. Additional details on each school's requirements are also listed in the school specific sections.

Once you have identified your potential referees, you need to organize a meeting with them. It is much better for you to meet with them rather than simply requesting a reference letter by email. When you meet with them, you should ask them if they think they can write a strong reference letter for you. This is important, as you do not want a bland, slightly positive letter. If the person hesitates or is not sure, try to find another referee.

Once you have found your referees, fill out all the envelopes for them including stamps. Include your personal statement and your CV as well as any other information you think may help them write a strong letter for you. This may include a description of your extracurricular activities, your academic transcripts, any papers you have published or even a bullet point list of key elements you believe should be included in the reference letter. If you have had a bad semester, it may be appropriate to explain to your referee why that happened and efforts you have put forward to improve since.

Between your personal statement, a letter you may have written and the conversations you have with your referees, it is important to convey the reasons why you want to go to medical school. It is rare that even a referee who knows you well will know all about your motivations, inspirations, and reasons for going into medical school. It can significantly strengthen your reference letter if in fact the referee does know all about these elements of your character prior to writing the letter.

Returning home to practice

One of the most important considerations for medical school applicants when deciding if they want to study medicine abroad, and if so, where they will go, is how difficult it will be to come back and practice as a doctor at home. This section aims to give some answers to applicants who want to study medicine abroad and plan to come back to either Canada, the US or the UK after their studies.

This section includes information about which medical schools are accredited and the steps to take to return home to practice, including additional examinations. This section also provides some information about how competitive it is for international medical graduates to secure residency positions and employment positions in Canada, the US and the UK.

Returning to Canada

Because Canada has a patient to doctor ratio among the lowest of any industrialized nation, there is a perceived doctor shortage by many. This, combined with the very competitive entrance to medical school has convinced many students to apply abroad with the plan to come back to practice in Canada.

Some facts about Canadians studying abroad (CSAs)

CaRMS (The Canadian Resident Matching Service) released a comprehensive report last year about Canadians studying abroad. Some key findings are outlined here for your consideration. The full report is available on www.carms.ca

- Almost all Canadians studying medicine abroad desire strongly to come back and practice in Canada.
- There are approximately 3500 canadians studying in foreign medical schools (outside US and Canada), with the largest number in the Caribbean (about 2000).
- Canadian international graduate may contribute to up to 700 graduates per year applying to residency training in Canada. This is about 30% of the total Canadian medical school output.
- Many Canadians studying abroad are residents of British Columbia and Ontario where the success rates of medical school applicants are the lowest.

- Canadians studying abroad expressed a lot of frustration not being able to arrange clinical experience in Canada during their medical training. The Caribbean school respondents reported the most difficulty, while students in Australia and Ireland reported some success there.

There is a general consensus amongst published books, journal articles, online blogs, medical professionals and many medical school students that returning to Canada to practice after studying abroad is very difficult. Some will say it is not worth trying. We think that many international medical school graduates come back to Canada each year and with that in mind, it seems unreasonable to say that it is impossible. However, it is very very difficult and possibly a lot more difficult than getting into medical school in Canada in the first place for many specialties. If Canada is where you want to be, there is a way, but prepare yourself for a lot of hard work and fierce competition for a limited number of places. Many students consider going to the United States for residency as their backup plan.

Medical schools that are accredited

To be eligible for participation in the first iteration of the residency match in Canada, you must be either a medical student, or a graduate having obtained or in the process of obtaining a medical degree by July 1 of the match year from:

1. A Liaison Committee on Medical Education / Committee on Accreditation on Canadian Medical Schools (LCME/CACMS) accredited school (http://www.lcme.org/directry.htm)
2. A school of osteopathic medicine
3. An international medical school listed with the International Medical Education Directory (IMED), published by the Foundation for the Advancement of International Medical Education and Research (FAIMER)

To see if your school is on the FAIMER list, visit: http://imed.ecfmg.org/

Applicants who are attending or have graduated from a school of osteopathic medicine, or who are attending or have graduated from a school listed with the International Medical Education Directory (IMED), published by the Foundation for the Advancement of International Medical Education and Research (FAIMER), must also have

1. Written and passed the Medical Council of Canada Evaluating Examination (MCCEE)
2. Or be scheduled to write the September OR November MCCEE

Steps in obtaining a residency in Canada

We have detailed below a step by step process and information for IMGs who wish to obtain a residency position in Canada. **Please note that if you obtain a residency position, you are legally obliged to attend.**

Important information:
1. Make sure you are eligible by checking your medical school is accredited according to the criteria detailed in the previous section.
2. You can then test your readiness for the Medical Council of Canada Evaluating Examination (MCCEE) through the Medical Council of Canada Self Administered Evaluating Examination (SAE - EE). More information on this test can be found at http://www.mcc.ca/en/exams/self_admin.shtml. IMGs who take the SAE - EE will receive the number of questions correctly answered as well as a percentile table that compares their performance to the results achieved by other MCCEE candidates. Fees are CAD62 per examination.
3. You must then write and pass the Medical Council of Canada Evaluating Examination (MCCEE) or be scheduled to write the September OR November MCCEE.
4. If you are an IMG who has already completed post graduate training outside Canada, note that most IMGs need to repeat some post graduate training in Canada to obtain provincial licensure to practice.
5. In addition to the criteria above, some programs will have additional criteria. To find out the details of those criteria, please visit the following link: http://www.carms.ca/eng/r1_eligibility_prov_e.shtml.
6. Note that provincial funded position are only open to permanent residents and Canadian citizens.

Step by Step process:
1. IMGs do not have an automatic registration number and thus need to register online to get an AWS token. This token will then allow the IMGs to complete an online application for a residency position.
2. At this stage, IMGs need to pay the fee to access the online application.
3. You then have to complete an application form
4. The next step is to prepare and submit all the documentation that is required. This includes transcripts, medical school performance record or Dean's letter, letters of references, personal letters and other additional documents you may wish to submit. Note that if you do not have a medical school performance record or Dean's letter because your medical school does

not provide them, you can explain this in your personal letter. Also, it is not a good idea to send masses of additional documents as they may count against you in your application if they are not deemed relevant.

5. In the next step, applicants select the programs they wish to apply to and assign the documents to the correct programs.

6. The final stage is very important. It consists of ranking the programs in your order of preference. If this is not done before the deadline, the application will be removed and the fees will not be refunded.

How are IMGs considered?

How IMGSs are considered varies significantly from province to province. For complete information, please visit the CaRMS website or the provincial websites. We have summarized some key information regarding the provincial differences below:

1. In most provinces, IMGs are automatically eligible to apply for the first iteration (or first round) of the residency match. However, in British Columbia, IMG's must have an assessment from the BC IMG Assessment Program to be eligible for the first iteration. Find more information on this assessment at http://www.imgbc.med.ubc.ca/Home.htm In Alberta, IMGs are not eligible for the first iteration of the residency match.

2. In the majority of provinces, IMGs apply to a separate stream of positions than Canadian graduates in one or more disciplines. This is called a parallel system. The provinces using this system in the first iteration are Newfoundland, Nova Scotia, Ontario, Saskatchewan and British Columbia.

3. Quebec and Manitoba use what is known as a "competitive" system in the first iteration where IMGs apply to the same positions as Canadian graduates in all disciplines.

4. For the second iteration (an additional round in which applicants compete for positions not filled during the first iteration), all provinces use the "competitive" system described above, and all provinces allow IMGs to apply. Note that to apply in Alberta, applicants first need to go through the Alberta International Medical Graduate Program (AIMG).

5. It is also important to note that students with previous creditable post-graduate training are not eligible in the first iteration in any province. These students can apply in the 2nd iteration in most provinces except Quebec.

MCCEE and MCCQE

The MCCEE is a 4-hour computer based exam offered both in English and French that consists of 180 multiple choice questions, each listing five possible answers of which only one is the correct or best answer. It is a general assessment of the applicant's basic medical knowledge in the principal disciplines of medicine: Child Health, Maternal Health, Adult Health, Mental Health, Population Health and Ethics required at the level of a new medical graduate who is about to enter the first year of supervised postgraduate training practice.

The MCCEE is offered up to five times per year in January, March, May, September and November, during two-to three-week testing windows. For more information on how to register for the test, the fees and the sites at which the text can be taken, visit http://www.mcc.ca/en/exams/ee/scheduling.shtml.

All candidates then need to pass the MCCQE part 1 exam and the MCCQE part 2 exam, just like Canadian medical graduates do. To write the exam, the applicants' school must be listed in the World Health Organization (WHO) directory or the Foundation for Advancement of International Medical Education and Research (FAIMER) International Medical Education Directory (IMED) directory [20]. The MCCQE part 1 exam is a one day, computer based test. Candidate are allowed up to 3½ hours in the morning session to complete 196 multiple-choice questions [21]. Candidates are allowed 4 hours in the afternoon session for the clinical decision making component [21]. This exam is usually written before medical students graduate from medical school.

Before being authorized for independent clinical practice, all new doctors need to pass the MCCQE part 2 exam as well. This is usually done in the first two years of residency training. Once a doctor has passed the MCCQE part 2, he or she obtains a Licentiate of the Medical Council of Canada (LMCC) which is a pre-requisite for provincial licensure to practice medicine.

NAC OSCE

All provinces have the right to request additional assessments to qualify for residency positions in their province. These assessments may include the National Assessment Collaboration Objective Structured Clinical Examination (NAC OSCE), which is only administered in

Canada. Candidates must take the MCCEE before being eligible to take the NAC OSCE, and certain jurisdictions may add region-specific eligibility criteria or may require the Medical Council of Canada Qualifying Examination Part I for certain provincially funded training positions.

The National Assessment Collaboration (NAC) Objective Structured Clinical Examination (OSCE) assesses the readiness of an international medical graduate (IMG) for entrance into a Canadian residency program. It is a national, standardized examination that tests the knowledge, skills and attitudes essential for entrance into postgraduate training in Canada.

Comprising a series of clinical stations and an additional written therapeutic component, the NAC OSCE is a "hands-on" examination that simulates typical clinical scenarios. The examination may include problems in medicine, pediatrics, obstetrics and gynecology, preventive medicine and community health, psychiatry and surgery. Candidates are assessed for language usage and proficiency as well as basic knowledge of therapeutic management of common complaints.

The NAC OSCE is intended to help rank IMGs who apply to individual Canadian medical school graduate programs. Passing this examination does not guarantee a training position in Canada, but rather provides feedback to the program directors who are selecting trainees on the strengths and weaknesses of the individuals who take this examination.

IMG residency statistics

Match Results for IMGs by Discipline Preference
2010 First Iteration R-1 Match

Discipline	1st Choice Discipline	Matched to 1st Choice Discipline	Matched to Another Discipline	Number of Unmatched IMGs
Anatomical Pathology	16	6	0	10
Anesthesiology	62	9	4	49
Cardiac Surgery	2	0	1	1
Community Medicine	30	2	0	28
Dermatology	12	1	3	8
Diagnostic Radiology	36	5	4	27
Emergency Medicine	22	5	0	17
Family Medicine	733	108	7	618
General Pathology	3	1	0	2
General Surgery	48	6	3	39
Hematological Pathology	0	0	0	0
Internal Medicine	144	27	8	109
Laboratory Medicine	43	4	2	37
Medical Biochemistry	3	2	0	1
Medical Genetics	3	1	0	2
Medical Microbiology	1	0	0	1
Neurology	31	2	2	27
Neurology - Pediatric	7	1	1	5
Neuropathology	0	0	0	0
Neurosurgery	6	1	1	4
Nuclear Medicine	0	0	0	0
Obstetrics & Gynecology	41	3	2	36
Ophthalmology	15	2	0	13
Orthopedic Surgery	36	6	4	28
Otolaryngology	8	0	0	8
Pediatrics	67	12	3	52
Physical Med & Rehab	19	3	0	16
Plastic Surgery	12	1	0	11
Psychiatry	74	17	2	55
Radiation Oncology	5	1	0	4
Urology	16	1	0	15
Total	1497	227	47	1223

Table 16. Canadian residency match statistics for International Medical Graduates in 2010 [22]

Canadian residency match statistics are published every year on www.carms.ca. In 2010 there were 274 IMG applicants who secured Canadian residencies out of 1223 IMGs applicants. 212

of these filled positions were dedicated positions for IMGs, with 17 dedicated IMG positions going unfilled. These ratios differ from specialty to specialty. For example, for family medicine, 733 IMG applicants chose family medicine as their first choice, from which 108 matched in family medicine, 7 matched in a different specialty and 618 went unmatched, for a first choice success rate of 15%. 104 family medicine places were set aside that year specifically for IMGs. For anesthesiology, there were 62 IMG applicants listing anesthesiology as their first choice. 9 of those 62 IMGs matched in this specialty, and 4 of those 62 matched in another specialty. 49 of them did not match, for a first choice success rate of 15%. One IMG listing anesthesiology as their second choice matched in anesthesiology, accounting for the 10 places reserved in anesthesiology for IMGs that year. The number of designated IMG positions, the number of IMG applicants and the final IMG match results are all available on the CaRMS website at www.carms.ca/eng/operations_R1reports_10_e.shtml Many students who do not match in Canada complete their residency training in the US.

Returning to the UK

Schools that are accepted

The GMC (General Medical Council) defines an acceptable overseas qualification as one which meets the following criteria: it must be a primary medical qualification in allopathic medicine that has been awarded by an institution listed on the Avicenna Directory for Medicine. This directory can be found at the following link: http://avicenna.ku.dk/database/medicine/. The schools listed in the this directory but not accredited in the UK are listed below.

At the time of printing, **the GMC is not registering graduates** who hold primary medical qualifications obtained from the following medical schools:

Belize
St Matthew's University School of Medicine
Grace University School of Medicine
Cook Islands
St Mary's Medical School
Grenada
Keith B Taylor Global Scholars program - combined MD programme between St George's University, Grenada and Northumbria University, UK

Liberia
Saint Luke School of Medicine
Nigeria
Ambrose Ali University (this only applies to those who graduated after 10 December 2010)
Ebonyi State University (this only applies to those who graduated after 10 December 2010)
Igbinedion University College of Health Sciences (this applies only to those who graduated on or after 1 April 2010)
Ladoke Akintola University of Technology (LAUTECH) (this only applies to those who graduated after 10 December 2010)
Nnamdi Azikiwe University (this only applies to those who graduated after 10 December 2010)
University of Benin (this applies only to those who graduated on or after 1 April 2010)
University of Jos (this only applies to those who graduated after 10 December 2010)
University of Maiduguri (this only applies to those who graduated after 10 December 2010)
University of Nigeria (this only applies to those who graduated after 10 December 2010)
University of Port Harcourt (this only applies to those who graduated after 10 December 2010)
Senegal
St Christopher Ibrahima Mar Diop College of Medicine
Seychelles
University of Seychelles American Institute of Medicine (USAIM)
St Lucia
Spartan Health Sciences University (this only applies to graduates who started their course of study on or before 31 December 2008. Refer to case-by-case list for those who started their course of study on or after 1 January 2009)
St Mary's Medical School

For some international medical schools, medical graduates may be allowed to register with the GMC to practice in the UK, but they must apply to do so and will **have their applications reviewed on a case by case basis**. The GMC might require them to submit additional information, such as transcripts and details of clinical rotation arrangements, before a decision is made on whether they have an acceptable primary medical qualification. Medical graduates from these schools should contact the GMC before they apply for registration to practice in the UK. See below for the list of the school for which graduates are considered on a case by case basis:

Antigua
American University of Antigua
Aruba
All Saints University of Medicine (this only applies to graduates who transferred to All Saints following a period of study at another medical school)

Xavier University School of Medicine (this only applies to graduates who transferred to Xavier following a period of study at another medical school)

Cayman Islands
St Matthew's University School of Medicine

Commonwealth of Dominica
All Saints University School of Medicine

Guyana
American International School of Medicine

Netherlands Antilles
American University of the Caribbean (this only applies to graduates who transferred to the American University of the Caribbean following a period of study at another medical school)
St James's School of Medicine, Bonaire (this only applies to graduates who transferred to St James's following a period of study at another medical school)
University of Sint Eustatius School of Medicine

Philippines
University of the East Ramon Magasaysay Memorial Medical Centre

Russia
Nizhny Novgorod State Medical Academy
St Petersburg State Medical Academy
St Petersburg State I.P Pavlov Medical University
St Petersburg State Pediatric Medical Academy

Samoa
Oceania University of Medicine

Sri Lanka
Malabe Private Medical College (this awarding body for this degree is not clear - it is either Nizhny Novgorod University in Russia or by the South Asian Institute of Technology in Sri Lanka)

St Kitts and Nevis
Windsor University School of Medicine
International University of Health Sciences
St Theresa's Medical University
University of Medicine and Health Sciences

St Lucia
Destiny University School of Medicine and Health Sciences (formerly known as the College of Medicine and Health Sciences)
Spartan Health Sciences University (this only applies to graduates who started their course of study on or after 1 January 2009)

Tanzania
Hubert Kairuki Memorial University

Uganda
Kigezi International School of Medicine (this school is now believed to have closed down)

Ukraine
Lugansk State Medical University (this only applies to graduates who transferred to Lugansk following a period of study at another medical school)

There are also some medical schools which are accredited in the UK and which are considered appropriate by the GMC to lead to licensure but that are not listed in the Avicenna directory. These schools are the following:

Iraq
University of Dohuk
University of Sulaimani
Italy
University of Udine
Palestine
Al Quds University
Gumma University
Taiwan
Chang Gung University
China Medical College, Taichung
Chung Shan Medical and Dental College
Kaohsiung Medical College
Nat Defense Medical Centre
Taipei Medical College
National Taiwan University
National Yang Ming Medical College

Private, UK based medical schools

Several courses in the UK claim that completing a degree in part or in whole at their campus in the UK leads to a primary medical qualification (PMQ) awarded by an overseas university. The GMC does not register or license graduates who have been awarded PMQs in such circumstances nor does it give any entitlement to sit the PLAB test. The list below contains some of these PMQ institutions that the GMC is aware of, but it may not be exhaustive. Note that the GMC accepts no liability for the reliance placed on these institutions or for any action or decision taken.

1. European College of Medicine, London (ECM)
2. Grace University School of Medicine, London

3. London College of Medicine
4. London School of Medicine
5. London Medical School
6. School of Health and Neural Sciences, Nottingham
7. American International School of Medicine, UK satellite campus
8. St. Christopher's College of Medicine, Luton
9. Kigezi International School of Medicine, Cambridge
10.Medical College London, Montserrat

Steps in obtaining a post graduate training job in the UK

All doctors wishing to work in any capacity in the UK, whether in the NHS or elsewhere, must be registered and licensed to practice with the GMC. The license will need to be revalidated periodically if the doctor wishes to continue to practice in the UK. Within the EEA there is mutual recognition of equivalent training and qualifications and the right to free movement of workers between member states. Most international medical graduates, which include anyone who has graduated from a medical school outside the UK, EEA or Switzerland, need to sit the PLAB exam. The most up to date and accurate information on the PLAB exam can be found at www.gmc-uk.org/doctors/plab/index.asp.

If you have already completed post graduate qualifications, you may be exempt from sitting the PLAB if your qualification is recognized by the GMC. The complete list of recognized post graduate qualification from oversees and from the UK can be found at http://www.gmc-uk.org/doctors/registration_applications/img_pgq_p1.asp.

The other group of people who are exempt from sitting the PLAB are those who have been selected for sponsorship under an arrangement approved by the GMC. The full list of all approved sponsors can be found at http://www.gmc-uk.org/doctors/registration_applications/list_of_sponsors.asp.

Step 1: If you do not have an approved post graduate qualification or an approved sponsorship, you must write the PLAB exam as a first step.

Once you have passed the PLAB, you can apply for provisional registration with a license to practice.

Step 2: You can apply for the provisional registration online. This includes a fee.

Step 3: You then need to submit your evidence of primary medical qualification. The primary medical qualifications which are accepted are listed on page 100.

Step 4: You now need to provide evidence of fitness to practice. You will be asked to provide details of your registration and licensing for all the medical regulatory authorities of any countries where you have practised or have held registration or a license in the last five years, even if you have not practised there. If there is no medical regulatory authority in the country to issue certificates of good standing or past good standing, you will need to ask your employer(s) in each of those countries to complete the employer reference form. If you have undertaken any clinical attachments or observer-ships in the UK or overseas in the last five years that lasted longer than two months, you will need to obtain an employer reference form to cover each clinical attachment or observer-ship. If you have been employed in a non-medical capacity in the UK or overseas in the last five years, you will need to ask your employer(s) to complete the non-medical employer reference form.

Step 5: In addition to the evidence of fitness to practice, the GMC asks you to account for all periods in the last five years where you were not practicing medicine. This includes alternative employment, clinical attachments, vacation, study leave, maternity leave, career breaks, unemployment, etc with an employer references for every job.

Step 6: You also need to fill in a fitness to practice declaration.

The processing of the application normally take about 5 days, but can take longer so it is important to apply well in advance.

Step 7: With a provisional registration with license to practice, you can now complete what is called the "Foundation Program". With a provisional registration, you need apply to F1 (foundation year 1) posts. At the end of this year, you will obtain a certificate of experience that will provide the evidence that you meet the requirements for full registration. In order to undertake any other posts, including foundation year 2, you must hold a full registration with a license to practice. To apply to the foundation program or find out more about it, visit http://www.foundationprogramme.nhs.uk.

The PLAB

Part 1 is a computer-marked written examination consisting of extended matching questions (EMQs) and single best answer (SBA) questions. The paper contains 200 questions and may contain images. It lasts three hours. The proportion of SBA questions will vary from examination to examination. You can have an unlimited number of attempts but you must pass Part 1 within two years of the date of your IELTS certificate or the date they specify when accepting alternative evidence of your proficiency in English.

Part 2 is an Objective Structured Clinical Examination (OSCE). It takes the form of 14 clinical scenarios or 'stations', a rest station and one or more pilot stations run for statistical purposes, where the marks do not count towards your result. Each station lasts five minutes. You must pass Part 2 within three years of passing Part 1. You can have four attempts at Part 2. If you fail at the fourth attempt you will have to retake IELTS (unless they have accepted alternative evidence from you and it is still valid) and both parts of the PLAB test.

You must apply for and have been granted registration with a license to practice within three years of passing Part 2 of the test.

Competition of IMGs

The job market in the UK is very competitive and students should think very carefully about whether they are willing to take the risks involved in competing for posts. Competition in some specialties and locations is stronger than in others. Securing employment can be a lengthy process: statistics show it could take six months to a year (or even longer) to find a first post once you have passed the PLAB test. A significant number of doctors are still unemployed a year after passing the PLAB test. The NHS Jobs website (http://www.jobs.nhs.uk) allows doctors to search for posts for which immigration sponsorship is more likely to be available, because UK or EEA doctors have not been found in response to earlier advertisements. During 2010, many NHS organisations have reported that they need good quality 'middle grade' doctors – those that have completed or nearly completed basic specialty training or equivalent – particularly in specialties such as pediatrics, accident and emergency medicine, anesthesiology and obstetrics and gynecology.

Returning to the US

Schools that are accepted

To practice as a physician, in addition to meeting the national requirements, some states have their own process for accepting qualifications. California is reputed as being one of the most difficult states for medical schools to gain accreditation from. The list of medical schools that have gained accreditation there is available from www.medbd.ca.gov/applicant/schools_recognized.html

Steps in obtaining a residency in the US

Provided your medical school is eligible, here are the steps to practice in the US after graduating from an international medical school:

1. Pass USMLE step 1 and USMLE step 2 board examinations
2. Obtain the ECFMG (Educational Commission for foreign Medical graduates) certification
3. Complete a US residency program
4. Complete the USMLE step 3 board examination (usually after the first year of residency)

To obtain the ECFMG certification, students must have attended a medical school listed in the International Medical Education Directory available from www.faimer.org/resources/imed.html, with the graduation year of the applicant included in the years the program has been accredited. Students also need to pass the USMLE step 1 examination and the USMLE step 2 examination.

USMLE step 1 and step 2

The USMLE step 1 is a multiple choice examination testing basic science knowledge that most American medical students write at the end of their second year of medical school. Some questions test the medical information per se, but the majority of questions require the examinee to interpret graphic and tabular material, to identify gross and microscopic pathologic and normal specimens, and to solve problems through application of basic science principles. Sections focusing on individual organ systems are subdivided according to normal and abnormal processes, principles of therapy, and psychosocial, cultural, and environmental considerations. Each examination covers content related to the traditionally defined disciplines of anatomy, behavioral sciences, biochemistry, microbiology, pathology, pharmacology, and physiology, as well as to interdisciplinary areas including genetics, aging, immunology, nutrition, and molecular and cell biology.

The USMLE step 2 multiple choice: The first component is a multiple choice examination focusing on the clinical application of medical knowledge. The examination is constructed from an content outline that organizes clinical science material along two dimensions. Normal Conditions and Disease categories (Dimension 1) form the main axis for organizing the outline. The first section deals with normal growth and development, basic concepts, and general principles. The remaining sections deal with individual disorders. Sections focusing on individual disorders are subdivided according to Physician Task (Dimension 2). The first set of physician tasks, Promoting Preventive Medicine and Health Maintenance, encompasses the assessment of risk factors, appreciation of epidemiological data, and the application of primary and secondary preventive measures. The second set of tasks, Understanding Mechanisms of Disease, encompasses etiology, pathophysiology, and effects of treatment modalities in the broadest sense. The third set of tasks, Establishing a Diagnosis, pertains to interpretation of history and physical findings and the results of laboratory, imaging, and other studies to determine the most likely diagnosis or the most appropriate next step in diagnosis. The fourth set of tasks, Applying Principles of Management, concerns the approach to care of patients with chronic and acute conditions in ambulatory and inpatient settings. Questions in this category will focus on the same topics covered in the diagnosis sections.

The USMLE step 2 clinical skills: The second component also known as USMLE step 2 clinical skills is a one day exam where graduates are asked to demonstrate communication skills, physical examinations and taking histories from patients.

More information, including full booklets and sample questions, is available from the official website http://www.usmle.org

IMG residency statistics

The match statistics for US residency programs are published each year at www.nrmp.org/data/index.html. In 2011, approximately 94% of US medical students matched to a residency program, 50% of US citizens trained in international medical schools matched (1,884 matched out of 3,769 active applicants), and 41% of non-U.S internationally trained graduates matched in a US program (2,721 out of 6,659 active applicants). The top three specialties in which US graduates of foreign medical schools matched, as well as non-US graduates of international medical schools are: (1) internal medicine (2) family medicine (3) pediatrics.

In terms of coming to the US for residency, there are no formal restrictions on residency programs or nationwide restrictions that limit the number of international medical graduates residency programs can take [23]. In recent years there have been more than 7000 IMGs entering US programs.

It has been a recent trend that many states are becoming stricter about accreditation of foreign medical schools, so it is best to try and attend a medical school that has been established for a while and that has achieved accreditation in most states.

Some foreign medical schools have obtained accreditation in every US state, while other schools may be accredited in the state you wish to practice in, without being accredited in other US state. If you wish to practice in the United States after graduation, you need to check with the medical board of the state you wish to practice in to find out if they have accredited the medical school you are planning to attend. To contact the medical board of a state or to find out more information about accreditation of medical schools in the US, visit the website of the Federation of State Medical Boards at www.fsmb.org

Canada

Medical programs

The English taught medical programs are listed by region below:

Western Canada
University of Alberta
University of British Columbia
University of Calgary
University of Manitoba
University of Saskatchewan

Ontario
McMaster University
Queen's University
Northern Ontario School of Medicine
University of Ottawa
University of Toronto
University of Western Ontario

Quebec and Maritime
McGill University
Dalhousie University
Memorial University

GPA and MCAT requirements

Amongst other important qualities, medical schools are looking for academically bright students that will be able to cope with the high demands of medical school and the high demands of a medical career. With the high numbers of applicants every year, admissions committees need to use quick and fair methods to select candidates for interview. The GPA and the MCAT scores are quick and easy tools to use and as such are used by many medical schools who set a minimum GPA and MCAT scores for selection.

While at Queen's University and the University of Western Ontario, meeting the GPA and MCAT cutoffs usually guarantees an interview, other Canadian universities place significant weight on additional factors before selecting applicants for interview. At McMaster University, applicants are considered for interview based on a score comprise of 25% GPA, 25% MCAT verbal reasoning score and 46% on a Computer-Based Assessment for Personal Characteristics (CASPer) (see page 164 for more details). Up to 4% more can be given for completion of a masters degree or PhD. At the University of Toronto, 40% of the pre interview assessment is based on non-academic criteria. For some schools, the non academic criteria carry an even greater weight in the pre interview formula. The selection formula for each medical program in Canada, including pre interview weightings and post interview weightings, are available under the heading "selection formula" in each school specific section.

See below for a table summarizing the applicant statistics for each school, as well as the MCAT and GPA averages of the entering classes. Statistics for 7 or 8 of these schools are also available from the Medical School Admissions Requirements (MSAR) book and online database, which are updated every year by the American Association of Medical Colleges.

	University	Entering class GPA and MCAT statistics
Western Canada	University of Alberta	Average GPA and MCAT: 3.86/32.94Q for 4 year applicants and 3.92/34.11R for second and third year applicants
	University of British Columbia	Average GPA and MCAT: 84.98%/31.8Q
	University of Calgary	In 2008: Average overall GPA and MCAT of applicants with a degree: 3.62/32.14Q, average best 2 years GPA was 3.82
	University of Manitoba	Average AGPA* and MCAT for in-province students: 4.15 on a 4.5 scale/31.83 Average AGPA* and MCAT for out-of-province students: 4.01 on a 4.5 scale/36.78
	University of Saskatchewan	Median GPA (best 2 years): 89.0% Out-of-Province cutoff (best 2 years): 92.3% In 2009, median MCAT: 28
	McMaster University	Average GPA of entering class: 3.82 Average MCAT verbal reasoning score: 10.86

Ontario	Queen's University	In 2007: cumulative GPA cutoff of 3.68 or most recent 2 year's GPA cutoff of 3.78. Also MCAT scores of 10, 10, 10 and P were required for undergraduate applicants to be granted an interview
	Northern Ontario School of Medicine	Average weighted GPA of approximately: 3.66; MCAT not required.
	University of Ottawa	The WGPA cutoffs for the 2011-2012 application cycle were 3.7 for Ottawa applicants, 3.7 for Champlain district applicants, 3.85 for in province applicants and 3.87 for out-of-province applicants. These are expected to stay the same in the next application cycle. The MCAT is not required.
	University of Toronto	Average GPA and median MCAT: 3.88/32Q
	University of Western Ontario	GPA cutoff for all applicants was: 3.70 For applicants from Southwestern Ontario, MCAT cutoffs: minimum of 8 in each section and a minimum overall of 30O. For applicants from outside Southern Ontario, MCAT cutoffs: minimum of 10 in biological sciences, 9 in Physical sciences and 11 in verbal reasoning and an overall minimum of 30P.
Quebec and Maritime	McGill University	Approximate average GPA: 3.8
	Dalhousie University	Average GPA and MCAT: 3.8/29
	Memorial University	Approximate average GPA and MCAT: 85%/30Q

Table 17. Admissions statistics of English taught medical schools in Canada.
*AGPA calculated for each applicant by the University of Manitoba. See the school specific section below for more details on the University of Manitoba's admission system.

The above table also shows the MCAT and GPA averages for the entering classes in the English taught Canadian medical programs. Although averages may give some insight, there is a large range of scores in both the accepted and rejected applicant pools. To illustrate this, below are the acceptance and rejection statistics for the University of British Columbia, Faculty of Medicine.

Overall Premedical Averages of the Entering Class 2009 and 2010			
Letter Grade	Percentage grade	Number of applicants accepted in 2009	Number of applicants accepted in 2010
A+	90.00-100%	18	28

A	85.00-89.99%	88	102
A-	80.00-84.99%	117	103
B+	74.00-79.99%	31	21
B	70.00-74.99%	2	2
		256	256

Table 18. Overall premedical averages of the entering classes in 2009 and 2010 at the University of British Columbia [24]

Overall Averages of Refused Applicants* for 2009 and 2010					
Letter Grade	Percentage grade	Number of in province applicants rejected		Number of out of province** applicants rejected	
		2009	2010	2009	2010
A+	90.00-100%	7	14	17	17
A	85.00-89.99%	74	79	104	137
A-	80.00-84.99%	251	327	140	164
B+	74.00-79.99%	335	401	81	67
B	70.00-74.99%	152	157	28	20
		819	978	370	405

Table 19. Overall averages of refused applicants for 2009 and 2010 at the University of British Columbia [24]
*Total number of applicants minus those accepted and registered or deferred, rejected due to ineligibility, accepted and declined, eligible applicants who withdrew, alternates admitted by registration date
**There were 26 out of province students that received acceptance letters in 2009 and 20 that received acceptance letters in 2010 (12 students accepted the offer each year).

The University of British Columbia rejected 81 in-province applicants with an A average or higher in 2009 and rejected 93 in 2009. Academic credentials are important in the admissions process, but academic credentials alone are not enough to gain admission. What you have done outside the classroom and what your references say about your character carry significant weight. Your essays are also key in gaining admission to medical school.

The web locations of class statistics for the Canadian medical programs taught in English are given below.

	University	Location of class statistics
Western Canada	University of Alberta	http://ume.med.ualberta.ca/ProspectiveLearners/MDAdmissions/AdmissionStatistics/Pages/default.aspx
	University of British Columbia	www.med.ubc.ca/education/md_ugrad/MD_Undergraduate_Admissions/MD_Undergraduate_Admissions_Statistics.htm
	University of Calgary	In applicant manual available at www.ucalgary.ca/mdprogram/prospective/admissions/applicants1011
	University of Manitoba	www.umanitoba.ca/faculties/medicine/admissions/index.html under 'Statistics'
	University of Saskatchewan	http://www.medicine.usask.ca/education/medical/undergrad/admissions/Admission%20statistics%202010%20five-year%20summary.pdf
Ontario	Queen's University	Not found and not available in MSAR. The cutoffs written on page 167 are from 2007 and were found in a University of Waterloo premedical services document which is also no longer available online.
	McMaster University	fhs.mcmaster.ca/mdprog/selection_process.html
	Northern Ontario School of Medicine	www.nosm.ca/education/ume/general.aspx?id=1248
	University of Ottawa	Not found and not available in MSAR. WGPA cutoffs for the English taught program for Ottawa-outauais, in-province and out-of-province applicants in 2011 are listed on page 171
	University of Toronto	www.md.utoronto.ca/admissions/statistics.htm
	University of Western Ontario	Cutoffs available from www.schulich.uwo.ca/admissions/medicine/index.php?page=requirements. Averages available from MSAR
Quebec and Maritime	McGill University	Information on GPA expectations available from: www.mcgill.ca/medadmissions/what-are-we-looking/academics-university Information on MCAT expectations available from: www.mcgill.ca/medadmissions/applying/general-requirements/mcat%C2%AE
	Dalhousie University	admissions.medicine.dal.ca/class.htm
	Memorial University	www.med.mun.ca/Admissions/FAQ-s.aspx gives approximate averages of MCAT and GPA

Table 20: Location of admissions statistics for Canadian programs taught in English

GPA calculation by medical schools

Every applicant who has completed a year of university in North America has a Grade Point Average (GPA) out of 4.0 or 4.3. It is important to understand that medical schools do NOT use the GPA given to an applicant by his or her university. Instead, each admissions office recalculates an applicant's GPA according to their own guidelines, policies and formulas. With that in mind, an applicant might have a GPA of 3.2 at their university but this might be equivalent to a GPA of 3.7 using the GPA calculation formula at the medical school he or she wants to apply to.

The University of Alberta drops the lowest year's GPA for all applicants who have completed 4 or more years of post-secondary coursework provided the lowest GPA is not the most recent year and not the only year where the applicant completed a full credit course load. However, the University of Alberta does not include summer courses completed by an applicant in their GPA calculation. On the other hand, the University of British Columbia includes all courses in their GPA calculation including summer and graduate degree courses. The University of Saskatchewan only uses an applicant's best 2 years in their GPA cutoff calculation. A student who obtained really low grades in his or her first year but excelled afterwards can thus be very competitive at certain universities.

The exact GPA calculation policy for each medical school is available in the school specific sections below under "GPA requirement". Important differences include: including or excluding summer courses, including or excluding graduate coursework, allowing or not allowing students to drop their lowest grades under certain conditions, and using the GPA as a strict cutoff or as one of several elements considered in shortlisting applicants for interview. Some schools also give an advantage (bonus points) to applicants who hold a master's degree or a PhD while other schools give no advantage to those with advanced degrees in their pre-interview scoring. These rules can potentially give very different GPAs to the same applicant at different schools which is why it is essential that applicants know where they have the best chances of getting in. Use the section "what are your chances" on page 124 to find an applicant profile that matches yours and find out which medical schools may look at your circumstances and achievements most favorably.

Entrance Statistics

The selection ratios for each English taught Canadian medical program are provided below. Selection ratios can give some insight, but note that medical schools offer more places than their class size, since not everyone accepts the offers. For example, at the University of Manitoba, 102 offers of admission were made to fill the 98 in province places, and 39 offers of admission were made to fill the 5 out-of-province places. Thus, the true out-of-province selection is more like 437/39 = 11:1, rather than 437/5 = 87:1 as calculated below. Note that in Canada in 2009, there were 3825 offers made for 2865 positions available, meaning that on average, the true selection ratio is approximately 25% better than the calculated ratios in the table (for example, if the calculated selection ratio is 4:1, the true selection ratio might be close to 3:1).

	University	Entering Class Statistics	Calculated Selection Ratio
Western Canada	University of Alberta	In 2010: 1234 applicants for 167 places	7:1
	University of British Columbia	In 2010: 1793 applicants for 288 positions	6:1
	University of Calgary	In 2010: 950 IP* applicants for approximately 152 places and 900 OOP applicants for approximately 28 places	IP: 6:1 OOP: 32:1
	University of Manitoba	In 2010: 275 IP applicants for 98 places, 437 OOP applicants for 5 places, and 148 rural applicants for 60 places	IP: 3;1 OOP: 87:1 Rural: 3:1
	University of Saskatchewan	In 2010: 370 IP applicants for 80 positions, and 478 OOP applicants for 4 places.	IP: 5:1 OOP: 120:1
	McMaster University	In 2010: 2979 IP applicants for 194 places, 762 OOP applicants for 9 places, and 44 international applicants for 1 place.	IP: 15:1 OOP 85:1 Int'l: 44:1
Ontario	Queen's University	In 2010: 3136 applicants for 100 positions	31:1
	Northern Ontario School of Medicine	In 2010: 1748 applications received for 64 places	27:1
	University of Ottawa	In 2010: 2631 IP applicants for approximately 130 places, and 1007 OOP applicants for approximately 34 places.	IP: 20:1 OOP: 30:1
	University of Toronto	In 2009: 2956 applications received for 250 places	12:1
	University of Western Ontario	In 2010: approximately 2302 applications for 171 places	14:1
	McGill University	In 2010: Approximately 175 accepted, including 160 IP, 9 OOP, and 4 international. There will be 180 places next year.	N/A

Quebec and Maritime	Dalhousie University	In 2010: 355 IP applicants for 99 places, 380 OOP and international applicants for 9 places	IP: 4:1 OOP/Int'l: 42:1
	Memorial University	Approximately 400 IP applicants for roughly 60 places, approximately 400 OOP applicants for 2 places, and approximately 100 international applicants for roughly 2 places.	IP: 7:1 OOP: 200:1 Int'l: 50:1

Table 21: Table showing entrance statistics and selection ratios for all English taught Canadian medical programs

*IP: In province, OOP: Out-of-province, Int'l: International

University Rankings

One agency that ranks Canadian universities each year is Macleans Magazine. There are also a few global university rankings. These include the QS World University rankings, which ranks the top 640 universities overall each year, and also ranks the top 200 universities in the field of medicine. The Shanghai Consulting World University Ranking ranks the top 500 universities worldwide, as well as the top 100 universities in the field of medicine. More details on these rankings are provided below.

Macleans University Guide 2010 - Overall

This ranking gives each university an overall score based on the following criteria. Note that this is a general university ranking, not a medical school ranking.

1. Admissions score (includes high school averages, out-of-province and international students, graduation rates, and other factors) (22% - 23%)
2. Class sizes (smaller class sizes receive better scores) (17% - 18%)
3. Faculty (national awards, grant funding, etc.) (17%)
4. Budget per student (12%)
5. Library (12%)
6. Reputation (scored according to survey and number of gifts the university receives) (19%)

The top 10 Canadian universities in this ranking are:

1. McGill University	6. McMaster University
2. University of Toronto	7. Dalhousie University
3. University of British Columbia	8. University of Calgary

| 4. University of Alberta | 9. University of Western Ontario |
| 5. Queen's University | 10. University of Saskatchewan |

The full ranking is available at: http://oncampus.macleans.ca/education/2010/11/10/our-20th-annual-university-rankings/

QS Top Universities - World University Rankings 2010/2011 - Overall

This ranking also gives each university an overall score based on the following criteria. Note that this is a general university ranking, not a medical school ranking.

1. Academic peer review based on survey
2. Employer review based on survey
3. Faculty student ratio
4. Citations per faculty
5. Proportion of international faculty
6. Proportion of international students

The top 10 universities in Canada, as well as their overall world rankings, are shown below:

19. McGill University	162. McMaster University
29. University of Toronto	164. University of Western Ontario
44. University of British Columbia	165. University of Calgary
78. University of Alberta	212. Dalhousie University
132. Queen's University	231. University of Ottawa

The full world ranking is available at: www.topuniversities.com/world-university-rankings

QS Top Universities - World University Rankings 2010/2011 - Life Sciences and Medicine

This ranking gives each medical school a ranking based on similar criteria to the QS Top Universities overall ranking outlined above.

The top 10 universities in Canada according to this ranking are:

12. University of Toronto	101. University of Calgary
13. McGill University	101. Queen's University
31. University of British Columbia	151. Dalhousie University
42. McMaster University	151. University of Ottawa
51. University of Alberta	151. University of Western Ontario

The full world ranking is available at: www.topuniversities.com/university-rankings/world-university-rankings/2010/subject-rankings/life-science-biomedicine

Shanghai Consultancy World University Rankings 2010 - overall

This ranking also gives universities an overall ranking, not a medical school ranking, based on the following criteria:

1. Alumni (10%)
2. Nobel Prizes and Fields Medals (20%)
3. Highly cited researchers (20%)
4. Papers published in Nature and Science (20%)
5. Papers in Science-Citation Index-expanded and Social Science Citation Index (20%)
6. Per capita academic performance (takes into account the number of staff) (10%)

The top 14 universities with medical schools in Canada according to this ranking are:

27. University of Toronto	201. Dalhousie University
36. University of British Columbia	201. Laval University
61. McGill University	201. Queen's University
88. McMaster University	201. University of Western Ontario
101. University of Alberta	201. University of Manitoba
101. University of Montreal	201. University of Ottawa
151. University of Calgary	201. University of Saskatchewan

The full ranking is available at: www.arwu.org/ARWU2010.jsp

Shanghai Consultancy World University Rankings 2010 - Clinical Medicine and Pharmacy

This ranking gives universities worldwide a ranking for their medical and life science related faculties, based on the following criteria

1. Alumni winning Nobel Prizes in Physiology or Medicine (10%)
2. Staff with nobel prizes in Nobel Prizes in Physiology or Medicine (15%)
3. Highly cited researchers in medicine, pharmacology and social sciences (25%)
4. Publications indexed in Science Citation Index-expanded and MED fields (25%)
5. Percentage of papers published in the top 20% of journals in MED fields (25%)

The top 5 universities in Canada according to this ranking are:

29. University of Toronto	76. University of Alberta
34. McGill University	76. University of Manitoba
51. McMaster University	

Note that the other universities in Canada were not in the top 100 worldwide according to this source.

The full ranking is available at: www.arwu.org/FieldMED2010.jsp

Entry for 2nd and 3rd yr. undergraduate students

There are several universities that accept applicants who have not yet completed a bachelor's degree but are currently in their second or third year of university. These places are more competitive than places for applicants who have completed undergraduate degrees. Applicants also need to have completed the prerequisite courses to be eligible. See below for a table presenting each medical schools' policy on entry for second and third year university students. See the schools' websites for details on what constitutes a full-time year of study and what is counted toward the number of credits required.

	University	Degree, credits or years of education required
Western Canada	University of Alberta	2nd and 3rd year students are eligible to apply (60 credits minimum)
	University of British Columbia	Minimum of 90 university-transferrable credits
	University of Calgary	Applicants must have completed the equivalent of at least two years of full-time study by the time of admission
	University of Manitoba	Applicants must have or be eligible to receive their bachelor's degree by June 29th, 2012. Note that a three year bachelor's degree will fulfill this requirement (many bachelor's degrees at the University of Manitoba are 3 year degrees) [1]
	University of Saskatchewan	Saskatchewan residents are eligible to apply during their second year of university. Out-of-province applicants are eligible to apply during their third year of university.
Ontario	McMaster University	A minimum of three full-time years of undergraduate study is required before May 2012
	Queen's University	A minimum of 3 years of study (fifteen full credits per year) in any university program prior to June 30th of the matriculation year required
	Northern Ontario School of Medicine	Either completion of a 4-year undergraduate degree by the time of admission or, for applicants who are 25 years or older as of October 1st of the application year, the minimum requirement is a 3 year undergraduate degree
	University of Ottawa	Three years of full time study completed by June of the matriculation year
	University of Toronto	Students who have completed a minimum of three years (or are in the process of completing their third year) of undergraduate study are eligible to apply
	University of Western Ontario	Students must have completed or be in the final year of a program leading to a 4-year undergraduate degree

	McGill University	Students must have completed or be in the final year of a program leading to an undergraduate degree (120 credits)
Quebec and Maritime	**Dalhousie University**	The minimum requirement for entry is a bachelor's degree. "Although candidates with three-year degrees are occasionally admitted; a four-year degree is strongly preferred."
	Memorial University	Most applicants are required to have a bachelor's degree, however, an applicant who has "work related or other experience acceptable to the Admissions Committee" may be eligible to apply provided they expect to complete at least 60 credit hours before admission.

Table 22. Number of credits or years of university required for admission at Canadian medical schools taught in English

International and out-of-province statistics

In 2009, 7.4% of the 189 US students who applied in Canada were granted admission, and 11.4% of the 299 non-US foreign applicants were granted admission. Most schools in Canada have guidelines or quotas for the number of out-of-province and international positions available. The two Canadian medical schools that do not favor in-province applicants over out-of-province applicants are Queen's University and the University of Toronto.

	University	**Out-of-Province positions available for 2012**	**International Student positions for 2012**
Western Canada	**University of Alberta**	15%	None
	University of British Columbia	Up to 10% (29 total)	None
	University of Calgary	15%	None
	University of Manitoba	10 places	None
	University of Saskatchewan	Maximum of 8 seats	None
	Queen's University	No distinction is made between in-province and out-of-province applicants	None

Ontario	McMaster University	Up to 10% for out-of-province and international applicants combined [1]. 5% of matriculants were from this category in 2011.	Up to 10% for out-of-province and international applicants combined [1]. 5% of matriculants were from this category in 2011.
	Northern Ontario School of Medicine	6 from out-of-province rural areas accepted in 2010. No reserved places for out-of-province.	None
	University of Ottawa	There is no quota for out-of-province applicants, but a different WGPA cutoff is set for out-of-province applicants to qualify for an interview. Once met, both in-province and out-of-province students compete for the same positions in the English program [1]	None unless applicant is the child of a University of Ottawa, Faculty of Medicine alumnus [25]
	University of Toronto	No distinction is made between in-province and out-of-province applicants	Able to admit up to 7 international students each year. For entry in 2010, 39 international students applied, 3 students were interviewed and 1 international student was admitted.
	University of Western Ontario	Higher MCAT and GPA cutoffs are set for out-of-province students each year, but there is no defined quota	None
Quebec and Maritime	McGill University	Approximately 9 seats available	Approximately 4 seats available
	Dalhousie University	There are 9 seats in total for non-maritime and international applicants combined	There are 9 seats in total for non-Maritime and international applicants combined
	Memorial University	Roughly 2 out of province applicants admitted each year.	Roughly 1-2 international applicants admitted each year.

Table 23. Number of out-of-province and international applicants accepted at the English taught medical schools in Canada.

What are your chances...

Statistically, the more schools a student applies to, the greater his or her chances of gaining admission to medical school. However, even if an applicant decides to apply everywhere in Canada, it is important to recognize where his or her application may be stronger.

Applicant X has an undergraduate GPA of 3.4 and has completed a master's degree with a GPA of 3.9. If applicant X applies to McGill University for example, they will consider his GPA to be 3.4. However, if the same applicant applies to Memorial University or the University of British Columbia, the admissions committee will include all the graduate courses in the overall GPA calculation, which in this case would significantly increase student X's chances.

Applicant Y also has an undergraduate GPA of 3.4 but has completed additional courses with a GPA of 3.8. These additional courses did not lead to any degree. If applicant Y applies to the Northern Ontario School of Medicine, they will not consider the additional courses in the overall GPA calculation. However, if applicant Y applied to McMaster University for example, all his additional courses will be counted towards the overall GPA.

These two examples illustrate how significantly different the admissions policies can be between the different medical schools in Canada and how valuable it may be for applicants to have researched those differences before applying. This unique section considers applicant profiles and medical school admissions policies in Canada, and shows where in Canada students with certain profiles may be given strongest consideration. This is here to help applicants consider where they want to apply and perhaps where they want to focus their greatest efforts.

With a high GPA and a high MCAT score

With a high GPA and a high MCAT, your chances are looking pretty good. However, every year in Canada, hundreds of applicants with a GPA above 3.8 are refused medical school admission. Most medical schools in Canada look at the complete applicant profile to select applicants for interview, including biographical sketch, personal statement and reference letters. A few schools have a different system whereby a high GPA and a high MCAT practically guarantees an interview, and the non academic criteria are assessed during the interview and in the post-interview selection.

University of Saskatchewan

Out of province applicants are invited for interview based on the average of two full time years (an average of approximately 92% has been required in the past two application cycles). Although this average is high, almost all students with this average will receive an interview, regardless of the rest of their application. Note also that after the interview, the offer of admission is based solely on interview performance.

Queen's University

All applicants who meet the GPA and MCAT cutoffs are normally invited for an interview. Note also that Queen's University is one of the 2 medical schools in Canada that does NOT favor in province applicants.

University of Western Ontario

Uses MCAT and GPA cutoffs to select applicants for interview. Although meeting the cutoff does not guarantee an interview, almost all applicants meeting the cutoff are invited for an interview.

Memorial University

For out of province and international applicants, whether a candidate is invited for interview is based largely on the applicant's MCAT score and GPA. All in province applicants that meet the MCAT and GPA cutoffs are also invited for interview, as well as the top in province applicants who do not meet the MCAT and GPA cutoffs.

With a low MCAT score

Applicants with very low MCAT scores are not affected at all when applying to medical schools that do not use the MCAT. The universities in this category are the Northern Ontario School of Medicine, the University of Ottawa and the 3 French medical programs in Quebec. At McGill University, CEGEP students are exempt from taking the MCAT, and submission of MCAT scores is optional for students applying with degrees from Canadian Universities. The MCAT is mandatory, however, for students applying with a degree obtained outside Canada. This includes applicants who obtained a second bachelor's degree obtained outside Canada if they would like to be considered on the basis of the second degree. The University of Saskatchewan does not require the MCAT for in-province applicants, but in-province applicants can write the exam if they do not qualify for application based on their university grades.

Every other medical school in Canada requires the MCAT but each of them use the MCAT scores very differently in their selection process. Applicants with low MCAT scores may not be disadvantaged at the following three medical schools, in addition to those mentioned above.

University of British Columbia
The MCAT is used to rank applicants after the interview but is NOT used in the interview selecting stage. Also, if an applicant has written the MCAT more than once, the best test score will be used.

University of Toronto
The MCAT is used as a flag only; as such, marks higher than the minimum requirements do not improve an applicant's chance of admission. This also means that if an applicant has not excelled in their MCAT but meets the minimum cutoffs, they will not be disadvantaged at the University of Toronto compared to applicants with very high MCAT scores.

McMaster University
McMaster University only uses the MCAT verbal reasoning score in their selection process. The other sections of the MCAT are not considered, allowing applicants who did strongly on the verbal reasoning section but less well on the other sections to still have an advantage in their selection process. The verbal reasoning section score is weighted as 25% of the pre-interview score, and 15% of the post-interview score.

With a low undergraduate GPA and additional courses

While some schools like the Northern Ontario School of Medicine will not consider additional courses taken outside of a degree program in their GPA calculation, many universities calculate their GPA using all courses taken. Details on some of these schools are listed below, and additional details on each school's GPA calculation are available in the school specific sections.

University of Alberta
The GPA calculation includes full years completed after the undergraduate degree, provided they are completed between September and April and consist of 18 or more credits transferrable to the University of Alberta.

University of British Columbia
All university courses are counted in the gpa calculation, including those completed after the undergraduate degree.

University of Calgary
The GPA calculation includes full years completed after the undergraduate degree, provided they are completed between September and April and consist of 4 full-year courses, 8 half-year courses or 24 credits transferable to the University of Calgary

University of Manitoba
Undergraduate courses completed after the undergraduate degree are counted in the AGPA calculation.

University of Saskatchewan
Normally, courses taken after the undergraduate degree are only taken into account if they are leading to another degree, however, applicants planning to take an extra year after their undergraduate degree are encouraged to contact the admissions office to see if their extra year will be eligible for consideration.

McMaster University
The GPA is calculated using all undergraduate courses taken, including those that are not part of the undergraduate degree.

Queen's University

The GPA cutoff can be met by averaging all years of full time study, including supplemental courses that did not lead to a degree.

University of Toronto

The applicant's GPA is calculated using all undergraduate courses taken, including those that are not part of a degree.

University of Western Ontario

Applicants who have earned a degree from a recognized university may elect to continue in full-time undergraduate studies so that their academic standing may be improved for application to medical school. Only the first special year taken by the applicant will be considered for determination of GPA. A special year will only be considered if it contains five full courses or equivalent taken between September and April. First year courses, repeat courses, and second-year courses that do not require a first-year prerequisite are not acceptable in the special year.

Dalhousie University

If an applicant completes a full academic year after their undergraduate degree, this can count toward meeting the minimum GPA requirement (which is based on meeting a cutoff in each of the last two years of full-time study), provided the grades are available from the supplemental year at the time of application.

Memorial University

All courses taken are taken into account in the GPA calculation, including those that are not part of the undergraduate degree.

With a low GPA and a master's degree or a PhD

Although some schools like McGill University do not consider graduate degrees in their GPA calculation, most, if not all schools will give some advantage to students with graduate degrees. There are several universities that give significant advantages to those who have completed higher level degrees, and details on these schools are listed below.

University of Alberta
Courses taken during the PhD or master's program will be used in the calculation of the cumulative GPA if the unit of course weight during the academic year is 18 credits or higher. Graduate students also benefit from the deletion of the lowest year GPA in the same way that undergraduate applicants do. Also, applicants with a master's degree get a 1 point bonus on their application and applicants with a PhD get a 3 point bonus (out of a total of 70 points available in the pre interview scoring, and 100 points available in the post interview scoring).

University of British Columbia
Courses taken as part of a PhD or master's degree are counted in the GPA calculation.

University of Calgary
Courses taken as part of a PhD or master's degree can supplement undergraduate grades in the GPA calculation.

University of Saskatchewan
In considering graduate students, the average may be based on the following, or the two best full-time undergraduate years, whichever works to their advantage:
1. Course-based graduate program, which may or may not include a research project: the average of all grades in the program will count as one full year combined with the best two full-time undergraduate years. The postgraduate program must be comparable to at least one full-time academic year (30 credit units).
2. Master's thesis-based program: the average of all Master's grades (minimum 9 credits) will count as one full year combined with the best two full-time undergraduate years.
3. Ph.D. thesis-based program: The average of all graduate grades (minimum 15 credits) will count as one full year combined with the best full-time undergraduate year.

Masters and PhD students who do not have the minimum number of course credits outlined above will have their post-graduate courses average on a course-weight basis with their best two full time undergraduate years. PhD students with between 9 and 15 course credits will have their post-graduate work weighted as a full year and combined with their best two full time undergraduate years.

McMaster University
Applicants receive a bonus of 1 point for a master's degree and 4 points for a PhD, out of 100 points.

Northern Ontario School of Medicine
Graduate applicants who fulfill the minimum requirement of a GPA of 3.0 out of 4.0 will have 0.2 added to their GPA.

University of Toronto
Graduate applicants are given a separate review, and can occasionally be accepted with a GPA slightly lower than 3.6 out of 4.0 (lowest 3.0 out of 4.0).

Memorial University
Graduate courses are included in the calculation of the overall GPA.

If you had a bad year or a bad term

As explained in the "GPA section" above, the same applicant has a different GPA at each medical school. This is because each medical school uses their own unique formula to calculate an applicant's GPA. Here is the list of Canadian medical schools that drop some of the lowest grades for applicants who have taken full course loads.

University of Alberta

The school drops the lowest year's GPA from their calculation of the applicant's cumulative GPA, provided the lowest GPA year is not the most recent completed year and is not the only year where the applicant completed a full 30 credit course-load.

University of Calgary

If an applicant has 3 full time years of study completed at the time of application, the GPA of the worst year will be dropped from the overall GPA calculation. Thus, for applicants in their final year of a four year degree, only the best two years are counted.

University of Manitoba

Applicants are given what is called an AGPA (scale of 0 to 4.5) calculated based on all their courses including summer courses. Credits will be dropped to improve the applicants GPA as a function of the number of credits completed in total. If an applicant has completed 120 credits or more, the 30 credits with the lowest marks will be dropped in the calculation of the AGPA. See table 34 on page 156 for the number of credits dropped in the University of Manitoba AGPA calculation as a function of the number of credits completed.

University of Ottawa

Students in their third year of undergraduate study at the time of application will have their second year marks counted times two and their first year marks times one. The current year of study is not used to determine which candidates are invited for interview. Students in their fourth year of undergraduate study at the time of application will have their third year marks counted times three, their second year marks counted times two and their first year marks counted times one. For students who have completed more than three years at the time of application, only the three most recent years of undergraduate studies will be used to determine the WGPA. See the table below for two examples:

	WGPA calculation*
Students completing their third year of full time undergraduate study	Example: Year 1 3.85 x 1 = 3.85 Year 2 3.82 x 2 = 7.74 Total 11.49 ÷ 3 = 3.83 (WGPA)
Students who have completed three or more years of undergraduate study	Only the most recent three years considered. Example of 5th year student: Example: Year 1 3.85 Year 2 3.82 Year 3 3.90 x 1 = 3.90 Year 4 3.85 x 2 = 7.70 Year 5 3.89 x 3 = 11.67 Total 23.27 ÷ 6 = 3.88 (WGPA)

Table 25. WGPA calculation at the University of Ottawa [25]
*Supplementary courses taken outside the usual academic session and summer courses will not be included in the above calculations

University of Toronto

A student with four years of full time study (5 full year courses or equivalent) completed at the time of application can drop the four lowest full-year course marks, or the eight lowest semester course marks, or any combination. A student with three full years completed at the time of application can drop the three lowest full-year course marks, or the six lowest semester course marks, or any combination.

University of Western Ontario

Only the best two full time years are used by the school to determine eligibility for interview.

Queen's University

The cutoffs can be met by using the most recent 2 years of full time study.

Taking extra courses after graduating

Some students who do not gain admission before completing their undergraduate degree choose to do additional years of full-time undergraduate courses after graduating. This can be more or less advantageous than gaining work experience or completing a graduate degree depending on which schools they are applying to. Below is a table summarizing each school's policy on additional courses taken after an undergraduate degree.

	University	Policy on courses taken outside a degree program
Western Canada	University of Alberta	Full years completed after the undergraduate degree will be counted in the cumulative GPA, provided they are completed between September and April and consist of 18 or more credits transferrable to the University of Alberta.
	University of British Columbia	All university courses are counted in the gpa calculation, including those completed after the undergraduate degree.
	University of Calgary	Full years completed after the undergraduate degree will be counted in the GPA calculation, provided they are completed between September and April and consist of 4 full-year courses, 8 half-year courses or 24 credits transferable to the University of Calgary.
	University of Manitoba	Undergraduate courses completed after the undergraduate degree will be counted in the AGPA calculation. Note that courses taken toward master's degrees or PhDs are not counted.
	University of Saskatchewan	Normally, courses taken after the undergraduate degree are only taken into account in the GPA requirement if they are leading to another degree. However, applicants planning to take an extra year after their degree are encouraged to contact the admissions office to see if their extra year will be eligible for consideration. This should be done in the fall of their extra year or earlier.
Ontario	McMaster University	Full years completed after the undergraduate degree, both in general studies or as part of another undergraduate degree, will be counted in the GPA calculation. Note that courses taken toward master's degrees or PhDs are not counted.
	Queen's University	Full years completed after the undergraduate degree, both in general studies or as part of another undergraduate degree, will be counted toward meeting the minimum GPA cutoff. Note that courses taken toward master's degrees or PhDs are not counted.
	Northern Ontario School of Medicine	Additional undergraduate courses completed after a degree is awarded are not used in the GPA unless these grades are part of a second undergraduate degree that will be completed prior to June 30th of the year of potential enrollment.
	University of Ottawa	Additional undergraduate courses completed after a degree is awarded are not used in the GPA unless these grades are part of a second undergraduate degree that is at least three years in length.

	University of Toronto	Full years completed after the undergraduate degree, both in general studies or as part of another undergraduate degree, will be counted in the GPA calculation provided the applicant is enrolled in full-time study.
	University of Western Ontario	Applicants who have earned a degree from a recognized university may elect to continue in full-time undergraduate studies so that their academic standing may be improved for application to medical school. Only the first special year taken by the applicant will be considered for determination of GPA. A special year will only be considered if it contains five full courses or equivalent taken between September and April. First year courses, repeat courses, and second-year courses that do not require a first-year prerequisite are not acceptable in the special year.
Quebec and Maritime	**McGill University**	Courses that are completed after the undergraduate degree are not counted in the GPA calculation. The only exception to this is if an applicant completes a second undergraduate degree. In this case, the highest degree GPA will be used.
	Dalhousie University	If an applicant completes a full academic year after their undergraduate degree, this can count toward meeting the minimum GPA requirement (which is based on meeting a cutoff in each of the last two years of full-time study), provided the grades are available from the supplemental year at the time of application.
	Memorial University	All courses taken are taken into account in the GPA calculation, including those that are not part of the undergraduate degree.

Table 26. Canadian medical school policies on additional courses taken after an undergraduate degree program. Information obtained from the schools' websites and from speaking with the admissions offices directly.

Dual degree programs

MD/Ph.D programs

The Ph.D portion of this degree can be completed in just about any field, ranging from humanities to biochemistry to medical physics depending on the school. The program usually requires 7-8 years in total, although some students take 6 years, while others may take 10 or more [26]. Some Canadian programs like the University of British Columbia expect students to complete both degrees in 7 years [27].

Students typically complete the first 1 and a half or 2 years of the medical program (the years that are spent mostly in the classroom), then complete their Ph.D, then return to complete the last two years of medical school (the clinical years).

In Canada, the sources of funding for MD/Ph.D programs vary from school to school, but most students receive a stipend throughout the Ph.D portion of their degree and potentially during some of their years in the MD portion of their program. Sources of funding include provincial organizations such as the Alberta Heritage Foundation for Medical Research (AHFMR), private institutions such as the National Cancer Institute of Canada, the Heart and Stroke Foundation and the Canadian Lung Association, university graduate fellowships and funding from the student's supervisor. Some universities like the University of Alberta will also add additional funding for those students who were not able to secure a certain amount of funding per year (for the University of Alberta, up to a maximum of $24,000) [28].

Some very competitive awards such as the Canadian Institute of Health Research Scholarship may offer sufficient funding to cover tuition and provide an additional stipend for almost the full duration of the MD/Ph.D.

There are usually three ways that applicants can enter MD/Ph.D programs. Students can apply to the programs before entering the MD program, which usually involves applying to both the graduate school and the medical school simultaneously. Students can also enter the MD program and then apply to the MD/Ph.D program once they have started medical school. This can be done as late as the middle of their second year of medical school, or even later sometimes depending on the school. The third possibility is for applicants who are currently in a master's or Ph.D program, who can gain admission to the medical school and have the research work they are currently doing counted toward the Ph.D component of their MD/Ph.D. See the schools' websites for specific application procedures.

MD/Ph.D programs are generally more competitive both for the grades required and the potential that applicants need to show for a research based career. Most schools have a panel mostly made up of researchers that interviews applicants along with the normal medical school interviews.

MD/MBA programs

McGill University, the University of Alberta and the University of Calgary offer an MD/MBA program. Students who wish to apply to these three programs are required to hold an undergraduate degree.

Students applying to the MD/MBA program at the University of Alberta and the University of Calgary apply to the business schools and the medical schools separately, while those applying to the MD/MBA program at McGill University submit the same application, only with different essay instructions and reference letter requirements.

Please note that students applying to the University of Alberta and the University of Calgary are required to have obtained a score of 550 on the GMAT. This GMAT is recommended, but not required at McGill University [29]. At the University of Alberta, students without work experience can be considered for MD/MBA program [1]. Students applying to the program at the University of Calgary are recommended to have 3 years of relevant employment [30].

At most schools in North America, students begin their MBA after their second or third years of medical school and then return to the medical school to complete their medical degrees. This is the case at the University of Alberta. At McGill, students start with one year in the Faculty of Management, and then begin their medical training. At the University of Calgary, most students do their MBA before beginning medical school, but students also have the option of taking a break during their MD degree to do the MBA [1].

Finding information on dual degree programs

A quite complete listing of dual degree programs in Canada and the US is available from the AAMC at services.aamc.org/currdir/section3/start.cfm although there are still several programs not listed on this page.

Another good website for MD/Ph.D programs is www.aamc.org/students/considering/research/mdPh.D which brings you directly to the school's MD/Ph.D websites when you click on the links.

The handout available at ucs.yalecollege.yale.edu/sites/default/files/MD-PhD-programs.pdf is also a useful summary.

Some information is available in the Medical School Admissions Requirements (MSAR) book published by the AAMC each year [31]. For additional information as well as information on dual degree programs not covered in either of these sources such as MD/MS programs, the best place to look is on the schools' websites.

Course requirements

One very important thing to know before applying is whether prerequisites need to be completed before application or before admission to the medical school. For the University of Toronto, the applicant is disqualified unless all prerequisites are complete or will be completed before the beginning of June preceding registration [25]. This means that applicants cannot plan to finish their prerequisite requirements during the summer in case they are admitted to the program. Some schools like McMaster University, the Northern Ontario School of Medicine, the University of Western Ontario and Dalhousie University do not have any prerequisite courses in 2012. For other universities like the University of Calgary, courses are recommended to serve as a guideline for the coursework that will help an applicant succeed on the MCAT and succeed in medical school, rather than giving the applicant an advantage in the admissions process [1]. There are several prerequisites frequently required or recommended by many Canadian schools. These include organic chemistry, biochemistry, biology, inorganic chemistry, physics, statistics, English, social sciences and humanities. Most science courses, with the exception of biochemistry, are required to have a laboratory component to satisfy the prerequisite requirements. It is important that you check the prerequisites for the schools you are applying to. The prerequisite course requirements for each of the English taught medical programs in 2012 are summarized in the table below and listed in the school specific sections with additional details.

	University	Course Requirements
Western Canada	University of Alberta	Half year of biochemistry, half year of statistics and a full year of the following: biology, English, general chemistry, organic chemistry and physics. When possible, a full year of biochemistry is encouraged. Some of these requirements can be met using AP and IB credits
	University of British Columbia	1 full of year of biochemistry, biology, English, general chemistry and organic chemistry are required. Courses in behavioral sciences, biometrics, statistics and physics are recommended, but not required. AP and IB credits may be used to fulfill part of these requirements.
	University of Calgary	There are no course requirements. See the school specific section for a list of recommended courses.
	University of Manitoba	1 full year of biochemistry and 3 full years of humanities. Applicants who complete a 4-year major may waive up to 12 credit hours of the humanities prerequisite, however, applicants with a general BSc or BA must complete the full requirement. It is possible to have AP and IB courses considered to fulfill the courses requirements.

	University of Saskatchewan	The required prerequisites are not for every applicant. Refer to the school specific section for details on who needs to complete the prerequisite courses. The required courses are: 1 full year of biochemistry, biology, physics, English and social sciences/humanities as well as half a year of general chemistry and organic chemistry.
Ontario	McMaster University	There are no course requirements.
	Queen's University	1 full year of biological sciences, 1 full year of humanities or social sciences and 1 full year of physical sciences.
	Northern Ontario School of Medicine	There are no course requirements. See the school specific section for a list of recommended courses.
	University of Ottawa	The course requirements are the following: 1 full year of biology, 1 full year of humanities/social sciences and the equivalent of two full-year courses of the following chemistry courses: i) general biochemistry without laboratory session; ii) general chemistry with laboratory session; iii) organic chemistry with laboratory session.
	University of Toronto	Applicants are required to complete at least two full year courses or four half-year courses in life sciences, and at least one full year course or two half year courses in humanities, social sciences or languages. Applicants are also recommended, but not required, to take one course in statistics and two courses that require expository writing.
	University of Western Ontario	There are no course requirements.
Quebec and Maritime	McGill University	1 full year of biology, chemistry and physics as well as half a year of organic chemistry. Distance or correspondence education courses are not acceptable. The university accepts AP and IB credit toward course requirements at the discretion of the admissions office
	Dalhousie University	There are no course requirements. See the school specific section for recommended courses.
	Memorial University	The only prerequisite course requirement is a full year (6 credits) of English. AP and IB credit can be used toward this prerequisite.

Table 27. Course requirements for Canadian medical schools in 2012

AP and IB credit

Some universities like the University of Alberta have strict criteria that differ for AP and IB - for example, IB chemistry allows students to fulfill half of the chemistry requirement while students with AP chemistry need to write a 'Credit by Special Assessment' exam to earn half of the chemistry requirement. Additional details are available on the University of Alberta website [32]. Some universities such as McGill University only accept IB and AP credits at the discretion of the admissions office. Details on each school's policy regarding AP and IB credit can be found on the schools' websites or by contacting the admissions offices.

Extracurricular activities and volunteer work

Most admissions committees in Canada, if not all, consider the nature and depth of the extracurricular activities you have undertaken to be a significant factor in your application to medical school. Although to our knowledge, medical schools in Canada no longer publish the percentage of matriculants with different types of work and volunteer experience, this data is available from 2007. Below is a table listing the percentages of accepted applicants having done volunteer work, medically related work and research at several Canadian medical schools in 2007 [31].

Medical School	% of Matriculants having done volunteer work	% of Matriculants having dome medically related work	% of Matriculants having dome research
University of Calgary	99%	95%	35%
Memorial University	100%	75%	50%
McMaster University	94%	82%	71%
University of Toronto	80%	75%	50%
University of Western Ontario	100%	75%	25%

Table 28. Percentages of matriculating students having done volunteer work, medically related work and research at a few Canadian medical schools in 2007 [31].

For more information on getting involved in volunteer work, medically related work, research and other extra-curricular activities, see page 69.

Essays and personal statement requirements

The 2011 essay requirements for the 14 Canadian medical schools taught in English are outlined below. Note that although some schools may not ask for personal statements, they will usually require an autobiographical sketch in which students enter their volunteer and work experience as well as any awards they have received. The autobiographical sketches may ask for detailed descriptions and may require a significant time commitment to complete.

	University	Essays
Western Canada	**University of Alberta**	No personal statement, but applicants submit 5 short descriptions regarding their awards and activities
	University of British Columbia	No personal statement, but applicants submit a report of non-academic experience is required
	University of Calgary	No personal statement, but applicants submit impact statements for their top 10 extracurricular activities.
	University of Manitoba	No personal statement, but applicants submit a brief description of all activities, awards and publications .
	University of Saskatchewan	No personal statement
Ontario	**McMaster University**	No personal statement, but applicants are required to submit the OMSAS autobiographical sketch and complete the CASPer online questionnaire (see page 164 for more details)
	Queen's university	No personal statement, but applicants are required to submit the OMSAS autobiographical sketch
	Northern Ontario School of Medicine	No personal statement, but applicants are required to submit the OMSAS autobiographical sketch as well as an additional questionnaire specific to the Northern Ontario School of Medicine [1].
	University of Ottawa	More detailed autobiographical sketch (in addition to the OMSAS autobiographical sketch)
	University of Toronto	1 personal statement (1000 words). As a general guideline, the statement should address and discuss the applicant's personal background, including particular interests and extracurricular experiences. Candidates should outline their choice of and preparation for a career in medicine. Applicants should also describe their premedical studies, expanding on what they have chosen to pursue and how this has prepared them for their future, including a career in medicine. In addition, applicants are required to complete the OMSAS autobiographical sketch
	University of Western Ontario	No personal statement, but applicants are required to submit the OMSAS autobiographical sketch

Quebec and Maritime	**McGill University**	Also, applicants are required to submit a personal narrative, personally written, reflecting their usual means of expression, as well as an abstract of the personal narrative. The essay prompt is: "Tell us about the journey that has brought you to the decision to apply to Medicine and your understanding of what being a good physician means." The letter cannot be longer than 1000 words. If applicants are applying for dual degrees or as Quebec Non-Traditional Students, their answers should reflect this. Students also submit a 900 character (about 150 word) abstract, summarizing what they said in their personal narrative for initial screening purposes. Applicants also need to submit a curriculum vitae, as well as a 1900 character CV highlights submission, answering the following prompt: "Highlight three elements of your c.v. that you believe best demonstrate your motivation and suitability for medicine, including an explanation of why you chose these three elements."
	Dalhousie University	The application includes a 1500 word personal essay describing how the applicant's experiences have shaped their desire to become a physician. Out-of-province and international students must also explain why they are applying to Dalhousie, including their connection to the maritime provinces. The application also includes sections covering applicants' extracurricular activities, medically related experience, volunteer work, employment, awards and publications.
	Memorial University	Applicants answer the following 3 prompts in the autobiographical sketch: (1) Write an autobiographical sketch about who you are, how you spend your time and why. (2000 character maximum) (2) Why do you wish to become a physician? (500 character maximum) (3) What do you expect from your day to day life as a physician? (500 character maximum). Applicants also list their awards, employment and extracurricular activities. There is also 3000 characters set aside for applicants to discuss any section of the application if they wish.

Table 29. Essay and personal statement requirements for Canadian medical schools in 2011. Information obtained from the schools' websites and by calling the admissions offices.

For information on writing effective personal statements and essays, please see page 76.

Reference letter requirements

Most Canadian schools require two to three reference letters. Most require all applicants to submit reference letters, however, some schools like Dalhousie University [33], the University of Saskatchewan [34] and the University of British Columbia [35] only require reference letters from applicants invited for interview.

Some schools like the Ontario medical schools require referees to complete a confidential assessment form and submit it with their letters. Some schools like the University of Calgary send your referees a confidential link that they can access to fill in and submit your reference letters online [36].

Each university may have different guidelines on who to ask for reference letters. For example, OMSAS advises applicants to ensure that referees have extensive personal knowledge of the applicant and are able to reasonably make statements about the applicant's character, personal qualities and academic capabilities. While referees may not be in a position to evaluate all the characteristics requested, applicants should ensure that, in choosing their referees, all subject areas are covered [25]. The University of Toronto adds that "applicants are encouraged to submit at least one letter of reference from an individual able to comment on non-academic accomplishments" [37]. In addition, they suggest that "at least one letter be from a referee who can provide a comparative perspective on your character and strengths with a number of your peers, for example someone who has had occasion to interact with a number students interested in medicine" [38].

At some schools like Memorial University, although it is strongly recommended to have at least one academic reference, the school recognizes that it can be difficult for some applicants to find an academic referee who knows them well. In such circumstances, some schools like Memorial University advise applicants to still submit an academic reference letter and outline their concern in their application [39]. Additional details are available on the schools' websites and in the school specific sections below.

Some schools such as the Ontario medical schools allow the submission of a University Premedical Advisory report along with their required number of reference letters [25]. Other universities such as Memorial University accept a pre-health professions advisory report instead of reference letters [39].

"Pick people that know you well and that can speak about your character. That is what we look for. We have your grades, activities and all that other stuff - the last thing we need is a referee discussing how well you did in a class...we already know all that. For most schools, big names don't matter much unless they are at the level of the common media as directors of admissions programs aren't generally MDs. So unless the chair of your department who you met once and barely remembers your name is Paul Farmer, Kofi Annan, or the guy who discovered SARS, go with people that might know you more than people that might have a bigger name. Oh, and try and make sure they are MDs/professors/etc." (admissions advisor)

For information on obtaining the best reference letters, see page 92.

Timeline of the application

The application deadlines for most Canadian schools are in October and November, however, for some schools like the University of British Columbia and the Ontario medical schools, applicants are required to complete part of the application process as early as September [25, 35]. The opening dates for application, as well as the application and transcript submission deadlines are available in the school specific sections. Below is a table showing the application deadlines in 2011 for medical programs taught in English.

University	Deadlines for entry in 2011
University of Alberta	November 1st, 2011
University of British Columbia	The application and all supporting documents, including transcripts, are due August 15th, 2011. Note, however, that reference letters are not due at this time. Only applicants invited for interview need to submit reference letters later in the year. MCAT scores must be received by October 1st, 2011.
University of Calgary	October 15th, 2011
University of Manitoba	The deadline for submission of the application form is October 7th, 2011, and transcripts will need to be received by the university at the by November 1st, 2011. Letters of reference do not need to be submitted until the university asks for them. For in-province applicants, they are due December 1st, 2011 and for out-of-province applicants, they are due February 10th, 2012.
University of Saskatchewan	October 31st, 2011

University		Deadlines for entry in 2011
OMSAS	- **McMaster University** - **University of Ottawa** -**Northern Ontario School of Medicine** - **Queen's University** - **University of Toronto** -**University of Western Ontario**	Applicants need to create an account by September 15th, 2011. The deadline for submitting the application, confidential assessment forms, supporting letters of reference and university transcripts is October 3rd, 2011. Applicants must release their MCAT scores to OMSAS by October 11th, 2010.
McGill University		The application for the MD program is due on November 1st, 2011, and the supplemental documents and reference letters is November 15th, 2011. The application deadline for CEGEP students is March 1, 2011.
Dalhousie University		August 15, 2011 is the deadline to submit the application form. The supplemental application form, which includes a personal essay as well as activity and award descriptions, is due September 1st, 2011. For applicants that are invited for an interview, the deadline to have reference letters submitted has been early January in previous years, and will be provided later in the application cycle.
Memorial University		October 17th, 2011

Table 30. Application deadlines for Canadian medical schools taught in English
Information obtained from the schools' websites and by calling the admissions offices

Deferring entry

The deferral policies vary significantly from school to school. Many schools like Queen's University only grant deferral if the applicant firmly accepts their admissions offer. Some schools like the University of Ottawa will not consider students for admission if they were accepted at another medical school the previous year and deferred their matriculation. See below for details on each school's policy on deferring entry.

	University	Deferred entry policies
	University of Alberta	Deferrals are generally only granted in exceptional circumstances
	University of British Columbia	Deferrals are only granted under exceptional circumstances. Students must have completed their first degree.
Western Canada	**University of Calgary**	Students who are admitted directly into the program can apply for deferred entry (usually five applicants per year can be granted deferral). Those who were admitted off the waiting list cannot request a deferral. Requests must be made within the first 15 days after acceptance. Deferrals can be granted for academic and non academic reasons, provided the reasons are not seen as trivial by director of admissions.

	University of Manitoba	Deferrals are only granted for health reasons, to finish a master's degree that has already been started, or for other reasons the admissions committee deems acceptable.
	University of Saskatchewan	Usually for Saskatchewan residents only. Applicants may be granted a deferral for up to two years, normally to complete a master's degree or a PhD. Applicants can occasionally be granted deferrals for other reasons as well, such as completing humanitarian projects.
Ontario	McMaster University	Deferrals are only granted under exceptional circumstances
Ontario	Queen's University	Usually only for applicants wishing to finish the requirements for their degrees (undergraduate or graduate). Students usually need to accept their offer before asking for deferral.
Ontario	Northern Ontario School of Medicine	Deferrals are only granted under exceptional circumstances
Ontario	University of Ottawa	May be granted for special circumstances. Requests must be made before June 8, 2012.
Ontario	University of Toronto	Some applicants can be granted deferrals for compelling academic or personal circumstances. Applicants should specify that they wish to defer at the time of acceptance of their offer. Deferrals are not granted to allow students to complete their degrees.
Ontario	University of Western Ontario	Deferrals are only granted under exceptional circumstances
Quebec and Maritime	McGill University	Deferrals can be granted for one year to obtain an advanced degree (note, however, that students currently enrolled in graduate programs are expected to apply in the final year of their programs). The deadline to request a deferral is July 1st of the matriculation year. CEGEP students are not eligible for deferral.
Quebec and Maritime	Dalhousie University	Deferrals are only granted under exceptional circumstances
Quebec and Maritime	Memorial University	Students who are admitted directly into the program can apply for deferred entry (usually two applicants per year are granted deferral). Those who are admitted off the waiting list cannot request a deferral.

Table 31. Deferred entry policies for Canadian medical programs taught in English.
Information obtained from the schools' websites and by calling the admissions offices.

Interview structures

The table below lists the interview styles for each Canadian medical school in 2012.

Medical Schools in Canada	Interview format
University of Alberta	MMI
University of British Columbia	MMI
University of Calgary	MMI
Dalhousie University	MMI
University of Manitoba	MMI
McGill University	MMI
McMaster University	MMI
Memorial University of Newfoundland	One hour interview with a panel of two interviewers.
Northern Ontario University	MMI
University of Ottawa	45 minutes interview with a 3 person panel
Queen's University	MMI and a standard, panel interview
University of Saskatchewan	MMI
University of Toronto	45 minute interview with a member of the faculty and a student
University of Western Ontario	45 minute interview with three interviewers: one physician, one community member and one senior medical student

Table 32. Interview structure for medical schools in Canada for entry in 2012

For information on how to prepare for the interviews, see page 447.

School by school
Western Canada

University of Alberta

Nationality restrictions
International students are NOT eligible to apply.

Degree requirement
Successful completion of at least two full years of undergraduate studies (60 credits).

Course requirements
Half year of biochemistry, half year of statistics and a full year of each of the following: biology, English, general chemistry, organic chemistry and physics. When possible, a full year of biochemistry is encouraged. Some of these requirements can be met using AP and IB credits: http://ume.med.ualberta.ca/ProspectiveLearners/MDAdmissions/AdmissionRequirements/Pages/default.aspx

GPA requirement
The minimum cumulative GPA requirement for applicants with four or more years of undergraduate study is 3.3 out of 4.0 for Alberta residents and 3.5 out of 4.0 for non-Alberta residents. For second and third year university students, the minimum GPA required is 3.7 out of 4.0. However, note that the average entering GPA in 2010 was 3.86 for fourth year applicants and 3.92 for second and third year applicants. Note also that for students who have completed 4 or more years of post-secondary study, the University of Alberta will drop the lowest year's GPA from their calculation of the applicant's cumulative GPA, provided the lowest GPA year is not the most recent completed year and is not the only year where the applicant completed a full 30 credit course-load. Also note that courses taken during spring and summer sessions are not counted in the full-time study requirements nor in the cumulative GPA requirements. They are not counted when calculating the GPA, but they can be used to satisfy prerequisite requirements. Full years completed after the undergraduate degree will be counted in the cumulative GPA, provided they are completed between September and April and consist of 18 or more credits transferrable to the University of Alberta [1].

MCAT requirement
There is a minimum requirement of 7 or better in all categories of the MCAT. The average entering MCAT scores were 32.94Q for fourth year applicants and 34.11R for second and third year applicants for entry in 2010.

MCAT requirement (Cont'd)

For admission in September 2012, applicants must have written the MCAT by September 2011, and no earlier than November 2006. For students that have written the MCAT more than once, the University of Alberta will only consider the best scores.

Selection Formula

Applicants are separated into 3 pools, each with different entrance cutoffs: Albertan, Non-Albertan and second/third year undergraduate applicants. There are also 10 places for rural applicants and 5 for aboriginal applicants. Applicants are then ranked for interview based on a pre interview score. See table 33 below for details on how the pre interview score is calculated. After the interview, applicants are ranked for admission based on their pre interview scores, the interview and their reference letters.

Applicants with a PhD or master's

The course requirements are the same as above with no course exemptions. Courses taken during the PhD or master's program will be used in the calculation of the cumulative GPA if the unit of course weight during the academic year is 18 credits or higher. Graduate students also benefit from the deletion of the lowest year GPA in the same way that undergraduate applicants do. Applicants who have obtained a master's degree or PhD by thesis may be asked to provide the name and address of the Chair of their Defense Committee so that an

evaluation of their thesis may be obtained. Additional points may be allocated to the application as shown in table 33.

Application documents

The University of Alberta does not require any essays but does require 5 descriptions related to the applicant's extracurricular activities: 1. Employment recored, 2. Awards and achievements, 3. Leadership roles, 4. Volunteer work, 5. Diversity of experience. Each of these should include a brief description as well as contact details of someone in charge such as the employer or a mentor. The application also requires 2 reference letters from people who know the applicant well. Referees are asked to answer specific questions on the form: 1) Should the applicant admitted and why 2) Would you have the applicant as your physician and why 3) Please address the applicants moral and ethical characteristics? 4) Please comment on any outstanding strengths or weaknesses of the applicant.

Interview

The interview is MMI format which includes approximately eight stations taking 10 minutes each. At each station, the interviewee will be provided with a question and allocated two minutes to read the question and formulate an appropriate response. After these two minutes, the interviewee will discuss their response with an interviewer for the remaining eight minutes before moving to the next station.

Application deadline

All application materials including reference letters, MCAT scores and transcripts are due on November 1st, 2011. The final transcripts of the current year of study need to be submitted by June 15, 2012.

Application cost

The application fee is $75 for University of Alberta students, $115 for all other students.

Cost of studies 2011-2012

Tuition fees of $11,750 per year

Statistics

Approximately 85% of the 167 seats available are assigned to Albertan applicants while the remaining 15% are assigned to non-Albertans. In 2010, there were 1,234 applicants for the 167 places available; 125 fourth year applicants, 27 second/third year applicants, 10 rural applicants and 5 aboriginal applicants were admitted.

Contact

2-45 Medical Sciences Bldg.
114 Street & 87 Avenue
Edmonton, Alberta, Canada. T6G 2H7
Tel: (780) 492-9524/6769
admission@med.ualberta.ca

		Alberta	Non-Albertan	2nd and 3rd year applicants**
Minimum Cutoffs		3.3 on 4.0 scale*	3.5 on 4.0 scale*	3.7 on 4.0 scale
All Applicants				
Pre interview score (max 70 points)	Cumulative average of University years	30 points		
	MCAT	15 points		
	MCAT Writing Sample	5 points		
	Personal Activities	20 points		
	Completion of: master's degree PhD	+1 point +3 points		
Overall rank score for selection (max 100 points)	Pre Interview score (see above)	70 points		
	Interview	25 points		
	Letters of Reference	5 points		

Table 33. Minimum cutoffs and selection factor weightings at the University of Alberta.
*The lowest year's GPA is dropped under certain conditions for students with 4 or more years of post-secondary education.
**Students applying in their second or third year of full-time undergraduate study.

Ref: 124. *University of Alberta*. Available from: http://www.med.ualberta.ca/education/ugme/admissions/dofm.cfm.

University of British Columbia

Nationality restrictions
International students are NOT eligible to apply.

Degree requirement
Successful completion of at least 90 credits at a post-secondary institution.

Course requirements
1 full of year of biochemistry, biology, English, general chemistry and organic chemistry are required. Courses in behavioral sciences, biometrics, statistics and physics are recommended, but not required. AP and IB credits may be used to fulfill part of these requirements. Additional details including information on the grades and course levels required to use IB and AP credits toward prerequisite requirements are available from: www.med.ubc.ca/education/md_ugrad/ MD_Undergraduate_Admissions/ Admission_Requirements.htm

GPA requirement
The minimum requirement for in-province applicants is an overall GPA of 75%, and for out of province applicants is 80%. The average GPA of the 2010 entering class was 84.98%. Note that in 2011, the average GPA of interviewed candidates was 83.91% for in province and 89.92% for out-of-province. Applicants who have completed university-level courses ten years or more years before the date of application may request in writing to have these grades excluded from the overall average. Note that in calculating an applicant's GPA, UBC includes summer courses and graduate courses with grades, if applicable, and uses the conversion scale available from: www.med.ubc.ca/__shared/assets/ Grade_Conversion_Table21093.pdf

MCAT requirement
The minimum MCAT requirement is a score of no less than 7 in any of the multiple choice sections and no less than M in the writing sample. It is suggested that applicants look at admissions statistics from previous years for an indication of competitive scores. In 2010, the mean MCAT scores for the entering class were 9.78 in verbal reasoning, 10.79 in physical sciences, 11.27 in biological sciences and Q in the writing section. The overall average MCAT score for the 2010 entry class was 31.8Q. Test results for the last five years, inclusive, are considered valid. If an applicant has written the MCAT more than once, the best eligible overall total score will be used. The admissions office will look at each individual score to produce the overall total converted score which will be the one used for evaluation.

Selection Formula

Applicants are given a pre interview score based on the combination of their GPA and their non-academic qualities score, both of which are weighted 50% at this stage. Applicants who have completed 90 credits at the time of application are eligible to have the academic year with the lowest GPA dropped from the calculation (if the lowest academic year had more than 30 credits, the 30 lowest credits are dropped). Note that the MCAT is not a factor at this stage and will only be considered after the interview. After the interview, all aspects of the file are considered including grade trends and graduate work, the MCAT, the interview and non-academic criteria.

Applicants with a PhD or master's

Students with a master's or PhD must complete the program in which they are registered by June 30th of the admission year. Graduate students in non-thesis based programs must complete all required courses, projects, etc. and have grades submitted by June 30th. Graduate students who are invited for an interview will be required to have their thesis supervisor, or department head complete an electronic form stating that the applicant will likely finish their program by June 30th. This deadline is firm.

Application documents

The application includes a report of non-academic experiences, however, it does not include reference letters. Applicants invited

for interview will receive notification early in December and will be asked to have their referees submit reference letters online. All applicants must also arrange to have one set of official transcripts from all post-secondary institutions attended sent directly to the admissions office.

Interview

The interviews follow the MMI format in which each applicant rotates through approximately 10 different interview stations. The interview at each station is roughly 7 minutes in duration, with a 2 minute transition period, which allows the applicant to advance to the next station, read a question or a scenario and prepare themselves before entering the next interview room. The entire interview cycle is approximately 2 hours in length and applicants may have up to two "rest" stations per cycle. The interviewer pool is diverse: clinicians, academics, community members and UBC 3rd & 4th year medical students from a variety of geographical areas across BC.

Application deadline

The application for the University of British Columbia opens on June 1st, 2011. The application and all supporting documents, including transcripts, are due August 15th, 2011. Note, however, that reference letters are not due at this time.

Application deadline (Cont'd)

Only applicants invited for interview need to submit reference letters later in the year. MCAT scores must be received by October 1st, 2011.

Application cost

The application fee is $107 for BC residents, $158 for out-of-province residents, and $31 for out-of-province transcripts (any number).

Cost of studies 2009-2010

Tuition fees of $14,900 per year.

Statistics

There will be a total of 288 positions available in 2012, of which up to 29 are available for out-of-province applicants. Approximately 700 students will be interviewed. 192 students will be placed in Vancouver, 32 in Victoria, 32 in Northern BC and 32 in Kalowna. Students indicate their site preferences at the interview [35]. In 2010, 256 students were admitted out of a total of 1793 applicants. Out of those, 35 students did not have a degree (had completed 3 years of undergraduate study) and 25 had a master's degree.

Contact

MD Undergraduate Admissions
Faculty of Medicine, Dean's Office
University of British Columbia
317 - 2194 Health Sciences Mall
Vancouver, BC V6T 1Z3
Tel: (604) 875-8298
admissions.md@ubc.ca

Ref: 35. *University of British Columbia, MD undergraduate Webpage.* Available from: http://www.med.ubc.ca/education/md_ugrad.htm.

University of Calgary

Nationality restrictions
International students are NOT eligible to apply.

Degree requirement
Applicants must have completed at least two years of full-time study.

Course requirements
The university recommends several courses for preparation for medical school, but completion of these courses is no longer graded as part of the application evaluation [1]. The courses recommended to prepare for medical school are: 1 year of biochemistry, biology, calculus or statistics, English, general chemistry, organic chemistry, physics, physiology and half a year of either psychology, sociology or anthropology.

GPA requirement
The GPA cutoff is 3.20 out of 4.00 for Albertans and 3.60 out of 4.00 for non-Albertans. The overall GPA of an applicant is used for eligibility and not the best 2 years' GPA. This is a slight change from previous years when applicant eligibility was determined based on the best two years, but note that if an applicant has 3 full time years of study completed at the time of application, the GPA of the worst year will be dropped from the overall GPA calculation. Thus, for applicants in their final year of a four year degree, only their best two years will be counted. For applicants with completed graduate degrees at the time of application, the overall GPA in their graduate degree will be counted as equivalent to one full time year of undergraduate studies. For applicants with multiple graduate degrees, the GPA for each separate degree will be added to the undergraduate degree. Note that the graduate GPA does not replace the undergraduate one, but only supplements it. Applicants who are admitted still need to maintain a GPA above 3.2 during the application year for the admission offer to remain valid. The average overall GPA of the class of 2011 was 3.62 and the average "best 2 years" GPA was 3.82. To learn how the GPA is calculated, you can find the university's GPA conversion scale in the applicant manual available from their website. Note that unlike some schools, AP and IB grades are not converted to percentage grades and are thus not included in the GPA calculation.

MCAT requirement
The average MCAT score for the class of 2011 was 32.14Q, however, unlike some other medical programs, there is no cutoff for the MCAT. If an applicant has written the MCAT more than once, the best set of scores will be used by the admissions office. You can find the university's MCAT conversion scale in the applicant manual available from their website.

MCAT requirement (Cont'd)

Note that only the VR score is used in the pre-interview formula but the full MCAT may be considered in the subjective assessment of academic merit, so the other components of the MCAT score still do make a difference.

Selection Formula

In the admissions process, there are three pre-interview stages for out-of-province applicants and two pre-interview stages for in-province applicants. The first stage for both in-province and out-of-province applicants is to attain the minimum GPA requirements. For out-of-province students, once these minimums are met, applicants are given a score according to the following formula: 2 x GPA + MCAT VR. They are ranked according to these scores and the top 250 applicants advance to the file review stage (the third stage). For in-province applicants, all applicants meeting the minimum requirements advance automatically to the file review stage. All applicants who qualify for the full file review are then given a score based on their entire application according to the following breakdown: 40% academics (consisting of 20% GPA, 10% MCAT VR, 10% Subjective Assessment of Academic Merit and 10% for each of the following:

- Evidence of communication skills
- Evidence of excellent interpersonal skills and collaboration

- Evidence of high ethical standards and professionalism
- Commitment to communities and advocacy on behalf of others
- Intellectual curiosity, scholarship and research
- Evidence of organizational/management skills and leadership

To assess the attributes above, the admissions committee will look at the entire file. The highest scoring applicants at this stage are then offered an interview. The applicants are then given a post interview score and ranked for admission based on the following: 50% pre-interview score and 50% MMI.

Applicants with a PhD or master's

See GPA section to see how applicants with a graduate degree can get extra points.

Application documents

Applicants submit impact statements for their top 10 extracurricular activities. Applicants also need to submit 3 reference letters, each of which should assess a distinct attribute of the applicant. The 3 attributes to be covered are:

1. Organizational/management and leadership skills
2. Commitment to communities and advocacy
3. Interpersonal behaviour and collaboration

Applicants may also need to fill in some information to help create an applicant timeline for the assessors.

Application documents (Cont'd)

This will be a visual timeline including where the applicants lived, their education, their employment and their primary extra curricular activity.

Interview

The interview is MMI format with nine stations. The written MMI is not part of the application process anymore.

Application deadline

For entry in 2012, the application opens August 1st, 2011 and closes on October 15th, 2011.

Application cost

The application fee in previous years has been $150, and is not expected to change substantially in the 2012-2013 application cycle [1].

Cost of studies 2010-2011

Tuition fees of $14,385 per year.

Statistics

In the 2010-2011 application cycle, there were approximately 950 in-province applicants, of which 440 were interviewed for the 152 places available. There were also 900 out-of-province applicants, of which 120 were interviewed for the 28 places available. Of the 180 seats available for entry in 2012, approximately 85% are for Albertans and 15% for non-Albertans.

Additional information

The University of Calgary is one of the two 3-year medical programs in Canada.

Contact

Office of Admissions
University of Calgary
Faculty of Medicine
3330 Hospital Drive NW
Calgary AB T2N 4N1
Tel: 403-220-4262
ucmedapp@ucalgary.ca

Ref: 128. *University of Calgary Admissions.* Available from: www.ucalgary.ca/mdprogram/prospective/admissions.

University of Manitoba

Nationality restrictions
International students are NOT eligible to apply.

Degree requirement
Applicants must have or be eligible to receive their bachelor's degree by June 29th, 2012.

Course requirements
The prerequisite courses are as follows: 1 full year of biochemistry and 3 full years of humanities/social sciences. Applicants who complete a 4-year major or honors program may waive up to 12 credit hours of the humanities/social sciences prerequisite, however, applicants with a general BSc or BA must complete the full requirement. It is possible to have AP and IB coursework considered to fulfill the course requirements. Details on the conversions are available from the school's website. In general, an AP grade of 5 translates to a grade of A, and 4 to a grade of B. For IB courses, a grade of 7 translates to an A+, 6 to an A, 5 to a B+ and 4 to a B.

GPA requirement
Applicants are given what is called an AGPA (scale of 0 to 4.5) calculated based on all their coursework including summer courses. Credits will be dropped to improve the applicants GPA as a function of the number of credits completed in total. If an applicant has completed 120 credits or more, the 30 credits with the lowest grades will be dropped in the calculation of the AGPA. See table 34 for the number of credits dropped in the University of Manitoba AGPA calculation as a function of the number of credits completed. Note, however, that courses used to fulfill the biochemistry requirement will always be included in the AGPA calculation. The minimum requirement is 3.30 out of 4.5 for in-province and out-of-province students, however, most successful applicants have an AGPA over 4.0. For entry in 2010, the average AGPA was 4.15 for in-province applicants and 4.01 for out-of province applicants who were granted admission.

Number of Credit hours the applicant has completed	Credit hours that the admissions committee will drop
90-95	15
96-101	18
102-107	21
108-113	24
114-119	27
120 or more	30

Table 34. Number of credits dropped in the University of Manitoba AGPA calculation as a function of the number of credits completed.

GPA requirement (cont'd)

Note that undergraduate courses completed after the undergraduate degree are still counted in the AGPA calculation, however, courses taken toward master's degrees or PhDs are not counted.

MCAT requirement

A minimum of 7 is required on each section of the MCAT as well as a minimum score of M on the written section. Once these cutoffs have been met, applicants are given an operative MCAT score equal to 0.3(Verbal Reasoning) + 0.2(Physical Science) + 0.3(Biological Science) + 0.2(Written Sample). The writing sample score is converted to a scale where T=14 and M=7. For entry in 2010, the average MCAT scores were 31.83 for in-province applicants and 36.78 for out-of-province applicants. Note that the University of Manitoba only accepts MCAT scores from April 3 years prior to the application date. Thus, for entry in 2012, the earliest acceptable MCAT date is April, 2008.

Selection Formula

Applicants are also given a personal assessment score (PAS) based on their personal attributes assessed using reference letters, the application, the list of publications, the interview, etc. Applicants who have competitive AGPAs, MCAT scores and pre interview PAS scores are invited for interview. After the interview, in-province and out-of-province applicants are scored according to the following formula: 15% AGPA, 40% MCAT and 45% post interview PAS.

Applicants with a PhD or master's

Graduate students are screened using the same formula as undergraduate students on the basis of undergraduate coursework and MCAT criteria. However, applicant's accomplishments during graduate studies will be taken into account in determining the Personal Assessment Score (PAS).

Application documents

Three reference letters written by supervisors (or equivalent) should be submitted when the university requests these documents. The secondary application in the 2012-2013 application cycle will include information about applicants' extracurricular activities, awards, and publications [1].

Interview

The interview is MMI format with approximately 12 stations. Immediately before the MMI, applicants will be given specific instructions. Each group will go through a set number of stations (approximately 12), spending 2 minutes reading a question or situation, and 8 minutes discussing the station with one interviewer. Applicants will be sequestered for approximately five hours to maintain confidentiality regarding that day's stations.

Application deadline

The deadline for submission of the application form is October 7th, 2011, and transcripts will need to be received by the university by November 1st, 2011. Letters of reference do not need to be submitted until the university asks for them. For in-province applicants, they are due December 1st, 2011 and for out-of-province applicants, they are due February 10th, 2012.

Application cost

Application fee of $95 before September 23rd, 2011, and $125 after this date.

Cost of studies 2011-2012

Annual tuition fees were $7,575 for year 1 and $7,259 for years 2-4.

Statistics

In the 2010-2011 application cycle, there were 275 in province applicants, of whom 236 were interviewed and 102 were offered admission for the 98 places available. There were also 437 out-of-province applicants, of whom 49 were interviewed and 39 were offered admission for the 5 places available (there were approximately 10 out-of-province students accepted in total including the aboriginal applicant pool [1]). 148 applicants were considered to have rural attributes, and among them 104 were interviewed, with 60 offers of admission for the 54 places available to these applicants.

Contact

Admissions, Faculty of Medicine
University of Manitoba
260-727 McDermot Avenue
Winnipeg MB R3E 3P5
Tel: 204-789-3929
ugadmit@cc.umanitoba.ca

Refs: 129. *University of Manitoba.* Available from: http://www.umanitoba.ca/faculties/medicine/.

University of Saskatchewan

Nationality restrictions

International students are NOT eligible to apply.

Degree requirement

Saskatchewan residents are eligible to apply during their second year of university. Out-of-province applicants must be in their third year of undergraduate study to apply.

Course requirements

There are two ways to qualify to apply to the University of Saskatchewan. The courses below are required for applicants meeting the qualification requirements using their prerequisite courses, but are only recommended for applicants meeting the qualification requirements using their MCAT scores (see "selection formula" section for explanation of how applicants can qualify to apply): 1 full year of biochemistry, biology, physics, English and social sciences/humanities as well as half a year of general chemistry and organic chemistry.

GPA requirement

To meet the competitive average requirement, in-province applicants must attain a minimum of 78% in the two-year average, and out-of-province residents a minimum of 80%. In recent years, the cutoff for out-of-province students offered an interview has been >90% for the best two years (92.3% in 2010). Courses taken during summer (May to August) are not considered in the two-year average. For in-province applicants, the current year of study will factor into the best two years' gpa calculation. The median entering GPA for the best 2 years in 2010 was 89.0%. For out-of-province applicants, only the years completed at the time of application are considered in the best two years' gpa calculation. Normally, courses taken after the undergraduate degree are only taken into account in the GPA requirement if they are leading to another degree. However, applicants planning to take an extra year after their degree are encouraged to contact the admissions office to see if their extra year will be eligible for consideration. This should be done in the fall of their extra year or earlier [1]. Applicants taking more than 3 or 4 years to complete a 3 or 4 year degree must also contact the admissions office for pre-approval of their additional years of study.

MCAT requirement

The minimum MCAT requirement is an overall score of 26 with no section score below 8. The MCAT average in 2009 entering class was 28, with 84.5% of accepted applicants having achieved above N on the writing section.

Selection Formula

First, in-province applicants and students who attended the University of Saskatchewan or the University of Regina must either have achieved an overall average of 78% on their prerequisite courses with no prerequisite grade less than 60%, or have achieved a minimum score of 26 on the MCAT with no section score less than 8. If they achieve one of these criteria, they will be considered for the next step. Out-of-province students who did not attend one of these universities can only qualify for the next step based on achieving an MCAT score of 26 overall with no section score below 8. If they did not achieve the necessary MCAT score, they will not be considered further. The next step for all applicants is to have their best two full-time years averaged, and be ranked for interview according to this average. In-province and out-of-province applicants are ranked separately, and in previous years, in-province applicants have needed averages >82% and out-of-province applicants have needed averages >92% to be competitive for interview. After the interview, Saskatchewan residents are ranked for admission with 35% of the score based on academic performance and 65% based on the interview. For out-of-province applicants, after the interview, the offer of admission is based solely on interview performance. Note that reference letters are not scored, but rather are used on a rule in/rule out basis.

Applicants with a PhD or master's

In considering graduate students, the average may be based on the following, or the two best full-time undergraduate years, whichever works to their advantage:

1. Course-based graduate program, which may or may not include a research project: the average of all grades in the program will count as one full year combined with the best two full-time undergraduate years. The postgraduate program must be comparable to at least one full-time academic year (30 credit units).

2. Master's thesis-based program: the average of all Master's grades (minimum 9 credits) will count as one full year combined with the best two full-time undergraduate years.

3. Ph.D. thesis-based program: The average of all graduate grades (minimum 15 credits) will count as one full year combined with the best full-time undergraduate year.

Masters and PhD students who do not have the minimum number of course credits outlined above will have their post-graduate courses average on a course-weight basis with their best two full time undergraduate years. PhD students with between 9 and 15 course credits will have their post-graduate work weighted as a full year and combined with their best two full time undergraduate years.

Application documents

Only applicants invited for interview need to send reference letters. They will be sent forms by the university when they are offered an interview. Three references will be required. Appropriate references include undergraduate or graduate instructors or research supervisors. Also, official transcripts from all universities attended must be sent directly to the College of Medicine by the application deadline. Note that there is no autobiographical sketch/essay required with the application.

Interview

The interview is MMI format which includes approximately 10 stations taking 10 minutes each. At each station, the interviewee will be provided with a question and allocated two minutes to read the question and formulate an appropriate response. After these two minutes, the interviewee will discuss their response with an interviewer for the remaining eight minutes before moving to the next station.

Application deadline

The application deadline is October 31st, 2011.

Application cost

The application fee is $125.

Cost of studies 2012-2013

Tuition fees of $13,649 per year.

Statistics

In the 2011-2012 application cycle, there were 84 places available, but this may increase to 100 in the 2012-2013 application cycle. There were 370 in-province applicants in 2010, of which 286 were interviewed for 80 places. That year there were also 478 out of province applicants, of which 56 were interviewed for the 4 places available. A maximum of 8 seats are available for out-of-province applicants.

Contact

Admissions Office
College of Medicine, U of S
A204 Health Sciences Bldg.
107 Wiggins Rd
Saskatoon SK S7N 5E5
Tel: (306) 966-4030
med.admissions@usask.ca

Refs: 130. *University of Saskatchewan, Medical School Admissions.* available from: http://www.medicine.usask.ca/education/admissions/.

The Ontario Medical Schools

OMSAS

The six Ontario medical schools use a centralized application service called the Ontario Medical School Application Service (OMSAS). Applicants to Ontario medical schools submit only one set of application materials and academic documents, regardless of the number of schools to which they are applying. OMSAS will process and forward applications to all requested medical schools regardless of the qualifications of the applicant or the completeness of the application.

Application Deadline

Applicants need to create an account by September 15th, 2011. The deadline for submitting the application, confidential assessment forms, supporting letters of reference and university transcripts is October 3rd, 2011. Applicants must release their MCAT scores to OMSAS by October 11th, 2010.

GPA requirements

The application service converts all grades onto a 4.0 scale using the OMSAS conversion scale available at www.ouac.on.ca/omsas/ – under "Grade Conversion Table" on the right. The GPA requirements and statistics of the Ontario medical schools are listed in the school specific sections. Canadians and international applicants who have not met the minimum course credit requirements for a university using Canadian or US courses, and who require inclusion of international courses to meet the course credit requirements, need to submit foreign transcripts to the World Education Service for assessment, as well as to OMSAS [2, 4, 28]. The WES converts grades to their Ontario educational equivalents. More information on submitting transcripts to the WES is available in the OMSAS instruction manual: www.ouac.on.ca/omsas.

OMSAS Autobiographical sketch

The application includes a common section requiring applicants to fill in their personal and academic background as well as to list all pertinent awards and activities since age 16 (this section is called the autobiographical sketch). The elements to be included are:

Ref: 131. *OMSAS Information.* Available from: http://www.ouac.on.ca/omsas/omsas-answers.html

- Formal Education (name of institution, dates, program, degree)
- Employment
- Volunteer Activities
- Extracurricular Activities
- Awards and Accomplishments
- Research
- Other

Application documents

The autobiographical sketch described above will be sent to each Ontario medical school. Three reference letters with confidential assessment forms (an extra sheet that referees fill in and include with their reference letters) also need to be sent directly by the referees to OMSAS [25]. Most schools have additional questions or essays to fill in as outlined in the school specific section below. Official transcripts of all post-secondary institutions other than Ontario universities for all courses completed before the current academic year also need to be sent by October 3rd, 2011. Transcripts from Ontario universities and colleges must be requested through OMSAS. Fees are $10 per transcript requested, with some exceptions.

Application fees

The application service fee is $210 plus the following institutional fees for each medical school selection.

McMaster University	$105
Northern Ontario School of Medicine	$75
University of Ottawa	$75
Queen's University	$75
University of Toronto	$85
University of Western Ontario	$75

Applying to all 6 schools costs $700.

McMaster University

Nationality restrictions
International students ARE eligible to apply.

Degree requirement
By May 2012, applicants must have completed 15 full year credits or 30 half year credits (equivalent to three full time years of undergraduate study). Applicants who have completed the requirements for a bachelor's degree in less than three years by the application deadline, and who meet the 3.00 GPA requirement, are also eligible to apply.

Course requirements
There are no prerequisite course requirements.

GPA requirement
By October 3, 2011 applicants must have achieved an overall OMSAS converted average of 3.0 on the 4.0 point scale. The average GPA of applicants matriculating in 2010 was 3.82 (it was 3.89 in 2009). An overall simple average will be calculated using the grades from all undergraduate degree level courses ever taken. Courses from different years are treated equally. This average is calculated by the applicant on the OMSAS academic record form and verified on the OMSAS verification report which is sent to applicants. McMaster University may also review and revise this average. The marks from supplementary and summer courses are included in the GPA calculation.

MCAT requirement
A minimum score of 6 on the verbal reasoning section is required. Other sections of the MCAT are NOT considered in the selection process and thus there is no overall minimum score required for the MCAT. The score from the verbal reasoning section of the MCAT is used in the formula to select applicants for an interview and the formula used after the interview. The most recent test result (not the best) is used. For the class matriculating in 2010, the average MCAT verbal reasoning score was 10.86. 176 students scored 10 or above, while 23 students scored 9 and 4 students scored between 6 and 8.

Other requirements
There is a 90 minute Computer-Based Assessment for Personal Characteristics (CASPer) that applicants need to complete on either Wednesday October 19, 2011, or Sunday, October 23, 2011. Applicants will receive an email around October 7th, 2011 with more detailed instructions. The questionnaire has 12 sections with 2 or 3 short questions in each. Eight of the 12 are prompted by situational challenges shown in one minute video clips, and the other four sections are for self-descriptive questions. It is an assessment of interpersonal skills and decision making.

Selection Formula

In selecting applicants for interview, 90% of interview positions will be given to those who qualify as Ontario residents. The remaining 10% will be given to all others. Applicants were ranked for interview according to the following formula: 25% undergraduate GPA, 25% MCAT verbal reasoning, 46% CASPer Score, 1% completion of a master's degree, 4% completion of a Ph.D (maximum 4% for graduate work). After the interview, applicants are ranked according to the following formula: 70% MMI score, 15% undergraduate GPA and 15% MCAT verbal reasoning score. The best scoring applicants are offered admissions.

Applicants with a PhD or master's

An applicant's graduate experience will be considered in the admissions process if it is complete and the degree has been conferred by the application deadline of October 3rd. Individual grades received for courses taken as part of a graduate degree will not be included in the GPA calculation. Applicants with a graduate degree will receive bonus points in their pre interview score (master's degree = +1 point; PhD = +4 points, for a maximum of 4 points out of a possible 100), providing a significant, albeit not decisive, advantage for graduate degree holders.

Application documents

In 2011, along with the OMSAS application, McMaster requires CASPer to be completed in October 2011. See section above "Other requirements" for more information on CASPer.

Interview

Several hundred applicants will be invited to Hamilton in March or April 2012 of the interviews (554 in last year's application cycle). During the MMI, applicants will move between interview "stations" in a 10-station circuit. Each station lasts eight minutes and there is a two minute break between each one. At each station, applicants will interact with, or be observed by, a single rater. The stations deal with a variety of issues, which may include but are not limited to, communication, collaboration, ethics, health policy, critical thinking, awareness of society health issues in Canada and personal qualities. Applicants are not assessed on their scientific knowledge.

Application deadline

See application deadline through OMSAS above.

Application cost

See application fees through OMSAS above.

Cost of studies 2011-2012

For Canadian students, tuition fees of $23,338 for the first year, $22,505 for the second year and $21,703 for the third year. For international students, tuition fees of $95,841 per year.

Additional information

McMaster University is one of the two 3-year medical programs in Canada.

International applicants

All non-Canadians can apply through the regular stream, via OMSAS. International applicants who have not met the requirements through American or Canadian universities must have their foreign transcript assessed by World Education Services (WES). Those requiring WES assessment must also ensure that their transcripts are received by WES in time for their assessment to reach OMSAS by October 3, 2011. Students who meet the requirements with Canadian and US courses do not need to have a WES assessment, and foreign grades will not be used in the GPA calculation, but they must still have the foreign university send transcripts to OMSAS.

Statistics

In the 2011-2012 application cycle, 3,549 applications were submitted for the 204 places available: 28 at their Waterloo Regional campus, 28 at the Niagara Region Campus and 147 at the main campus in Hamilton. Applicants can rank their preferences at the interview, and the offers of admission are binding to a specific site. In the 2010-2011 admission cycle, there were 2,979 in-province applicants, of whom 477 were interviewed and 194 admitted. There were also 762 out of province applicants, of whom 48 were interviewed and 9 admitted. Finally, there were 44 international applicants, of whom 1 was interviewed and admitted. Each year, up to 10% of places are available for out-of-province and international students combined [1], although only 5% of matriculants came from these categories in 2011.

Contact

MD Admissions Office
McMaster University, Michael G. DeGroote School of Medicine
1200 Main Street West, MDCL - 3104
Hamilton, ON L8N 3Z5
Tel: (905) 525-9140 x22235
mdadmit@mcmaster.ca

Ref: 132. *McMaster University, Medical School Admissions.* Available from: http://fhs.mcmaster.ca/mdprog/admissions.html.

Queen's University

Nationality restrictions
International students are NOT eligible to apply.

Degree requirement
To qualify, candidates are required to have a minimum of 3 years of full time undergraduate study (90 credits).

Course requirements
The courses below are required: 1 full year of biological sciences, 1 full year of humanities or social sciences and 1 full year of physical sciences. Examples of biological science courses include anatomy, biochemistry, biology, botany, genetics, immunology, microbiology, physiology and zoology. Examples of humanities courses include classics, English, French, foreign languages, film studies, drama, music, history, philosophy and religion. Examples of Social Sciences include anthropology, economics, geography, political science, psychology and sociology. Examples of physical science courses include general chemistry, geology, organic chemistry and physics. It is strongly suggested that applicants complete courses in the humanities or social sciences that include an essay component. AP and IB credit can be used to meet the prerequisite requirements provided these courses appear on the applicant's university transcript.

GPA requirement
The GPA cutoffs for Queen's University have been posted in previous years but to our knowledge are no longer posted on their website. The cutoffs vary significantly from year to year. The cutoffs from 2007 were 3.68 cumulative GPA or 3.78 for the GPA of the most recent 2 years [125]. The GPA cutoff at Queen's University can be met by averaging all years of full time study (including summer and supplemental courses) or averaging the most recent two years of full-time study (summer courses are not taken into account in this calculation). Any year in which you have completed a minimum of 3 courses in each academic semester will be considered full time. You do not have to carry a full course load to be considered full time. Exceptions to meeting the GPA cutoffs may be made for students holding a master's degree, a PhD or another graduate degree on a case by case basis. Full years completed after the undergraduate degree, both in general studies or as part of another undergraduate degree, will be counted toward meeting the minimum GPA cutoffs. Note that courses taken toward master's degrees or PhDs are not counted.

MCAT requirement
The MCAT cutoffs for Queen's have been posted in previous years but to our knowledge are no longer posted on their website.

MCAT requirement (cont'd)

The cutoffs from 2007 were 30P with a minimum of 10 in each section [125].

Selection Formula

Sequential steps are used to select the applicants invited for an interview. The first cutoff is based on the GPA. Applicants who have completed a graduate degree and meet the MCAT cutoff but are slightly below the GPA cutoff will be reviewed on an individual basis by the admissions committee. The second cutoff is based on the MCAT results. Candidates who meet the GPA and MCAT cutoffs will be invited for interview. After the interview, the academic marks are no longer considered in the admission process. The interview is the main determinant of an admission offer at this stage. Offers will be made after the first round on a rolling basis until the class has been filled.

Applicants with a PhD or master's

Exceptions to meeting the GPA cutoffs may be made for students holding a graduate degree or on a case by case basis as long as the MCAT requirement is met.

Application documents

The documents required are those required by OMSAS for all Ontario medical schools (see above in OMSAS section).

Interview

Interviews consist of both an MMI and a standard, panel-type interview.

Application deadline

See application deadline in OMSAS section above.

Application cost

See application fees in OMSAS section above.

Cost of studies 2009-2010

Tuition fees of $19,438 per year.

Additional information

Note that Queen's University is one of the two Canadian schools that does not favor in-province students.

Statistics

There were 3,136 applicants in the 2011-2012 application cycle for the 100 seats available.

Contact

Undergraduate Medical Education
68 Barrie Street, Queen's University
Kingston, Ontario, K7L 3N6
Tel: (613) 533-3307
queensmd@queensu.ca

Ref: 134. *Queen's University, Medical School Admission.* Available from: http://meds.queensu.ca/undergraduate/prospective_students.

Northern Ontario School of Medicine

Nationality restrictions
International students are NOT eligible to apply.

Degree requirement
Applicants must have completed a four-year undergraduate degree. Mature applicants (25 years of age or older by the application deadline) may apply with a three-year degree.

Course requirements
There are no prerequisite course requirements, however, it is recommended that applicants who majored in science should complete at least 2 full-year course equivalents in arts, social sciences and/or humanities while those who have majored in arts, social sciences and/or humanities should complete at least 2 full year course equivalents in science subjects.

GPA requirement
A minimum GPA of 3.00 on the 4.00 scale is required to apply. The GPA is calculated using all undergraduate courses completed as part of the undergraduate degree. Additional undergraduate courses completed after a degree is awarded are not used in the GPA unless these grades are part of a second undergraduate degree that will be completed prior to June 30th of the year of potential enrollment. For an applicant, applying as a non-mature student applicant, who has completed two four-year undergraduate degrees, the GPA will be calculated on each of the degrees, and the best GPA will be used for scoring. This applies if the combination of degrees includes a three-year degree along with the completion of a four-year degree. The average GPA for the 2010 entering class (including the 0.2 points added for students with master's degrees and PhDs) was 3.66 on a 4.00 scale.

MCAT requirement
The MCAT is not required.

Selection Formula
Once the GPA cutoff is met, applicants are given a pre interview score based on their GPA, their autobiographical sketch from the OMSAS application, the admissions questionnaire (an additional section in the OMSAS application specific to the Northern Ontario School of Medicine) and their context - context being primarily based on the places in which they have lived for one year or more. Advantage is given to students from within Northern Ontario, rural and remote areas in the rest of Canada, and Aboriginal and Francophone applicants. There are a few ways that applicants can qualify as Francophone students including having a diploma from a secondary school taught in French. More details are available on the school's website. After the interview, the entire application is taken into account in selecting students for admission.

Applicants with a PhD or master's

Applicants who provide proof of convocation from a graduate degree prior to December 30th of the application year will be considered for admission based on the GPA of their undergraduate degree. However, applicants who fulfill the minimum GPA of 3.0 will have 0.2 added to their GPA. Applicants will not get additional points added to their GPA for having more than one graduate degree.

Application documents

The documents required are those required by OMSAS for all Ontario medical schools (see above in OMSAS section), as well as an additional questionnaire specific to the Northern Ontario School of Medicine [1].

Interview

Admission interviews are normally conducted in March and/or April in both Sudbury and Thunder Bay The Northern Ontario School of Medicine uses the Multiple Mini Interview format. Applicants invited to interview will receive a description of the interview process with their invitation to interview.

Application deadline

See application deadline through OMSAS above.

Application cost

See application fees through OMSAS above.

Cost of studies 2011-2012

Tuition fees of $17,920 per year.

Statistics

In the 2010-2011 application cycle, 1748 applications were received and 393 applicants were interviewed for a total of 64 places in the class. Of the 64 students admitted in 2010, 58 were from Northern Ontario and the other 6 were from rural or remote areas in the rest of Canada. Also, 14 of those student had a master's degree and one had a PhD. There are no positions reserved for out-of-province applicants, but they accept some out-of-province applicants each year. The 64 places include 36 at Laurentian University in Sudbury, Ontario (East Campus) and 28 are at Lakehead University in Thunder Bay, Ontario (West Campus). Applications are made to the school without designation of preference for a particular campus. Candidates who are invited for interview will be asked to indicate their preferred campus.

Contact

Tel: (807) 766 7463
nosmadmit@normed.ca.

Ref: 9. *Northern Ontario School of Medicine webpage.* Available from: http://www.normed.ca/education/ume/default.aspx?id=352&ekmensel=c580fa7b_96_0_352_1#.

University of Ottawa

Nationality restrictions

International students are NOT eligible to apply except children of alumni of the University of Ottawa, Faculty of Medicine.

Degree requirement

Applicants are required to have completed three years of full-time studies in any undergraduate program leading to a bachelor's degree. A full-time academic year where the equivalent of four full-year courses is taken is accepted and counted in the WGPA calculation only if the missing course is completed either as an additional course within another academic year or as a summer course. Any year with less than four full-year courses will not count as a full-time year of study. A full-time summer semester does not replace a semester of studies within an academic year.

Course requirements

The course requirements are the following: 1 full year of biology, 1 full year of humanities/social sciences and the equivalent of two full-year courses of the following chemistry courses: i) general biochemistry without laboratory session; ii) general chemistry with laboratory session; iii) organic chemistry with laboratory session. Candidates are allowed to complete missing prerequisite courses during the academic year preceding admission but not during the summer before their registration.

GPA requirement

Each year, a minimum weighted grade point average (WGPA) is set for the current application pool. Students in their third year of undergraduate study at the time of application will have their second year marks counted times two and their first year marks times one. The current year of study is not used to determine which candidates are invited for interview. Students in their fourth year of undergraduate study at the time of application will have their third year marks counted times three, their second year marks counted times two and their first year marks counted times one. For students who have completed more than three years at the time of application, only the three most recent years of undergraduate studies will be used to determine the WGPA. Marks obtained during a summer session will not be included in the WGPA calculation. WGPA cutoffs for admission in 2011 to the English taught program for Ottawa applicants and applicants from the Champlain district Local Health Integration Network was 3.7 out of 4.0, for in-province applicants was 3.85 out of 4.00 and for out-of-province applicants was 3.87 out of 4.00 [1]. These cutoffs are expected to remain the same for entry in 2012 [1]. Additional undergraduate courses completed after a degree is awarded are not used in the GPA unless these grades are part of a second undergraduate degree that is at least three years in length.

	WGPA calculation*
Students completing their third year of full time undergraduate study	Example: Year 1 3.85 x 1 = 3.85 Year 2 3.82 x 2 = 7.74 Total 11.49 ÷ 3 = 3.83 (WGPA)
Students who have completed three or more years of undergraduate study	Only the most recent three years considered. Example of 5th year student: Example: Year 1 3.85 Year 2 3.82 Year 3 3.90 x 1 = 3.90 Year 4 3.85 x 2 = 7.70 Year 5 3.89 x 3 = 11.67 Total 23.27 ÷ 6 = 3.88 (WGPA)

Table 35. WGPA calculation for the University of Ottawa [25]
*Supplementary courses taken outside the usual academic session and summer courses will not be included in the above calculations

MCAT requirement

The MCAT is not required.

Selection Formula

Interview invitations are based on meeting the minimum WGPA cutoff for the applicant's category that year and the committee's assessment of the detailed autobiographical sketch. See table 36 for the different applicant categories. Although the WGPA cutoffs are different for applicants in different regions, once these WGPA cutoffs are met, all anglophone applicants are competing for the same seats; that is, there are no regional quotas defined, only different WGPA cutoffs. After the interview, a composite score based on the interview assessment and the WGPA is calculated, and final selections are made for offers of admission.

Applicants with a PhD or master's

Graduate candidates who are registered in (or have recently completed) a master's or doctoral degree are allowed to apply to the MD program provided they meet the eligibility requirements, including the successful completion of the necessary prerequisites. These applications will be assessed like all other applications. All applications will be evaluated based on the grades obtained during the candidate's undergraduate studies.

Application documents

The documents required are those required by OMSAS for all Ontario medical schools (see above in OMSAS section). In addition, applicants submit a more detailed autobiographical sketch detailing extra-curricular activities and awards after high school.

Anglophone program Those applying to the Anglophone program will be split into the following categories	•Applicants who are sponsored by the Canadian Forces (CF) applying to the anglophone program •Residents from the LHIN (Local Health Integrated Network) Champlain district (as determined by the Ministry of Health) •Residents from the region (Ottawa–Outaouais) applying to the anglophone program •Residents from the province of Ontario applying to the anglophone program •Residents from other provinces applying to the anglophone program •Aboriginals applying to the Anglophone program
Francophone Program Those applying to the Francophone program will be split into the following categories	•Applicants who apply to the Consortium National de formation en santé (CNFS): residents from outside the provinces of Ontario and Québec applying to the Francophone program •Residents from Ontario and the Outaouais region applying to the Francophone program •Aboriginals applying to the Francophone program
Residents from the province of Quebec have the same WGPA cutoff regardless of whether they apply to the Francophone or Anglophone program	

Table 36. Applicant categories at the University of Ottawa. Each category has its own WGPA cutoff.

Interview
The interview is a panel interview, typically with a doctor, a person from the lay community and a senior medical student that lasts 45 minutes.

Application deadline
See application deadline through OMSAS above.

Application cost
See application fees through OMSAS.

Cost of studies 2011-2012
Tuition fees of $18,400 per year.

Additional information
The school offers their medical program in either English or French. Applicants choose which of these two programs they wish to apply to and the interview will be conducted in this language.

Statistics
In the 2010-2011 application cycle, there were approximately 2,631 in-province applicants, of whom 573 were interviewed for 130 places. There were also 1,007 out-of-province applicants for the 34 places available.

Contact
Admissions
Faculty of Medicine University of Ottawa
451 Smyth Road, Room 2046
Ottawa, ON, Canada. K1H 8M5
Tel: 613-562-5409
admissmd@uottawa.ca

Ref: 8.   *University of Ottawa, school of Medicine webpage.* Available from: http://www.medicine.uottawa.ca/eng/.

University of Toronto

Nationality restrictions
International students ARE eligible to apply.

Degree requirement
Applicants are required to have completed at least 3 years of study toward a bachelor's degree in any discipline.

Course requirements
Applicants are required to complete at least two full-year courses or four half-courses in life sciences, and at least one full-year course or two half-courses in humanities, social sciences or languages. It is recommended, although not required, that applicants complete a university-level course in statistics, and two courses that require expository writing. IB courses can be used to meet prerequisites. If you have completed AP credits or CLEP credits and would like to know which subjects can count toward prerequisite courses, you can contact Leslie Taylor (admissions officer) by email at ld.taylor@utoronto.ca or by phone at (416) 978-2729. Note that applicant are usually disqualified unless all prerequisites are complete or are showing as current registrations on their transcript at the time of application [135].

GPA requirement
The GPA is calculated using grades from all courses taken at an undergraduate level on a full-time basis. Grades from courses taken during part-time study are not counted in the GPA, but can be used toward prerequisite requirements. Grades from multiple degree programs and/or from full-time non-degree study (e.g. a fifth year of courses taken following a four-year degree) are counted, as are grades from full-time summer sessions. Grades are not weighted differentially based on the year of study. For undergraduate applicants, a minimum GPA of 3.6 out of 4.0 on the OMSAS scale is required. For graduate applicants, slightly lower GPAs are acceptable (lowest 3.0 out of 4.0). A GPA weighting formula is used for students who have completed at least three years of undergraduate study and have taken a full course load (i.e. five full credits), during the regular academic session, in each of their academic years. A student with four full years completed at the time of application can drop the four lowest full-year course marks, or the eight lowest semester course marks, or any combination. A student with three full years completed at the time of application can drop the three lowest full-year course marks, or the six lowest semester course marks, or any combination. Note that taking four courses during the regular academic year and one summer course will NOT be counted as a full course load, and the advantages above will not be applied. This is also the case for students who took full course loads some years but not others. All years must have a full course load.

GPA requirement (cont'd)

If a student has a good reason for not taking five courses one year, this should be included in the section of the OMSAS application explaining why their transcript does not reflect their true abilities. A letter can also be written to the admissions office explaining extenuating circumstances. These will be reviewed and the above advantages may be granted. The calculated GPA used to fulfill the academic requirement will not include the candidate's current year of study. The average GPA required for admission in 2011 was 3.88.

MCAT requirement

The expected minimum MCAT score is 9 in each section and N on the writing sample - lower marks in any section will significantly decrease an applicants chance of admission. Only the most recent MCAT score is considered in the application process. Applicants who fall slightly below the minimum requirement but who believe their file is extremely competitive can apply and will have their files assessed. Those with any section below 8 (used to be 7) are not recommended to apply. The MCAT must have been written before the application deadline, and within the past 5 years. Also note that only the most recent MCAT scores will be considered in the application process. The MCAT is used as a flag only; as such, marks higher than the minimums do not improve the chances of admission. The average MCAT score of applicants in the

2011-2012 application was 32Q. Note that there were applicants accepted who had MCAT scores as low as 7 on verbal reasoning, 7 in physical sciences, 8 in biological sciences and M in the writing section.

Selection Formula

Students meeting the cutoffs will have their files fully reviewed (including autobiographical sketch, reference letters and personal statement) by 2 faculty and 1 student. The pre interview assessment is weighted as follows: 60% academics and 40% nonacademic qualifications. Note that the MCAT is not included in the academics calculation, but is used as a "flag" - "less than minimum marks will jeopardize the success of the application."

Applicants with a PhD or master's

Graduate candidates must have completed all program requirements for their graduate degree by June 30th in the proposed year of entry, including successful defense of the thesis, if applicable. A GPA slightly lower than the minimum of 3.6 out of 4.0 (lowest 3.0 out of 4.0) can be accepted, but the MCAT and course requirements are the same as for undergraduate applicants. In the selection process, graduate applications are given a separate review.

Applicants with a PhD or master's (cont'd)

Graduate students are assessed based on undergraduate marks, graduate course marks, letters of reference, MCAT results, non-academic assessment, publications and performance in the interview. There is an emphasis on academic achievement in graduate level study, particularly research productivity. Graduate applicants are also required to submit a supplemental package of information directly to the medical school (not OMSAS). This package includes a cover sheet completed by the applicant's supervisor or graduate director, a CV, up to three additional letters of reference (along with the three letters submitted through OMSAS) and the first page of published or ready-to-publish articles). For articles submitted or "in press", applicants should provide a copy of the letter or email from the editor/journal about the paper. One of the letters submitted (whether with the OMSAS application or with the supplemental package) must be provided by the graduate supervisor, and must comment on the applicant's progress in his or her graduate program.

Application deadline

See application deadline through OMSAS above.

Application documents

The documents required are those required by OMSAS for all Ontario medical schools (see above in OMSAS section). In addition applicants are required to submit a 1000 word personal statement. As a general guideline, the statement should address and discuss the applicant's personal background, including particular interests and extracurricular experiences. Candidates should outline their choice of and preparation for a career in medicine. Applicants should also describe their premedical studies, expanding on what they have chosen to pursue and how this has prepared them for their future, including a career in medicine. Note that the computer space of 8000 characters is not the limit of the essay. The essay limit is 1000 words, regardless of number of characters. If it is obvious that an applicant has substantially exceeded the limit, this lack of attention will be a factor in the evaluation process.

Interview

All interviews take place in person at the faculty of medicine, over three weekends from late February to mid-April. The interview panel usually consists of one faculty member and one medical student.

Application cost

See application fees through OMSAS above.

Cost of studies 2011-2012

For Canadian students, $19,833 in tuition fees per year. For international students, $51,051 in tuition fees per year.

International Applicants

Up to 7 positions are offered to international applicants every year. Regardless of citizenship, applicants attending non-Canadian universities must complete a bachelor's degree, equivalent to a four-year honors bachelor's degree obtained in Canada. Transcripts of study undertaken at universities outside Canada or the USA must be submitted to World Education Services (WES) for assessment. A course-by-course evaluation that includes an overall GPA is required. Provision of the WES assessment does not replace the requirement for submission of official transcripts. If this information is not contained in the official transcript, applicants are required to supply the faculty with a certified academic record containing individual course grades for all academic work in each year of study. In other respects, admissions requirements and application procedures are the same for international applicants as they are for domestic applicants (i.e. minimum GPA, prerequisite courses, MCAT scores, non-academics, etc.)

Additional information

Note that the University of Toronto is one of the two Canadian schools that does not favor in-province students [1].

Statistics

In the 2010-2011 application cycle, there were 2956 applicants. 528 candidates were interviewed for approximately 250 positions available. There are a maximum of 7 positions available for international students. For entry in 2010, 39 international students applied, 3 students were interviewed and two international students were admitted. There will be approximately 259 places available in the 2012-2013 application cycle, including 205 at the St. George campus and 54 at the Mississauga campus. More details on the campuses are provided at the interview.

Contact

Medical Sciences Building, Rm 2135
1 King's College Circle
Toronto, Ontario, M5S 1A8
Tel: 416-978-7928
medicine.admiss@utoronto.ca

Ref: 7.   *University of Toronto, Medical School webpage.* Available from: http://www.facmed.utoronto.ca/site4.aspx.

University of Western Ontario

Nationality restrictions
International students are NOT eligible to apply.

Degree requirement
Applicants must have completed or be in the final year of a program leading to a 4-year undergraduate degree at a recognized university and expect to have completed a minimum of 20 full courses by the end of the academic year in which the application is being made. Also, students must have registered in courses in such a way that there have been at least two full-time academic years (taken during September - April) in which a minimum of 5 full or equivalent courses have been taken concurrently. There are no exceptions for this. Applicants who complete the requirements of a four year honors degree or equivalent in less than four years may apply to the medical program without penalty.

Course requirements
There are no prerequisite courses. A mixture of biological/medical science courses and social science/humanities courses is recommended.

GPA requirement
The GPA cutoff for all students in 2011 was 3.7 out of 4.0. Applicants must achieve the minimum GPA in EACH of their best two full-years (if only one year meets the cutoff,

an admission can be granted contingent on meeting the requirement during the current year). Only those years in which at least 5 full or equivalent courses are taken between September and April will be used in the calculation of the GPA. Note that students cannot take more than 2 full-year courses (or four half-year courses) below their university level in these two years. This means that first year students must take 3 of 5 courses at 1st year level or above, second year students must take 3 of 5 courses at 2nd year level or above, etc. Note that in fourth year (and possibly fifth year if applicable), any courses above third year level count toward the 3 out of 5 requirement. When students are required to take more than 5 full courses during any academic year because of program requirements, the five best courses will be used in the calculation of the GPA. Summer courses are not counted in the overall GPA. Applicants who have earned a degree from a recognized university may elect to continue in full-time undergraduate studies so that their academic standing may be improved for application to medical school. Only the first special year taken by the applicant will be considered for determination of their GPA. A special year will only be considered if it contains five full or equivalent courses taken between September and April. First year courses, repeat courses, and second-year courses that do not require a first-year prerequisite are not acceptable in the special year.

GPA requirement (cont'd)

Also note that if a course is repeated, the course is not counted in the course load for that year, nor is it factored into the GPA calculation for that year. Thus, if you take 5 full or equivalent courses but one of them is a repeat course, the university will consider this year as having only 4 full courses, and that year will not be considered for your GPA calculation. Students who have one undergraduate degree already and are working towards a second degree are not eligible to apply before the final year of their program. Their program must be an honors degree or equivalent program to be considered. 60% of the courses (3 out of 5 full courses or equivalent) taken in each of the upper years of the second degree program must be senior-level courses. The applicant's GPA in this case is calculated only based on the two best years of the second degree program. Applicants who are offered a conditional acceptance must complete all second degree program requirements before registration in the MD program.

MCAT requirement

The MCAT cutoffs for Southwestern Ontario applicants in 2011 were 8 minimum in each section and a minimum overall of 30 with O in the written section. The MCAT cutoffs for non-Southwestern Ontario applicants in 2011 were a minimum of 10 in biological sciences, a minimum of 9 in physical sciences, a minimum of 11 in verbal reasoning and a minimum of P in the writing section. All of these minimums were the same as those in 2010. If the MCAT is written more than once; the most recent MCAT score is used. MCAT scores are valid for 5 years, and are used both to screen applicants for interview and subsequently to assist in ranking applicants for admission.

Selection Formula

The university uses MCAT and GPA cutoffs to determine which applicants are invited for interview. Note that achieving the minimum GPA and MCAT cutoffs does not guarantee an invitation for an interview, however, nearly all students who achieve these cutoffs will be invited for interview. The minimum GPA and MCAT requirements may vary for each applicant pool as described in the GPA and MCAT sections. The definition of each applicant pool is in the "additional information" section. After the interview, applicants are given a total score based on the following weighting: 25% GPA (best 2 years), 25% MCAT and 50% interview [1].

Applicants with a PhD or master's

Graduate students are required to have completed all course requirements for their degree before matriculation late in August or early in September. Their thesis, if applicable, must be submitted for defense to their examination committee before their registration in the medical program. The university does not count graduate courses in the GPA calculation; only undergraduate years are used.

Applicants with a PhD or master's (cont'd)

Applicants who are currently enrolled in a master's program are encouraged to make inquiries about their MD/PhD program.

Application documents

The documents required are those required by OMSAS for all Ontario medical schools (see above in OMSAS section).

Additional information

Applicants in the Southwestern Ontario category include applicants from Grey, Bruce, Huron, Perth, Oxford, Middlesex, Lambton, Chatham-Kent, Elgin, Essex and Norfolk Counties. Attending high school in one of these counties allows students to be considered as SWOMEN applicants. Applicants from elsewhere in Canada are placed in the non-Southwestern Ontario category and are required to meet the higher GPA/MCAT cutoffs.

Interview

Applicants are invited for a panel interview conducted by a faculty member, a senior medical student and a member of the lay community which lasts approximately 45 minutes.

Application deadline

See application deadline through OMSAS above.

Application cost

See application fees through OMSAS above.

Cost of studies 2011-2012

Tuition fees of $20,183 for the first year, and $19,474 per year in subsequent years.

Statistics

In the 2010-2011 application cycle, there were 2,302 applicants, of whom approximately 450 were interviewed for the 171 places available, including 133 places at the London campus and 38 at the Windsor campus. Although non-Southwestern Ontario applicants are required to meet higher cutoffs, there are no quotas defined for how many of these applicants can be accepted.

Contact

Admissions & Student Affairs
Schulich School of Medicine & Dentistry
Room K1
Kresge Building
The University of Western Ontario
London ON N6A 5C1
Tel: (519) 661-3744
admissions.medicine@schulich.uwo.ca

Ref: 93. *The University of Western Ontario - Medicine admission webpage.* Available from: http://www.schulich.uwo.ca/education/admissions/medicine/.

Quebec and Maritime Provinces

McGill University

Nationality restrictions
International students ARE eligible to apply.

Degree requirement
Applicants must have completed an undergraduate degree in any discipline consisting of 120 credits minimum. The degree must have been conducted with an average credit load of 15 credits throughout each regular session and applicants are expected to take every opportunity to complete the program in the prescribed time. Applicants who feel that their previous undergraduate degree is uncompetitive may choose to complete a second undergraduate degree consisting of at least 45 consecutive grade credits. If this is the case, the highest degree GPA will be used (with the expectation that it is the most recent degree). If the basis of admission is on the academic performance of the second degree, it is understood that the applicant will have that degree completed before matriculation at medical school. Note that applicants completing their final year of CEGEP in Quebec can apply to the MED-P program. These students complete one year of science courses with humanities and social science electives. If they achieve a minimum GPA of 3.5 with no grades less than B in the mandatory courses, they join the incoming 4-year medical program students the next year.

Course requirements
The prerequisite courses are as follows: 1 full year of biology, chemistry and physics as well as half a year of organic chemistry. Distance or correspondence education courses are not accepted without permission from the admissions office. Prerequisite courses completed more than eight years prior to the date of application are not accepted. Exceptions may be made for applicants with advanced degrees in the material concerned. University level courses in biochemistry, cell and/or molecular biology, and statistics are recommended, but are not required for admission. The university accepts AP and IB credit toward course requirements at the discretion of the admissions office. As a rule of thumb, students with a score of 4 or better on AP exams and 5 or better on IB exams are eligible to receive credit provided they have completed sufficient laboratory work and course work in their AP and IB courses.

GPA requirement
It is recommended that applicants have a minimum 3.50 cumulative GPA on a 4.00 scale to be considered competitive.

GPA requirement (cont'd)

Successful applicants have an average cumulative GPA of 3.8 out of 4.00 with roughly two-thirds of admitted students having their GPA in the range of 3.67 to 3.98. The GPA of applicants' basic science courses tend to be similar. Courses that are completed after the undergraduate degree are not counted in the GPA calculation.

MCAT requirement

The MCAT is optional for applicants applying with degrees from Canadian universities. CEGEP applicants are exempt from taking the MCAT. Students who are applying with a degree obtained outside of Canada must submit MCAT scores. This includes students who completed their first bachelors degree in Canada and a second bachelor's degree outside Canada, who would like to be considered on the basis of their second degree. MCAT results must be from no more than 5 years prior to the application deadline. Competitive applicants generally have written the exam only once or twice, with a minimum MCAT score of 30, with no science section with a score of less than 9 and verbal reasoning section less than 8. The highest overall MCAT results out of all attempts are used for the application. The average score is approximately 33, and applicants with scores below 27 are not usually considered. When the sub-components are reviewed individually, the average biological sciences score tends to be 12, the physical sciences section 11, and the verbal reasoning section 10. If you have the option of submitting your MCAT scores, the university advises that you do so if you "are confident that these scores provide stronger evidence of [your] abilities in the basic sciences."

Selection Formula

Applicants are first divided into categories (in-province traditional, in-province non-traditional, CEGEP graduates, out-of-province students and international students). The students are given a preliminary ranking based on academic criteria. Those who rank well in their cohort in this stage of the application have their non-academic qualities scored through their CV and personal statement, and the top ranking group from each category is invited for interview. After the interview, applicants are given a final score with a weighting of 80% for the MMI and 20% for the personal narrative (the only exception is non-traditional Quebec residents, whose weighting is 75% MMI and 25% personal narrative).

Applicants with a PhD or master's

While completed graduate degrees are considered in the review of an application, applicants should know that the undergraduate cumulative GPA scores are the major consideration in measuring academic performance.

Applicants with a Ph.D or Master's (cont'd)

There are no special admissions criteria or special consideration for students who have completed a master's degree or a PhD.

International applicants

International applicants must submit with their application a letter or official statement issued by the responsible authorities in their country indicating that their country recognizes the medical degree awarded by the faculty of medicine at McGill University and that this degree will enable them to practice medicine in their country. This is generally the case even for US applicants [1].

Application deadline

The application for entry in 2012 opens September 1st, 2011. The application for the MD program is due on November 1st, 2011, and the supplemental documents and reference letters are due November 15th, 2011. The application deadline for CEGEP students is March 1, 2011.

Application cost

Application fee is approximately $85.

Application documents

Applicants are required to have official academic transcripts of every post-secondary educational institution attended sent to the admissions office. In addition, applicants are required to submit their post-secondary academic history according to the instructions presented on McGill University's website. Also, applicants are required to submit a personal narrative, personally written, reflecting their usual means of expression, as well as an abstract of the personal narrative. The essay prompt is: "Tell us about the journey that has brought you to the decision to apply to Medicine and your understanding of what being a good physician means." The letter cannot be longer than 1000 words. If applicants are applying for dual degrees or as Quebec Non-Traditional Students, their answers should reflect this. Students also submit a 900 character (about 150 word) abstract, summarizing what they said in their personal narrative for initial screening purposes. Applicants are also required to submit a standard CV categorized using the following headings: 'Education & Training'; 'Work Experience (remunerated and non-remunerated)'; 'Research, Publications, Scholarly Activities'; 'Service to Community'; 'Awards, Honours, Accolades'; 'Certificates, Licenses, Special Memberships'; 'Skills, Interests, Hobbies'; 'Other extracurricular activities'. A one page appendix is allowed to include contacts who can verify the information in your CV, especially work, research, and community service.

Application documents (cont'd)

A second one page appendix is allowed for students with several entries under the "Research, Publications and Scholarly Activities" heading", especially for students applying to the MDCM/PhD program. In addition, applicants must submit a 1900 character (approximately 300 word) CV highlights submission, answering the following prompt: "Highlight three elements of your c.v. that you believe best demonstrate your motivation and suitability for medicine, including an explanation of why you chose these three elements." Applicants are also required to ask three referees to submit web based reference forms by the application deadline. People with a professional rapport with the applicant (not family and friends) can submit a letter, provided they are well positioned to evaluate the personal qualities relevant to studying medicine. For some students, a pre-medical advisory committee reports can meet the reference letter requirement as well. MD/MBA must have two additional referees submit an MBA recommendation form from their website.

Interview

The interview is conducted in the MMI format. There are approximately 10 stations.

Cost of studies 2011-2012

Quebecois: Approximately $2050 - $5050 per year.
Other Canadians: Approximately $5560 - $13,700 per year.
International: Approximately $15,400 - $37,900 per year.

Statistics

In the 2012-2013 application cycle, there will be approximately 180 students accepted in total. The places are divides as follows: approximately 4 places for international applicants; approximately 9 places for out-of-province Canadians; approximately 160 places for residents of Quebec (split roughly equally between students with university degrees and students graduating from CEGEP); a maximum of 2 places for first nations and Inuit students.

Contact

Admissions Office, Faculty of Medicine
McGill University
3708 Peel Street
Montréal, QC H3A 1W9
Tel: 514-398-3517
aed.med@mcgill.ca
Submit questions at: www.mcgill.ca/medadmissions/contact-us

Ref: 136. *McGill University Admission webpage.* Available from: http://www.mcgill.ca/medicine/admissions/criteria/selection/evaluations/.

Dalhousie University

Nationality restrictions
International students ARE eligible to apply.

Degree requirement
Applicants are required to have completed an undergraduate degree to be eligible. Although candidates with three-year degrees are occasionally admitted; a four-year degree is strongly preferred.

Course requirements
There are no required courses for admission in 2011, however, applicants who have pursued a broad academic background are more likely to gain admission as the admissions committee believes that coursework in humanities, physical sciences and social sciences "cultivate desirable personal qualities for students and physicians." Applicants are also encouraged to gain sound training in the basic sciences and gain more than the basic level of training in at least one field, whether it be a social science, physical science, life science or humanities subject.

GPA requirement
Maritime applicants are required to achieve a minimum of 3.3 on a 4.0 scale in each of the last two years of full-time study. Non Maritime students are required to achieve a minimum of 3.7 on a 4.0 scale in each of the last two years of full-time study. The GPA is calculated using the OMSAS conversion scale. For the purpose of assessing transcripts, full time study is deemed to be 5 full credits per academic year. If an applicant completes a full academic year after their undergraduate degree, this can count toward meeting the minimum GPA requirement, but note that the grades from this year must be available at the time of application in order for the additional year to be counted toward the gpa requirements [1]. The average GPA score for the 2010 entering class was 3.8 out of 4.0.

MCAT requirement
Maritime students are required to achieve a minimum score of 24 on the MCAT. These applicants can have one section below 7, but must compensate on another section to achieve a total score of 24. Non-Maritime students are required to achieve a minimum score of 30 on the MCAT. These applicants can have one section with a score of 9, but must compensate on another section to achieve a total score of 30. The mean MCAT score for the 2010 entering class was 29. MCAT scores are valid for 5 years.

Selection Formula
Dalhousie sets competitive baseline cutoffs each year, particularly for out-of-province students. Alongside this, applications are evaluated before inviting students for interview. For out-of-province students, only 55-65 of the ~150 applicants meeting the GPA and MCAT cutoffs are invited for an interview.

Selection Formula (Cont'd)

"Since the academic standards are already set at a high level, it is the essay & supplementary sheet which determine whether you will be competitive enough to receive an interview". For maritime applicants, those meeting the cutoffs who are felt to have "a reasonable chance of admission" will be invited for interview. After the interview, applicants are given a score on each component of the application including the interview and ranked for admission [1].

Applicants with a PhD or master's

Graduate students must complete and submit their thesis prior to starting medical school and thus graduate students should not apply until there is a firm end point established to their graduate work. If a student has completed their graduate degree, all of the courses will be counted as one full year, and this average must meet the minimum GPA requirement mentioned above, in addition to the last two full-time years of undergraduate study [1]. In this sense, applicants with graduate degrees must meet an additional requirement compared to those with only undergraduate degrees.

International applicants

International applicants are in the same applicant pool and have the same requirements as out-of-province applicants.

Application deadline

The online application for Dalhousie opens July 1st, 2011 and closes on August 15th, 2011. The supplemental application form, which includes a personal essay as well as activity and award descriptions, is due September 1st, 2011. Transcripts and MCAT scores are also accepted up to September 1st, 2011 (the last accepted MCAT sitting is July 29th, 2011). For applicants that are invited for an interview, the deadline to have reference letters submitted has been early January in previous years, and will be provided later in the application cycle.

Application cost

The application fee is approximately $70

Application documents

The application includes a 1500 word personal essay describing how the applicant's experiences have shaped their desire to become a physician. Out-of-province and international students must also explain why they are applying to Dalhousie, including their connection to the maritime provinces. The application also includes sections covering applicants' extracurricular activities, medically related experience, volunteer work, employment, awards and publications. The admissions office requires 2 reference letters for applicants that are selected for an interview. Other students do not need to submit reference letters. Official transcripts must also be submitted.

Interview

Interviews are MMI format with 10 stations. Each station lasts eight minutes and there is a two minute break between each one. At each station, applicants interact with or are observed by a single rater, who is usually a faculty member, medical student, community person or allied health care professional.

Cost of studies 2012-2013

For Canadians, tuition is $15,200 per year [1]. For international students, tuition is approximately $25,000 per year.

Statistics

In the 2010-2011 application cycle, there were approximately 355 maritime applicants, of whom 250 were eligible for interview, and 380 Non-Maritime applicants, of whom 75 were eligible for interview. Roughly 99 seats are reserved for in-province applicants. This includes approximately 30 seats for New Brunswick applicants, 63 for Nova Scotia and 6 for Prince Edward Island. There are approximately 9 positions available for out-of-province and international students combined, as well as 1-3 positions for military applicants this year. Approximately 300 Maritime and 60 non-Maritime applicants will be invited for an interview. There are two campuses: the New Brunswick campus will accommodate 30 students and the remaining 78 will study at the Halifax campus.

Contact

Room C-124
CRC Building
5849 University Avenue
Halifax, Nova Scotia. B3H 4H7
Tel: (902) 494-1874
medicine.admissions@dal.ca

Ref: 94. *Dalhousie University Medical School webpage.* Available from: http://dlm.cal.dal.ca/_MEDI.htm#3.

Memorial University

Nationality restrictions
International students ARE eligible to apply.

Degree requirement
Applicants are generally required to have completed an undergraduate degree to be eligible. In exceptional circumstances, those with "work related or other experience acceptable to the admissions committee" may be eligible to apply provided they expect to complete at least 60 credit hours including the 6 hour english prerequisite requirements prior to admission.

Course requirements
The only prerequisite course requirement is a full year (6 credits) of English. AP and IB credit can be used toward this prerequisite.

GPA requirement
The academic average of matriculating students has been about 85% (GPA of approximately 3.70). Note that all courses taken during all years of study are taken into account (including graduate courses). If a student fails a course and successfully repeats it, the admissions committee will consider both grades. The grade conversion chart used by the school is available from http://www.med.mun.ca/Admissions/ApplicationEvaluationCompetitions.aspx under "Academic Record/MCAT Scores."

MCAT requirement
The average MCAT scores of matriculating students have been 10 on each section and Q on the writing sample. The admissions committee considers all writings of the MCAT and takes improvement into consideration. Students must submit all test scores.

Selection Formula
For in-province applicants at Memorial University, there is a combined MCAT and GPA cutoff determined each year to receive an automatic interview. All in-province students who do not meet the automatic interview cutoff will have their files fully reviewed and the top applicants from this group will also be invited for interview. For out-of-province and international students, whether or not a candidate is invited for interview is determined largely based on the applicant's MCAT score and GPA, but the full file is often reviewed [1]. Although all in-province applicants may be considered for interview, high MCAT scores and high academic standing are essential. The scores from the interview are then used by the admissions committee in conjunction with the rest of the application to select the entering class.

Applicants with a PhD or master's
There is neither preference given to nor bias against students in a graduate program. Graduate courses are considered in the overall GPA calculation.

International applicants

International students are eligible to apply, and are assessed the same way as out-of-province applicants.

Application documents

All students applying for entry in 2012 are required to answer the following 3 prompts in the autobiographical sketch:

1. Write an autobiographical sketch about who you are, how you spend your time and why. (2000 character maximum)
2. Why do you wish to become a physician? (500 character maximum)
3. What do you expect from your day to day life as a physician? (500 character maximum)

Applicants also list their awards, employment and extracurricular activities. There is also 3000 characters set aside for applicants to discuss any section of the application if they wish.

Interview

The interviews are conducted by a panel of 2 interviewers and last approximately one hour. Panel members are not given information about the applicant beforehand.

Application deadline

The deadline for application and supporting documents will be October 17th, 2011.

Application cost

The application fee is approximately $75.

Cost of studies

Canadian students normally pay $6250 in tuition fees per year and non-Canadian students pay $30,000 in tuition fees per year.

Statistics

The are approximately 64 places available each year for approximately 900 applicants. Approximately 200-250 applications are received from Newfoundland and Labrador for about 44 places; 100 applications from New Brunswick for about 10 places and 50 applications from Prince Edward Island for about 4 places. There are also 10 applicants from the Yukon for 1 place, and 10 aboriginal applicants for approximately 2 places. Each year there are roughly 400 out-of-province applications for about 2 places, and approximately 100 international applications for 1-2 places [1].

Contact

Admissions Office, Faculty of Medicine
Memorial University of Newfoundland
Room 1751, Health Sciences Centre
300 Prince Philip Drive
St. John's, NL Canada   A1B 3V6
Tel: (709) 777-6615
munmed@mun.ca

Ref: 137. *Memorial University, medical school admission webpage.* Available from: http://www.med.mun.ca/Admissions/Home.aspx

UK
Medical Programs

4 year programs for graduate applicants

The 4 year programs available for graduate applicants are listed below:

1. Barts and the London School of Medicine and Dentistry
2. University of Birmingham
3. University of Bristol
4. Cambridge University
5. Imperial College London
6. Keele University
7. King's College London
8. University of Leicester
9. University of Liverpool
10. University of Newcastle
11. University of Nottingham
12. University of Oxford
13. University of Southampton
14. St George's, University of London
15. Swansea University
16. University of Warwick

5 year programs for graduate applicants

The 5 year programs available for graduate applicants are listed below:

1. University of Aberdeen
2. Barts and the London School of Medicine and Dentistry
3. University of Birmingham
4. Brighton and Sussex Medical School
5. University of Bristol
6. Cardiff University
7. Cambridge University (6 year program, but completed in 5 years by graduates)
8. University of Dundee
9. University of East Anglia
10. University of Edinburgh
11. University of Glasgow
12. Hull York Medical School
13. Keele University
14. King's College London
15. University of Leeds
16. University of Leicester
17. University of Liverpool
18. University of Liverpool, Cumbria and Lancashire Medical and Dental Consortium
19. University of Manchester
20. University of Newcastle
21. University of Nottingham
22. University of Oxford (6 year program, but completed in 5 years by graduates)
23. Peninsula Medical School
24. Queen's University Belfast
25. University of Sheffield
26. University of Southampton
27. University College London (6 year program, but completed in 5 years by graduates)

6 year programs for graduate applicants

The 6 year programs available for graduate applicants are listed below:

1. University of Bristol
2. Cardiff University
3. University of Dundee
4. Imperial College London
5. Keele University
6. University of Liverpool
7. University of Manchester
8. University of Sheffield
9. University of St Andrews
10. University of St. Andrews, North American Program

Programs with no entrance exams

The programs open to graduate applicants that do not require an entrance exam are listed below:

1. University of Birmingham, 4 and 5 year programs
2. University of Bristol, 4, 5 and 6 year programs
3. Cambridge University, 4 year program
4. University of Liverpool, 4 year program, two 5 year programs and a 6 year program

Note that Cambridge University and the University of Birmingham are actively considering introducing an entrance exam requirement in the future.

Medical schools requiring the GAMSAT, UKCAT and BMAT are listed in the exam specific sections on pages 50, 57 and 64.

Entrance Statistics

Interpreting selection ratios

The selection ratios for each program are provided below. Note that medical schools offer more places than their class size, since not everyone accepts the offers. For example, the true "acceptance ratio" for the King's College Graduate Entry Program is roughly 45:1, rather than 66:1, since more students are offered admission than the 24 who eventually accept. Similarly, the true "acceptance ratio" at Imperial College London 6 year program is roughly 4:1, rather than 7:1, because roughly 500 applicants are offered admission for the 286 places available.

4 year program selection ratios

University	Applicants to Graduate Entry Program	Class size	Ratio	Year
Barts and the London School of Medicine	1000	45	22:1	2010
University of Birmingham	2200	330	7:1	2011
University of Bristol	513	19	27:1	2010
Cambridge University	200	22	9:1	2009
Imperial College London	500	50	10:1	2009
Keele University	2700	130	21:1	2011
King's College London	1600	24	66:1	2010
University of Leicester	619	64	10:1	2010
University of Liverpool	300	32	9:1	2009
University of Newcastle	880	25	35:1	2010
University of Nottingham	Over 1000	93	>10:1	2010

University	Applicants to Graduate Entry Program	Class size	Ratio	Year
University of Oxford	240	30	8:1	2009
University of Southampton	1415	40	35:1	2011
St. George's University	980	118	8:1	2010
Swansea University	680	70	10:1	2011
University of Warwick	1818	178	10:1	2010

Table 37. Selection ratios at 4 year medical programs in the UK.

5 year program selection ratios

University	Applicants to 5-year program	Class size	Ratio	Year
University of Aberdeen	2400	175	14:1	2011
Barts and the London School of Medicine	2050	282	7:1	2010
Brighton and Sussex Medical School	2170	144	15:1	2011
University of Birmingham	2200	350	6:1	2010
University of Bristol	3200	235	14:1	2011
Cambridge University	1700	288	6:1	2010
Cardiff University	3200	250	13:1	2011
University College London	2500	330	8:1	2011
University of Dundee	1680	140	12:1	2011
University of East Anglia	2000	130	15:1	2010

University	Applicants to 5-year program	Class size	Ratio	Year
University of Edinburgh	2350	202	12:1	2010
University of Glasgow	2000	223	9:1	2011
Hull York Medical School	1200	140	9:1	2011
Keele University	2700	130	21:1	2010
King's College London	3400	300	10:1	2010
University of Leeds	3600	223	16:1	2011
University of Leicester	2400	162	15:1	2010
University of Liverpool	2500	292	9:1	2010
University of Manchester	2500	380	7:1	2011
University of Newcastle	2057	327	6:1	2010
University of Nottingham	2400	249	10:1	2010
University of Oxford	1490	150	10:1	2010
Peninsula Medical School	1809	215	8:1	2011
Queen's University Belfast	800	255	3:1	2010
University of Sheffield	2500	230	11:1	2011
University of Southampton	2675	260	10:1	2011

Table 38. Selection ratios at 5 year medical programs open to graduate applicants in the UK.

6 year program selection ratios

University	Applicants to 6 year program	Class size	Ratio	Year
University of Bristol	309	10	31:1	2010
Cardiff University	250	16	16:1	2011
University of Dundee	124	15	8:1	2011
Imperial College London	2000	286	7:1	2010
Keele University	190	10	19:1	2010
University of Liverpool	70	12	6:1	2010
University of Manchester	250	20	13:1	2011
University of Sheffield	200	20	10:1	2011
University of St. Andrews	1000	160	6:1	2011

Table 39. Selection ratios at 6 year medical programs open to graduate applicants in the UK.

University Rankings

All medical schools in the UK have a high standard of education. Each university's curriculum and examinations are overlooked and regulated by the General Medical Council (GMC).

Several ranking agencies rank medical schools according to specific criteria.

TIMES ONLINE - Good University Guide 2011 - Medicine

This ranking gives each medical school an overall score out of 100 depending on:

1. Student satisfaction
2. Research quality
3. Entry standards
4. Graduate prospects

The top 10 medical schools in this ranking are:

1. University of Oxford	6. University of Aberdeen
2. Cambridge University	7. University of Newcastle
3. University of Edinburgh	8. University of St. Andrews
4. University College London	9. Hull-York Medical School
5. Imperial College London	10. University of Leeds

The full ranking is available at: extras.thetimes.co.uk/gooduniversityguide/subjects/medicine Students must sign up for an online membership (£1 for 1 day trial) to access this link.

Guardian.co.uk - University Guide 2011 - Medicine

This ranking gives each medical school an overall score out of 100 depending on:

1. % satisfied with the course
2. % students satisfied with teaching
3. % students satisfied with feedback
4. Student/Staff ratio
5. Spending per student
6. Average entry tariff
7. Value added score out of 10 (comparing student's degree results with their entry qualifications)
8. Career prospects (% with job 6 months after graduation)

The top 10 medical schools in this ranking are:

1. University of Oxford	6. University of Dundee
2. Cambridge University	7. University of Leicester
3. University of Edinburgh	8. Peninsula Medical School
4. University College London	9. University of Newcastle
5. Imperial College London	10. University of Nottingham

The full ranking is available at: http://www.guardian.co.uk/education/table/2010/jun/04/university-guide-medicine?INTCMP=ILCNETTXT3487

The Complete University Guide Ranking - Medicine

This ranking gives each medical school an overall score out of 100 depending on:

1. Student satisfaction
2. Research quality
3. Entry standards
4. Graduate prospects

The top 10 medical schools in this ranking are:

1. University of Oxford	6. University of Newcastle
2. University of Edinburgh	7. University of Aberdeen
3. Imperial College London	8. Hull-York Medical School
4. University of Durham	9. University of Birmingham
5. Cambridge University	10. University of Glasgow

The full ranking is available at: www.thecompleteuniversityguide.co.uk/single.htm?ipg=8727

QS Top Universities - World University Rankings 2010/2011 - Overall

This ranking gives each university an overall score based on several factors including academic peer review, employer review, research and faculty. More details are available on page 118.

The top 10 UK universities with medical schools in this ranking are given below:

1. University of Cambridge	22. University of Edinburgh
4. University College London	27. University of Bristol
6. University of Oxford	30. University of Manchester
7. Imperial College London	53. University of Warwick
21. King's College London	59. University of Birmingham

The full world ranking is available at: www.topuniversities.com/world-university-rankings

QS Top Universities - World University Rankings 2010/2011 - Medicine

This ranking gives each medical school a ranking based on similar criteria to the QS Top Universities overall ranking outlined above.

The top 15 UK universities with medical schools in this ranking are given below:

2. University of Cambridge	51. Cardiff University
4. University of Oxford	51. Queen Mary, University of London
9. Imperial College London	51. University of Aberdeen
25. University College London	51. University of Dundee
27. University of Edinburgh	51. University of Glasgow
30. Kings College London	51. University of Leeds
32. University of Manchester	51. University of Sheffield
48. University of Bristol	

The full world ranking is available at: www.topuniversities.com/university-rankings/world-university-rankings/2010/subject-rankings/life-science-biomedicine

Shanghai Consultancy World University Rankings 2010 - overall

This ranking also gives universities an overall ranking, not a medical school ranking, based on Nobel Prizes, Fields Medals and research. More details are available on page 119.

The top 10 UK universities with medical schools in this ranking are given below:

5. University of Cambridge	54. University of Edinburgh
10. University of Oxford	63. King's College London
21. University College London	66. University of Bristol
26. Imperial College London	84. University of Nottingham
44. University of Manchester	88. University of Sheffield

The full ranking is available at: www.arwu.org/ARWU2010.jsp

Shanghai Consultancy World University Rankings 2010 - Clinical Medicine and Pharmacy

This ranking gives universities worldwide a ranking for their medical and life science related faculties, based on research, as well ass alumni and faculty awards in medicine. More details are available on page 120.

The top 10 UK universities with medical schools in this ranking are given below:

11. University College London	30. University of Nottingham
13. University of Oxford	50. University of Bristol
14. University of Cambridge	51. University of Glasgow
23. Imperial College London	51. University of Manchester
27. King's College London	76. University of Sheffield

The full ranking is available at: www.arwu.org/FieldMED2010.jsp

Medical Courses' Structures

Although the main factor in deciding where one goes to medical school is, for most applicants, where one can get in, it may be that you have the option to choose between a few medical schools for your training. Particularly if you have a very strong academic background and a strong application, you may want to consider which medical school suits your style of learning the best when choosing where to apply.

In some universities, graduate students form a separate class and follow an entirely separate program than the undergraduate students whereas in other medical schools, graduate students and undergraduate students are together as one class for most of the program.

In addition to the class structure, the styles of teaching vary significantly between programs with some having more didactic sessions including lectures and seminars, compared to other curricula being more clinically focused and requiring students to study the core material from textbooks independently.

There are four main course structures:

1. Problem based learning (6 graduate entry programs)

This is a relatively new type of program, where students are taught through a series of patient cases. For example, during the neurology module, the first case might be a case of paralysis following trauma in a motorbike accident. The case would be discussed in small group sessions, and there would be lectures, workshops, self-study modules and independent assignments focused on the important issues in this case, such as neuroanatomy, pain-control, and the neurological examination. The way these modules are structured differs from place to place, but in each case there is a significant focus on group learning and self-directed study.

2. System based learning (8 graduate entry programs)

System based learning is more similar to the traditional undergraduate learning experience during the classroom years, and focuses on teaching medicine through a series of modules related to patient care, such as anatomy, physiology, cardiology, pulmonology, etc. As is the case in many problem based learning curricula, students often get a chance to interact with patients early in the program to see how what they are learning relates to the patients they will be treating after graduating. The teaching is done primarily through lectures, workshops and self-directed study.

3. Combined system based and problem based learning (2 graduate entry programs)

Some programs have a combination of both learning types, either by starting with system based learning and then moving to problem based learning, or by using system based learning for some subjects and problem based learning for others.

4. Traditional classroom learning (no 4 year graduate entry programs use this method, but it is still used at a few 5 and 6 year programs in the UK)

This learning method is used at medical schools such as the 6 year programs at the University of Cambridge and the University of St. Andrews. These programs structure the first two or three years very similar to a BSc, with the courses focusing more on the science underlying medical practice. Students usually get some patient contact in the first years, but there is a stronger divide between the classroom years and the clinical years.

The course structures of each of the 16 graduate entry programs are summarized in table 40:

University	Class structure	Course structure
Barts and the London School of Medicine	Students in the 4 year program are in a separate class until the clinical years.	Problem Based Learning
University of Birmingham	Students in the 4 year program are in a separate class for year 1, join the 5 year program students for some classes in year 2, and join the 5 year program students for the clinical years.	Problem Based Learning
University of Bristol	Students in the 4 year program join the 5 year program students for their pre-clinical and clinical training.	System Based Learning
Cambridge University	Students in the 4 year program are in a separate class until the clinical years.	System Based Learning
Imperial College London	Students in the 4 year program are in a separate class until the second year of the course.	Problem Based Learning and System Based Learning
Keele University	Students in the 4 year program join the 5 year program students for their pre-clinical and clinical training.	Problem Based Learning
King's College London	Students in the 4 year program join the 5 year program students for their pre-clinical and clinical training. Some classes are with the 5 year program first year class, some with the 5 year program second year class, and some lectures are only for 4 year program students.	Problem Based Learning and System Based Learning
University of Leicester	Students in the 4 year program are in a separate class until second year of the course.	System Based Learning

University	Class structure	Course structure
University of Liverpool	Students in the 4 year program have their own PBL groups and some of their own classes for the first year, but also join year 1 and year 2 students from the 5 year program for some of their first year classes. They join the 5 year program students for the second year and for the clinical years.	Problem Based Learning
University of Newcastle	Students in the 4 year program are in a separate class until the second year of the course.	System Based Learning
University of Nottingham	Students in the 4 year program are in a separate class until the clinical years.	Problem Based Learning
University of Oxford	Students in the 4 year program are in a separate class until the clinical years.	System Based Learning
University of Southampton	Students in the 4 year program are in a separate class until the second year of the course.	System Based Learning
St. George's University	Students in the 4 year program are in a separate class until the second year of the course.	Problem Based Learning
Swansea University	The only medical program at the university is the 4 year graduate entry program.	System Based Learning
University of Warwick	The only medical program at the university is the 4 year graduate entry program.	System Based Learning

Table 40. Course structures of graduate entry medical programs
Information obtained from the medical schools' websites and by contacting the admissions offices directly.

Undergraduate science degree vs. non-science degree

Some programs accept any degree as a first degree, others require applicants to have an undergraduate degree in a scientific background to be eligible, and some programs only accept applications from students who have a biomedical or health science related undergraduate degree. See below for a table that summarizes the degree requirements of the medical programs in the UK that are open to graduate students.

University	Accepts any degree	Requires a science or health related degree
University of Aberdeen	For the 5 year program	

University	Accepts any degree	Requires a science or health related degree
Barts and the London School of Medicine and Dentistry (Queen Mary)	For the 5 year program, a degree in any discipline is accepted provided the applicant has a satisfactory level in chemistry and biology	For the 4 year program, applicants require a degree in a science or health related field.
University of Birmingham	For the 5 year program, a degree in any discipline is accepted.	For the 4 year program, applicants require a degree in a life sciences discipline
Brighton and Sussex Medical School	For the 5 year program	
University of Bristol	For the 5 year and 6 year programs	For the 4 year program, applicants require a degree in a bio-medical science
Cardiff University	For the 5 year and 6 year programs	
Cambridge University	For the 4 year and 5/6 year programs	
University of Dundee	For the 6 year program, only degrees in non-scientific disciplines are accepted	For the 5 year program, applicants require a degree in a scientific discipline
University of East Anglia	For the 5 year program	
University of Edinburgh	For the 5 year program	
University of Glasgow	For the 5 year program	
Hull York Medical School	For the 5 year program in previous years, currently under review	
Imperial College London	For the 6 year program, applicants can apply with any degree provided they have satisfactory A-levels	For the 4 year program, applicants require a degree in a biological subject
Keele University	Graduates with any degree and acceptable GAMSAT score or acceptable A-levels will be considered for the 5 year program. However, for non-science graduates with non-science A-levels, the usual option is the 6 year Health Foundation Program (requiring UKCAT), or possibly the 4 year route having passed the GAMSAT. For the 4 year program, a degree in a biological science is preferred but other degrees can be considered as well	
King's College London	For the 5 year program	
University of Leeds	For the 5 year program, a degree in a scientific discipline is generally required, but those with non-science degrees can qualify with A-levels or an Access to Medicine course, and are encouraged to contact the admissions committee with any concerns	

University	Accepts any degree	Requires a science or health related degree
University of Leicester	For the 4 year and 5 year programs	
University of Liverpool		For the 4 year and 5 year programs, applicants require a degree in biology or health sciences
University of Manchester	For the 5 year and 6 year programs	
Newcastle University	For the 4 year and 5 year programs	
University of Nottingham	For the 4 year program	For the 5 year program, applicants require a degree in a scientific discipline
University of Oxford	Students with any undergraduate degree are eligible for the 6 year program and may be exempted from the first year.	For the 4 year program, applicants require a degree in an experimental science. The list of accepted degrees is provided on their website
Peninsula College of Medicine and Dentistry	For the 5 year program	
Queen's University Belfast	For the 5 year program	
University of Sheffield	For the 6 year program	For the 5 year program, applicants require a degree in a scientific discipline.
University of Southampton	For the 4 year and 5 year programs	
University of St. Andrews	For the 6 year program and the 6 year North American Program	
St George's, University of London	For the 4 year program	
University College London	For the 5/6 year program	
Swansea University	For the 4 year program	
University of Warwick		For the 4 year program, applicants require a degree in a biological, natural, physical or health sciences discipline

Table 41. Degree requirements at UK medical schools open to graduate applicants in 2012
Information obtained from the universities' websites and by contacting the admissions offices directly.

International Applicants

The only two medical schools that do not allow international graduate applicants to apply are Swansea University and St. George's University, both of which only offer a 4 year program for graduate applicants. All other universities allow them to apply to at least one of their programs. Some universities like the University of Manchester give special preference to non-E.U applicants from countries without medical schools or without sufficient training facilities.

International applicants submit their applications through UCAS as well. E.U and international applicants (normally excluding those from Ireland and Northern Ireland) are usually required to submit their transcripts to the National Academic Recognition Information Centre UK (NARIC UK) at www.naric.org.uk to ensure that they have met the basic degree requirements. Transcripts often need to be sent directly to the admissions offices as well.

Some universities require international applicants to submit other additional materials. For example, international students applying to the University of St. Andrews are asked to submit an additional reference letter.

In general, the government's imposed limit on non-E.U students is about 7.5% of their total class size [40]. Details on the exact policy of each medical school are listed in the table below.

University	Does not accept non-E.U applicants	Accepts non-E.U applicants
University of Aberdeen		Accepts roughly 13 non-E.U applicants to the 5 year program.
Barts and the London School of Medicine and Dentistry (Queen Mary)		Accepts roughly 4 non-E.U applicants to the 4 year program and 22 non-E.U applicants to the 5 year program.
University of Birmingham	Does not accept non-E.U applicants for the 4 year program.	Accepts some non-E.U students in the 5 year program.
Brighton and Sussex Medical School		Accepts roughly 10 non-E.U students in the 5 year program.
University of Bristol	Does not accept non-E.U applicants for the 4 year program.	Accepts approximately 19 non-E.U applicants in the 5 year program and some students in the 6 year program.
Cambridge University	Does not accept non-E.U applicants for the 4 year program.	Accepts roughly 22 non-E.U applicants in the 5/6 year program.

Cardiff University		Accepts roughly 24 non-E.U applicants in the 5 year and 6 year programs combined.
University of Dundee		Accepts roughly 11 non-E.U applicants in the 5 year and 6 year programs combined.
University of East Anglia		Accepts roughly 13 non-E.U applicants in the 5 year program.
University of Edinburgh		Accepts roughly 16 non-E.U applicants in the 5 year program.
University of Glasgow		Accepts roughly 18 non-E.U applicants in the 5 year program.
Hull York Medical School		Accepts roughly 10 non-E.U applicants in the 5 year program.
Imperial College London		Accepts roughly 10 non-E.U applicants for the 4 year program and 21 non-E.U students for the 6 year program.
Keele University	Does not accept non-E.U applicants for the 4 year program.	Accepts roughly 10 non-E.U applicants in the 5 year program, and some non-E.U applicants to the 6 year program.
King's College London		Accepts 2 non-E.U applicants to the 4 year program and approximately 30 non-E.U applicants to the 5 year program.
University of Leeds		Accepts roughly 20 non-E.U applicants in the 5 year program.
University of Leicester	Does not accept non-E.U applicants for the 4 year program.	Accepts roughly 19 non-E.U applicants to the 5 year program.
University of Liverpool	Does not accept non-E.U applicants to the 4 year program or the Medical and Dental Consortium 5 year program.	Accepts some non-E.U applicants to the 5 year program.
University of Manchester		Accepts roughly 29 non-E.U applicants in the 5 year program and 20 non-E.U applicants to the 6 year program.
Newcastle University	Does not accept non-E.U applicants to the 4 year program.	Accepts roughly 26 non-E.U applicants to the 5 year program.
University of Nottingham		Accepts roughly 2 non-E.U applicants to the 4 year program and 28 non-E.U applicants to the 5 year program.

University of Oxford		Accepts a few non-E.U applicants to the 4 year program and roughly 3 non-E.U applicants to the 5/6 year program.
Peninsula College of Medicine and Dentistry		Accepts roughly 15 non-E.U applicants to the 5 year program.
Queen's University Belfast		Accepts roughly 12 non-E.U applicants to the 5 year program.
University of Sheffield		Accepts roughly 18 non-E.U applicants to the 6 year/5 year program.
University of Southampton		Accepts 1 or 2 non-E.U applicants to the 4 year program and roughly 18 non-E.U applicants the 5 year program.
University of St. Andrews		Accepts roughly 40 non-E.U applicants to the 6 year program, including the North American Program.
St George's, University of London	Does not accept non-E.U applicants.	
University College London		Accepts roughly 24 non-E.U applicants each year to their 5/6 year program, but note that students generally need to have completed part of their education in the UK.
Swansea University	Does not accept non-E.U applicants.	
University of Warwick		Accepts roughly 14 non-E.U applicants to their 4 year program.

Table 42. UK medical schools' policies regarding non-E.U graduate applicants
Information obtained from the universities' websites and by contacting the admissions offices directly.

What Are Your Chances

In choosing which 4 medical schools to apply to on the UCAS application, many students factor in location, curriculum, reputation and medical school culture. For most students however, the main factor will still be where they have the greatest chances of getting in.

Applicant X has a lower second class honours degree but has good work experience and achieved a GAMSAT score of 65. If applicant X applies to the 4 year program at Keele University for example, he or she will automatically be rejected for not achieving the minimum requirement of an upper second class honours degree. However, if the same applicant applies to the 4 year program at the University of Nottingham or the 5 year program at Peninsula Medical School, he or she would automatically be invited for interview, and if the applicant had good work experience and prepared well for the interview, they would have a high chance of admission.

Applicant Y has an upper second class honours degree, strong work experience and a score of 2350 on the UKCAT. If applicant Y applies to the University of St. Andrews, his UKCAT score would likely be lower than the minimum cutoff score set each year (2457 for 2011, with true cutoffs being higher depending on the strength of the applicant pool), and the applicant would almost certainly not get an interview invitation. However, if applicant Y applies to Keele University for example, the UKCAT would only be used as a tie-breaker after the interview, giving the applicant a chance to succeed at the interview and gain admission.

These two examples illustrate how significantly different the admissions policies can be between the different medical schools in the UK and how valuable it may be for applicants to have researched those differences before applying. This unique section considers applicant profiles and medical school admissions policies in the UK, and shows where in the UK students with certain profiles may be given strongest consideration. This is here to help applicants consider which universities they want to apply to.

With a 2:2 in your undergraduate degree

Although most medical programs in the UK open to graduate applicants require an upper second class honours degree, several programs accept students with lower second class honours degrees or third class degrees.

Peninsula Medical School, 5 year program
Graduates who meet the GAMSAT cutoff are granted an automatic interview, regardless of the grades they received in their first degree. This is one of the only options to apply to medical school in the UK for an applicant with a third in his or her undergraduate degree. Note, however, that because the grades in the degree are not considered, the GAMSAT cutoffs tend to be slightly higher than most other universities accepting the GAMSAT (usually around 62 to 65 compared to 58 to low 60s).

University of Nottingham, 4 year program
The minimum eligibility requirement is a lower second class honours degree in any discipline. After this has been met, the GAMSAT is the main determining factor in whether or not an applicant will be granted an interview. Applicants are expected to have gained healthcare experience before the interview. Those who do not have healthcare experience at this time can still be interviewed if they provide concrete plans for gaining healthcare related experience in the program's online questionnaire.

St. George's, University of London, 4 year program
The minimum eligibility requirement is a lower second class honours degree in any discipline. Applicants with third class honours degrees who have completed master's degrees or other higher degrees can also apply. After the minimum degree requirement is met, the GAMSAT is the sole determining factor in whether or not an applicant receives an interview.

University of Oxford, 4 year program
Applicants with lower second class honours degrees have been admitted, but this happens very seldom [1].

➡ Some universities allow applicants with lower second class honours degrees to apply if they have gained additional qualifications.

King's College London, 5 year program

Applicants with a lower second class honours degree can apply if they have a master's degree or a Ph.D.

University of Warwick, 4 year program

Applicants with a lower second class honours degree can apply if they have completed a Ph.D.

University of St. Andrews, 5 year program

Applicants with a lower second class honours degree can apply if they have work experience in a healthcare profession for a significant number of years.

With no healthcare experience

All medical schools in the UK will assess an applicant's healthcare experience during the selection process as part of the initial screening or during the interview. Some universities like the University of Nottingham and the University of Southampton say that applicants are expected to have experience relevant to a career in medicine. Although a few programs like the University of Leicester 4 year program require professional healthcare experience or experience within a formal healthcare setting, in many cases, any type of substantial work in a caring role can be considered. For example, at Keele University, appropriate experience can include caring for a sick family member for a significant period of time [1].

For applicants who are not able to gain significant experience related to a career in medicine before the application deadline, it may be beneficial to apply to medical schools that give automatic interviews based on grades and exam scores. This may give them sufficient time between the application deadline and the interview date to gain experience that will help them succeed in the interview.

Several universities only consider academic criteria in selecting applicants for interview. These programs include the 5 year program at Peninsula Medical School, the 4 year program at St. George's medical school and the 5 year program at Queen's University Belfast. Information on each medical school's selection formula is available in the school specific sections.

With a high GAMSAT score

There are several medical schools that automatically interview applicants with a high GAMSAT score.

University of Nottingham, 4 year program

Once the minimum requirement of a lower second class honours degree in any discipline is met, the GAMSAT is the main determining factor in whether or not an applicant is granted an interview. After the interview, the interview score is the main factor that determines whether applicants are offered admission. Applicants are expected to have gained healthcare experience before the interview. Those who do not have healthcare experience at the time of application can still be interviewed if they provide concrete plans for gaining healthcare related experience in the program's online questionnaire.

St. George's, University of London, 4 year program

Once the minimum academic requirements are met, the GAMSAT score is the sole determining factor in whether or not an applicant is granted an interview. After the interview, the interview score is the main factor that determines whether applicants are offered admission.

Peninsula Medical School, 5 year program

Applicants who meet the GAMSAT cutoff each year are automatically interviewed. After the interview stage, the admissions decision is based on the applicant's interview performance.

With a high UKCAT score

There are a few programs that weight the UKCAT heavily in their admission process. A few of them automatically give interviews to those scoring very well on the test. Some of the universities that give significant advantages to students with high UKCAT scores are listed below.

University of Newcastle, 4 year and 5 year programs:
In previous years, applicants to both programs have been granted an interview if they met the academic requirements and met the UKCAT cutoff. Once selected for interview, applicants have had their full applications assessed.

University of Oxford, 4 year program
Applicants scoring roughly in the top 25% of the applicant pool on the UKCAT are usually invited for interview. Those in the top 40% are interviewed as well if they have particularly strong academic backgrounds. After the interview, the full file is reviewed in combination with the interview performance to select applicants for admission.

University of Glasgow, 5 year program
Applicants are ranked solely on their UKCAT scores and the top scoring applicants are invited for interview.

With a low GAMSAT score

Of the five programs using the GAMSAT, four set cutoffs each year for interview. The 4 year program at Swansea University is the only program that does not have a set GAMSAT cutoff, and only uses the GAMSAT after the interview to help make a final decision. Thus, applicants who have a strong application in other aspects and perform well at the interview can still be admitted with a relatively low GAMSAT score.

With a low UKCAT score

While a few medical schools set rigid UKCAT cutoffs to rank applicants for interview, there are several medical programs that do not weigh this component of the application as heavily.

Keele University, 5 year and 6 year program
For the 5 and 6 year programs, the UKCAT is used only when there is a tie between applicants.

University of Leeds, 5 year program
Once the minimum academic criteria are met, applicants are ranked for interview based on their UCAS application only. The UKCAT is taken into account after the interview.

Queen's University Belfast, 5 year program
Graduates meeting the minimum requirements of an upper second class honours degree and BBB at A-level are automatically given 36 out of 36 points for academics in their pre-interview score. The UKCAT is scored out of 6 points, and thus each applicant is given a total score out of 42. Because qualifying graduate applicants automatically receive 36 out of 42 points for academics alone, they are routinely interviewed. After the interview, the UKCAT, academics, non-academic qualities and interview are considered in selecting students for admission.

University of East Anglia, 5 year program
There has previously been no UKCAT cutoff for the 5 year program. The UCAS application and UKCAT have been used to invite students for interview. The 2012-2013 selection formulas are being finalized at the time of this publication, and will be released in June, 2011 [1].

Hull York Medical School, 5 year program
The UKCAT is only given 10 points in the pre-interview score. This is substantially less than the weight given to the UCAS application. Note, however, that applicants with UKCAT scores below 2000 or individual section scores below 450 are unlikely to be interviewed. After the interview, the UKCAT still makes up only a small portion of the total score.

Brighton and Sussex Medical School, 5 year program
Although strong UKCAT scores are advantageous, low UKCAT scores can be overcome by other factors. Both academic and non-academic criteria are used in interview selection.

There are many universities that do not set a UKCAT cutoff. Details on each medical school's selection formulas are available in the school specific sections.

Access to Medicine Courses

Access to medicine courses are intended for students whose current qualifications do not allow them to gain admission to medical school. If your previous grades are too low or if your current courses do not allow you to apply to the programs you would like to attend, Access to Medicine courses may be a good option. Courses generally take one year and usually include human anatomy, physiology, math, chemistry and biochemistry.

In deciding whether to attend an Access to Medicine course and which one to attend, note that many universities set restrictions on how Access to Medicine courses can be used. For example, at Brighton and Sussex Medical School, an Access to Medicine course is normally only considered if the applicant passed at distinction level. At the University of St. Andrews, Access to Medicine courses are not acceptable for students who have previously completed an undergraduate degree. While some medical schools accept all approved Access to Medicine courses, many medical schools accept only a few courses. For example, only the access courses from City College Norwich, College of West Anglia and Sussex Downs Adult College, as well as the University of Bradford Foundation in Clinical Sciences course are accepted at the University of Leeds. The most commonly approved Access to Medicine course (last statistics taken in 2006) is the course at West Anglia [40]. Some of the Access to Medicine courses available are listed below [41]:

1. Birkbeck College, University of London
2. University of Bradford
3. City and Islington College
4. Lambeth College
5. University of Leeds
6. University of Lincoln
7. Manchester College of Arts and Technology
8. City College Norwich
9. St. Martin's College (Lancaster)
10. Sussex Downs College
11. College of West Anglia

Application Process in the UK

General information

If you are a student with an undergraduate degree, a healthcare professional or any other professional who wants to study medicine, you may have the option to apply to any of the 53 programs available in the UK. These programs can take 4, 5 or 6 years to complete. In general, 6 year programs tend to be for applicants who do not have a scientific background and 4 year programs tend to be the most competitive programs to gain admission to. However, this is not true for every medical school. The admissions policies and academic requirements for each medical school can be found in the school specific sections.

Most 4 year programs are open only to 'home applicants', which include UK and European Union applicants; however, a few of them, such as the University of Warwick and Imperial College London, also have some places reserved for non-E.U applicants. Most 5 year and 6 year programs are open to non-E.U applicants, although the number of allocated spaces are limited by a governmental quota. For information of international entrance statistics and number of places, refer to page 206.

About 50% of 4 year programs in the UK consider application from students who completed their first degree in a scientific discipline. The other half consider any undergraduate degree, including arts, social sciences or humanities. Most of the 5 year programs accept all undergraduate degrees. There are a few exceptions to this such as the University of Dundee or the University of Nottingham, which consider applications to their 5 year program only from students with an undergraduate degree in a scientific discipline. All 6 year programs open to graduate applicants allow students to apply with degrees from non-scientific disciplines. Each medical school's policy regarding which undergraduate degrees are accepted is outlined in the section "undergraduate science degree vs. non-science degree" on page 203.

The application process for most programs is centralized through UCAS and is exclusively online (www.ucas.co.uk). The application opens in mid-June. Applicants can only apply to 4 medical programs at a time. Making a well informed decision in choosing which medical schools to apply to significantly increases the chances of admission.

Note that the only program that does not use the UCAS application form is the University of Liverpool Foundation for Health Studies program (6 years). See the school specific section on page 265 for more details. Also note that the UCAS regulation limiting application to Oxford and Cambridge only applies to school leavers and thus if you are a graduate student, you can apply to both these medical schools at the same time.

Some medical schools like Cambridge and Oxford ask applicants to submit an additional personal statement and ask for additional reference letters. Alongside the UCAS application, most, but not all universities, require applicants to write either the GAMSAT, BMAT or UKCAT. The GAMSAT is only offered once a year in the UK so applicants should make sure not to miss the deadline for registration for their application year. Once the UCAS applications are submitted and the medical schools receive the applicants' GAMSAT, BMAT or UKCAT scores, applicants may be notified of an unsuccessful application or be invited for an interview. One exception is the University of Southampton, where graduate applicants are normally not interviewed (only international graduates are interviewed).

For details on the interview structures of each university, please refer to page 227. After the interview stage, applicants either receive a refusal, a notification that they are on the waiting list, a conditional offer or an unconditional offer.

Note that applying for entry in 2012 offers a small advantage for students compared to previous years. Normally, a fraction of places are already filled by students deferring entry from the previous year, however, the jump in fees this year has reduced the number of students from 2011 who deferred entry, leaving more spaces open in many programs for 2012.

The UCAS application

The University and College Admissions Service (UCAS) is the centralized system through which most full-time undergraduate applications in the UK are submitted, including all UK medical school applications (with the exception of the University of Liverpool 6 year program application). The UCAS application requires the following components:

1. Personal details including name, address, contact details, nationality, date of birth, etc.
2. Programs applicants wish to apply to: applicants may choose up to 5 programs. Only four of the five programs can be in medicine.
   Note that the admissions committees do not know which other universities applicants have applied to. The only exception to this is if a student applies to 2 programs in the same

university, in which case that particular university will be aware of the two programs the student has applied to.

3. Education: list of courses and qualifications
4. Employment history
5. Personal Statement: the applicant's opportunity to explain why he or she wants to do medicine and to talk about work experience and the qualities that would make them a good doctor. Note that several medical schools have specific recommendations on what to include and also note that some medical programs do not take the personal statement into account. See the personal statement section on page 221 for more details.
6. Reference: this is a recommendation from a lecturer, employer or another professional who knows the applicant well and can write about their suitability for the course. Again, several medical schools have specific recommendations regarding who the referee should be, and what they should include. See the reference letter section on page 223 for more details.

The application must be filled in online at www.ucas.co.uk before October 15th of the year before the applicant wants to start medicine. This means your application needs to be submitted about 11 months before you will start your medical course.

The cost of application in the 2012-2013 application cycle is £11 to apply to only one program and £21 to apply to 2-5 programs.

Extracurricular Activities and Volunteer Work

Almost all medical schools in the UK place significant weight on extracurricular activities, volunteer work and work experience, either during the selection for interview or at the interview itself. Some universities even grade the extent of these experiences in their evaluation. For example, at the University of Bristol, applicants are selected for interview based on 6 elements in their personal statements, four of which are for extracurricular activities (all elements carry equal weight):

1. Realistic interest in medicine.
2. Informed about a career in medicine.
3. Demonstrated commitment to helping others.
4. Demonstrate a wide range of interests.
5. Contribution to school and community activities.
6. Range of non-academic personal achievements.

Some universities like King's College London give the applicant's personal statement and reference letters to interviewers, which allow them to ask applicants about their experiences. Interviewers at the University of Sheffield also receive applicants' UCAS applications beforehand, and assess students on evidence of commitment to caring, depth of interests (achievements in specific fields) and medical work experience, among other criteria.

For more information on getting involved in volunteer work, medically related work, research and other extra-curricular activities, see page 69.

Personal Statement requirements

The UCAS application form requires applicants to write one personal statement that can be no longer than 47 lines and no longer than 4000 characters. Both limitations must be met for the application to be processed. The UCAS essays are screened for any evidence of plagiarism [42].

Although the same personal statement goes to all programs, it is important to note that many medical schools give guidelines on what they would like applicants to include in their personal statement. For example, the University of Warwick states that the two assessors grading the UCAS application are looking for evidence of the following: "consideration of reasons for studying medicine; discovering what it means to be a member of the medical profession in a health care environment; experiencing a caring role, particularly for individuals outside the family; team working and life beyond academic work. The personal statement should include some evidence of reflecting on the work experience so that it is clear what an applicant has learned in terms of their own abilities and what is required of someone aiming to be a doctor."

Here is how Hull York Medical School has assessed the UCAS application in previous years: "Using a standard assessment sheet, we score your UCAS form out of a maximum of 50 points. We assess the level of evidence you provide for each of the following personal attributes:

1. Academic ability
2. Motivation for medicine
3. A realistic understanding of medicine, including hands-on experience of caring and observing healthcare in hospital and community settings
4. Self-motivation and responsibility
5. Communication skills
6. Ability to work with others
7. Other unusual qualities or life-experience

When writing about your work experience, we look not only for a list of what you have done but also for your reflections on what you learned about yourself, or the medical profession, from that experience."

At the University of Bristol "The personal statement is scored on six parameters, each given a score out of four.

1. Realistic interest in medicine
2. Informed about a career in medicine
3. Demonstrated commitment to helping others
4. Demonstrate a wide range of interests
5. Contribution to school, university (if applicable) and community activities
6. Range of non-academic personal achievements"

At the University of St. Andrews, applicants are given the following guidelines: "The way that you present yourself is very important, as our only impression of you comes from your personal statement. The major areas you need to address are:

1. **Explain why you are choosing medicine**
   Why do you want to be a doctor? What influences have led you to consider a career in medicine?
2. **Work experience in a caring type role**
   You should research carefully what a career in medicine actually involves. We understand that medically related work experience, such as shadowing a GP or consultant may be difficult to obtain for some students. Any work that brings you into contact with the general public will improve your communication skills. If you have been able to gain work experience with ill, disabled or disadvantaged people, or have undertaken voluntary work, tell us what you feel you have gained from it.
3. **Interests/hobbies**
   We are interested to know more about you as a whole person. Tell us about how you choose to spend your spare time.
4. **Other information**
   This is a 'catch-all' for anything that you want to tell us about yourself that does not fit easily into one of the above categories."

Some of the criteria assessed are common to many medical schools including motivation or realistic understanding of what a career in medicine entails, as well as quality and range of non-academic experience. Applicants should visit the medical schools' websites to see what the medical schools they are applying to expect in their personal statements. If no criteria for the UCAS form are available, it may be useful to consider what criteria they look for in the interview.

For more information on writing personal statements, please see page 76.

Reference letter requirements

Applicants submit one letter in their UCAS form, which usually comes from a professor, tutor, or academic supervisor. Reference letters usually must include the following:

1. Assessment of your commitment for medicine, personal qualities (leadership, reliability, teamwork, humility, communication skills), extracurricular experiences and other non-academic factors.
2. Their opinion of your suitability for medicine
3. Information on your academic performance
4. Any extenuating circumstances that may have affected your academic performance if you wish for them to include this.

Note that graduate applicants can also use an employer as their reference in some cases, but should ensure that this is a satisfactory option at all the medical schools they apply to. For example, Keele University states that graduates <u>cannot</u> use employers as a referee: "We suggest that you give your employer's contact details to your academic referee. The employer may then be able to contribute to the reference that is submitted by your academic referee." For the 4 year program at the University of Nottingham, however, the reference "does not affect the outcome of the application", rather, it is used to check your identity and the information you provided in your personal statement. In this case, the criteria are much more liberal, and applicants who have not studied or graduated recently can obtain references from an employer, training officer or a senior colleague in employment or voluntary work.

Some universities like Queen's University Belfast give guidelines on what they would like the reference letter to focus on: A satisfactory letter should show support for the student's application "particularly relating to the applicant's character, suitability for the course, communication skills and initiative."

At the University of St Andrews, graduating applicants and graduates are given separate recommendations as to whom should supply their reference letters (note that applicants who have already graduated at the time of application supply an additional letter). "If you are graduating from a university you need to supply a reference from your university tutor which includes a prediction for your degree classification and that comments on your attitude and approach to academic ability and your suitability to become a doctor. If you are already a graduate, we would require an academic reference from your university tutor and a reference from someone you are currently working with. You could supply one as supplementary material."

Some medical schools like Hull York Medical School and the University of East Anglia may not outline specific criteria for what should be included in the reference letter, but do give their scoring criteria for the UCAS application, which includes the personal statement and reference letter (see the school specific sections for more details). Applicants are thus expected to address each of their criteria in one of the two components of their application.

For information on obtaining the best reference letters, see page 92.

Deferring Entry

Many universities in the UK allow applicants to defer for a year for personal or academic reasons (eg. wanting to complete a humanitarian project, or a one year master's degree). Applicants may also need to defer for family reasons.

See what the University of Birmingham says about deferring entry to their 5 year program (approximately 10% of their students each year take a gap year):

"Applying for deferred entry will in no way jeopardize your chance of an offer. If you intend to do this we recommend that the year is used to broaden your experience either by working, traveling, voluntary service or some other activity. We do not necessarily expect it to be in a field directly related to medicine."

Although most medical schools allow deferrals, a few universities are quite strict about not allowing students to defer entry for a year. Some universities strongly prefer that the intention to defer be specified on the UCAS form at the time of application or early in the application process, while at many other universities like Cardiff University, applicants can usually ask for deferral in writing after they have been accepted to the program. Each medical school's policy on differing entry is listed in the table below:

University	Allows deferred entry applications	Allows exceptionally but not recommended	Does not allow
University of Aberdeen	For the 5 year program		
Barts and the London School of Medicine and Dentistry (Queen Mary)	For the 5 year program		For the 4 year program
University of Birmingham	For the 5 year program	For the 4 year program	
Brighton and Sussex Medical School	For the 5 year program		
University of Bristol	For the 4, 5 and 6 year programs		
Cambridge University	For the 5/6 year program		For the 4 year program
Cardiff University	For the 5 and 6 year programs		
University of Dundee	For the 5 year and 6 year programs, applicants should indicate their intention to defer on the UCAS application, but the university can occasionally accommodate students who request deferral after admission.		
University of East Anglia	For the 5 year program, applicants should indicate their intention to take a gap year on the UCAS application, but the university can occasionally accommodate students who request deferral after admission.		
University of Edinburgh	For the 5 year program, applicants should indicate their intention to defer on the UCAS application, but the university can occasionally accommodate students who request deferral after admission.		
University of Glasgow	For the 5 year program		
Hull York Medical School	For the 5 year program		

University	Allows deferred entry applications	Allows exceptionally but not recommended	Does not allow
Imperial College London	For E.U applicants to the 6 year program.		All applicants to the 4 year program and non-E.U applicants to the 6 year program requesting deferral are not normally granted admission
Keele University	For the 4, 5 and 6 year programs, applicants need to indicate what they will do during the gap year in their UCAS form, or when they write to the university asking for deferral. Applicants are normally expected to ask for deferral on the UCAS form or early in the application process.		
King's College London	For the 4 year and 5 year programs		
University of Leeds	For the 5 year program		
University of Leicester	For the 5 year program, applicants can request deferral on the UCAS form, or can occasionally be granted deferral if they advise the admissions committee later in the application cycle.	For the 4 year program	
University of Liverpool	For the 5 year program, applicants can defer entry, particularly to gain work or academic experience.		Not normally possible for the 4 year program, or for international applicants.
University of Manchester	For the 5 year program		
Newcastle University	For the 4 and 5 year programs		
University of Nottingham	For the 5 year program, applicants are expected to use the time constructively: "Travel or work in a medically related field" are acceptable	For the 4 year program, deferred entry is only granted for exceptional reasons. This excludes financial considerations or the completion of a first or other degree	
University of Oxford	For the 5/6 year program, applicants wishing to defer entry are expected to discuss their plans at the interview. Should they gain admission, they should then write to the Director of Clinical Studies to request permission to defer entry.	For the 4 year program, deferred entry is possible but not encouraged	
Peninsula College of Medicine and Dentistry	For the 5 year program, requests must be indicated in the UCAS form. Applicants need to indicate what they will do during the gap year		

University	Allows deferred entry applications	Allows exceptionally but not recommended	Does not allow
Queen's University Belfast	For the 5 year program		
University of Sheffield	For the 5 and 6 year programs, applicants are expected to achieve something in the gap year. Plans for the gap year should be well thought out and included in the UCAS application. If students wish to defer mid-way through the application cycle, they can submit their request with gap-year plans to the admissions office. Most requests can be accommodated.		
University of Southampton	For the 4 and 5 year programs		
University of St. Andrews		For the 6 year program	
St George's, University of London	For the 4 year program		
University College London	For the 5/6 year program		
Swansea University			For the 4 year program
University of Warwick		For the 4 year program	

Table 43. Deferral policies at UK medical schools accepting graduate applicants
Information obtained from the medical schools' websites and by contacting the admissions offices directly.

Interview Structures

Below is a table summarizing the interview structures for each medical school. The information is correct for entry in 2012.

University	Interview format
University of Aberdeen	Panel interview
Barts and the London School of Medicine and Dentistry (Queen Mary)	For the 4 year program, a unique interview held in an assessment center where students are given different tasks to complete, some individually and some in a group. For the 5 year program, panel interview.
University of Birmingham	Panel interview

Brighton and Sussex Medical School	Panel interview
University of Bristol	Panel interview
Cardiff University	Panel interview
Cambridge University	Panel or one-on-one interviews, depending on the college
University of Dundee	MMI
University of East Anglia	MMI
University of Edinburgh	3 eight minute stations with two interviewers
University of Glasgow	Panel interview
Hull York Medical School	Panel interview last year
Imperial College London	Panel interview
Keele University	Panel interview
King's College London	For the 4 year program, MMI For the 5 year program, panel interview
University of Leeds	Panel interview
University of Leicester	Panel interview last year
University of Liverpool	Panel interview
University of Manchester	The interview has two steps, each taking 30 minutes. The first 30 minutes are spent with other applicants doing a group task. The first ten minutes are for individual reflection, then the rest of the time is spent coming to a consensus as a group, with three observers watching. The second 30 minutes are spent at three one-on-one stations covering the group discussion, the applicant's interest in medicine and other issues.
Newcastle University	Panel interview
University of Nottingham	For the 4 year program, MMI For the 5 year program, panel interview
University of Oxford	Panel interviews over two consecutive days

Peninsula College of Medicine and Dentistry	The interview has two parts. In the first part, students are asked to fill in a questionnaire aimed at investigating their motivation to study medicine. This section lasts approximately 20 minutes. Students will also be given 3 ethical scenarios related to medicine, one of which they will select as the basis of their interview. The second part of the interview process is the interview itself, which also lasts approximately 20 minutes.
Queen's University Belfast	MMI
University of Sheffield	Panel interview
University of Southampton	No interview for E.U applicants to the 5 year program. Non-E.U applicants and 6 year program applicants have a panel interview.
University of St. Andrews	Panel interview
St George's, University of London	MMI
Swansea University	Panel interview
University College London	Panel interview
University of Warwick	MMI type interview held at the university's selection center. The interview lasts approximately half a day. Trained assessors observe applicants completing a number of different tasks and grade them on criteria that assess their aptitude for studying medicine.

Table 44. Interview structures at UK medical schools in the 2012-2013 application cycle

School by School
England - East Anglia

University of Cambridge

Programs

Graduates can apply to a 4 year and a 6 year program. The 6 year program can be completed in 5 years by graduate applicants who meet the premedical requirements and have a good science honours degree.

Nationality restrictions

Non-E.U applicants are only eligible to apply to the 6 year program.

4 year program degree requirement

The minimum requirement is an upper second class honours degree in any discipline.

6 year program degree requirement

The minimum requirement is an undergraduate honours degree in any discipline. The university expects applicants to have an upper second class honours degree [1].

4 year program course requirements

A-levels in chemistry is required plus AS or A-level in two of the following: physics, biology, or maths. At GCSE, grades of A, B or C are required in double award science and math. Single awards in GCSE biology and physics may be substituted for double award science. If you do not meet some of the premedical requirements, you can write the BMAT exam instead. If this is the case for you, the university advises that you discuss it with a Cambridge admissions advisor first.

6 year program course requirements

The typical offer is A*AA at A-level. Although students can be admitted with only two science/mathematics A-levels, some Cambridge colleges require 3 science/mathematics A-levels, and most admitted students have completed three science/mathematics A-levels. Students must have completed three of the following at AS or A-level: biology, chemistry, physics or math. One of the subjects must be chemistry and at least one pass must be at A-level. Students must also have obtained grades of A, B or C in double award science and mathematics at GCSE level.

Admissions exam

The BMAT is required for the 6 year program. The test is only valid for one year.

4 year program selection formula

Approximately 90% of students who apply are invited for interview. After the interview, every part of the application is considered in selecting applicants for admission [1]. Reference letters are a very important part of the application.

6 year program selection formula

See 4 year program selection formula.

4 year program application documents

Students must complete the UCAS application and the Cambridge graduate course application form which is available from any Cambridge college, the Cambridge admissions office and in pdf format from the Cambridge website.

The Cambridge application form requires applicants to fill in all their grades since GSCE, O levels or equivalent. Applicants are also usually required to fill in their main activities in healthcare settings since leaving school, including all work experience, paid and unpaid. Applicants must select 2 referees to write about the following 4 topics:

1. Applicant's academic ability
2. Applicant's team work and communication skills
3. Any personal characteristics you feel make the applicant well suited for a career in the medical profession

4. Do you know of any reason why the applicant may not be suited for a career in medicine.

Finally, Cambridge University asks applicants to submit 2 essays. The first essay is a personal statement and should include the following information:

1. Why you want to be a doctor.
2. Why you feel you are ready to make this commitment to medicine at this particular stage in your life.
3. What attracts you to the course at Cambridge.
4. Information about any other interests, leisure activities or experience that you think are relevant to your application.

The second essay is usually a reflection on your healthcare experience. The guidelines are: "Reflect on one or more of the experiences in a healthcare setting that you mentioned in section D of the application form. Please explain how aspects of this experience (or these experiences) have informed your commitment to a career in medicine"

4 year program interview

There is a mandatory interview held at the university. The interview is a panel style interview lasting 40 minutes. A short guide to preparing for the interview is available from www.cam.ac.uk/admissions/undergraduate/interviews/

6 year program interview

Interviews can sometimes be scheduled in the applicant's home country. Countries in the past have included Malaysia, Singapore, Hong Kong, China and India. Applicants from some countries may have to submit their application a few weeks earlier to be considered for an overseas interview. Interviews at the university are often one on one interviews, but each college has slightly different interview policies [1]. Note that some colleges such as Emmanuel college have videos of mock interviews available on their website. For Emmanuel college, see http://www.emma.cam.ac.uk/admissions/videos/interviews/?showvideo=46 See the 4 year program interview section for the link to their interview preparation guide.

Cost of studies 2012-2013

£9,000 per year for UK/E.U students [2]. Those not eligible for tuition support (most students are eligible) must pay the £4000 - 5000 per year cambridge college fee in addition. Non-E.U: £14,073 - 26,028 per year, plus £4000 - 5000 per year college fees depending on the college in 2011.

Additional information

Graduate applicants can apply to the 4 year program and the 6 year program simultaneously, but they must do so at the same college for both courses. It is worth noting that the UCAS regulation limiting application to Oxford and Cambridge only applies to school leavers and thus if you are a graduate student, you can apply to both these schools at the same time. If you are an international student, you will need to send the Cambridge overseas application form to the admissions office of the college of your choice or, in the case of an open application, to the Cambridge Admissions Office.

4 year program statistics

In the 2010-2011 application cycle, there were roughly 200 applicants for the 22 places available. Statistics for each college are available from www.cam.ac.uk/admissions/undergraduate/statistics/

6 year program statistics

In the 2010-2011 application cycle, there were roughly 1700 applicants for the 288 places available, including 22 places for non-E.U applicants. Statistics for each college are available from www.cam.ac.uk/admissions/undergraduate/statistics/

Contact

Cambridge Admissions Office, Fitzwilliam House, 32 Trumpington Street
Cambridge, UK. CB2 1QY
Tel: +44 (0) 1223 333308
admissions@cam.ac.uk

Ref: 138. *University of Cambridge*. Available from: http://www.cam.ac.uk/admissions/undergraduate/courses/medicine/.

University of East Anglia

Programs
Graduates can apply to a 5 year program.

Nationality restrictions
None.

Degree requirements
The minimum requirement is an upper second class honours degree in any discipline. Note that those with an MSc. with a significant biology component or a nursing diploma can apply as well.

Course requirements
Students must have BBB at A-level, as well as significant knowledge of biology at A2 level (an equivalent qualification in their undergraduate degree may also be acceptable) [1].

Admissions exam
The UKCAT is required for all applicants. The test is only valid for one year.

Selection formula
In the 2011-2012 application cycle, there was no UKCAT cutoff. Once the academic requirements were met, personal statements and reference letters in the UCAS application were scored by two faculty, and the UKCAT was also taken into account. The following criteria were given a score between 0-5, for a total of 50 points between the two reviewers:
1. Capacity for self-directed learning
2. Capacity to work effectively in groups and with colleagues
3. Capacity to take responsibility
4. Motivation
5. Personal effectiveness

After the interview, the admissions decision was based solely on the interview [1].

Interview
There is a mandatory interview held at the university. The interview is MMI format with 5 stations, each with 1 interviewer [1].

Cost of studies 2012-2013
Annual tuition for UK/E.U students could be up to £9,000. Non-E.U: £23,250 in 2011

Statistics
In the 2011-2012 application cycle, there were roughly 2000 applications received for approximately 130 UK/E.U places, and approximately 200 applications received for the 13 non-E.U places [1]. Approximately 500-600 students are interviewed every year.

Contact
University of East Anglia
Norwich, UK. NR4 7TJ
Tel: +44 (0) 1603 591515
admissions@uea.ac.uk

Ref: 139. *University of East Anglia*. Available from: http://www.uea.ac.uk/med/course/mbbs.

England - Greater London

Barts and The London School of Medicine and Dentistry

Programs
Graduates can apply to a 4 year and a 5 year program.

Nationality restrictions
None.

4 year program degree requirement
The minimum requirement is an upper second class honours degree in a science or health related field. Note that North American applicants must hold a science degree with a GPA of 3.6 or higher.

5 year program degree requirement
The minimum requirement is an upper second class honours degree in any discipline, provided the applicant has achieved a satisfactory level in biology and chemistry. North American applicants must hold a degree with a GPA of 3.6 or higher to be eligible, and must demonstrate that they have reached an equivalent standard of chemistry and biology.

4 year program course requirements
UK applicants must have a significant component of chemistry and biology in their degree, at least equivalent to AS level. Alternatively, applicants must achieve a minimum of BB in AS/A-level chemistry and biology before starting their degree, or be in the process of completing AS/A-level chemistry and biology with grades of BB at the time of application. A list of which degrees requiring applicants to have AS-level chemistry and/or biology is available from: http://www.smd.qmul.ac.uk/admissions/medicine/gep/admissions/Acceptable degree course titles/18156.html

Those whose degrees are not listed should contact the admissions office. Note that no higher degrees such as master's degrees are taken into account unless the higher degree is the first degree completed by the applicant. International applicants must have taken chemistry and biology at university and should send their transcripts directly to the admissions office for evaluation.

5 year program course requirements
See 4 year program course requirements.

Admissions exam
The UKCAT is required for all applicants. The test is only valid for one year.

4 year program selection formula
Applicants must have met the minimum academic criteria and shown evidence of a commitment to medicine in their personal statement, as well as submit a satisfactory reference.

4 year program selection formula (cont'd)

They are then selected for interview based on their UCAS applications and their UKCAT scores. After the interview, the admissions decision is based on non-academic factors including the personal statement, reference letter and interview performance [1].

5 year program selection formula

Applicants must first meet the minimum academic criteria. They are then selected for interview based on the UCAS application. After the interview, the admissions decision is based on non-academic factors including the personal statement, reference and interview. [1].

4 year program interview

There is a mandatory interview, unique in style. It is held in an assessment center where students are given different tasks to complete, some individually and some in a group. One task for entry in 2009 asked applicants to watch a recording of a consultation and answer questions related to the video [1].

5 year program interview

There is a mandatory interview that lasts 15-20 minutes and usually consists of a panel of 2 members of the senior academic or clinical staff and a third or fourth year medical student. The panel may also include a trained selector from the lay community.

Cost of studies 2012-2013

£9,000 per year for UK/E.U students [1]. Non-E.U: £16,442 - 24,500 per year in 2011

4 year program statistics

In the 2010-2011 application cycle, there were roughly 1000 applications for 45 places, including 4-5 places for non-E.U applicants.

5 year program statistics

In the 2009-2010 application cycle, there were approximately 2050 applications. There are 282 places available, of which 22 are allocated to non-E.U applicants.

Contact

Barts and The London School of Medicine
Queen Mary, University of London
Garrod Building, Turner Street, Whitechapel,
London, UK. E1 2AD
Tel: +44 (0)20 7882 2244
gepmedicine@qmul.ac.uk
medicaladmissions@qmul.ac.uk

Refs: 140. *Barts and the London School of Medicine and Dentistry, Queen Mary, University of London.* Available from: http://www.smd.qmul.ac.uk/admissions/medicine/index.html.

King's College London

Programs

Graduates can apply to a 4 year and a 5 year program.

Nationality restrictions

None.

4 year program degree requirements

The minimum requirement is an upper second class honours degree. No advantage is given to applicants with a science degree. Applicants with a lower second class honours degree who hold a master's degree or a Ph.D will also be considered. Nurses qualified with a diploma of higher education and at least 2 years of work experience are also eligible. Other health professionals may be considered depending on their post-qualification experience.

5 year program degree requirements

Either an upper second class honours degree in any discipline and a pass at A/AS level chemistry and biology OR a lower second class honours degree in any discipline combined with a master's degree (with at least a merit). Graduates with only one A/AS level course in chemistry or biology will still be considered if they have successfully completed a unit/module in the other subject as part of their degree.

4 year program course requirements

No GCSE or A-level requirements.

5 year program course requirements

See 5 year program degree requirements.

Admissions exam

The UKCAT is required for all applicants. The test is only valid for one year.

4 year program selection formula

Normally, candidates must be within the top 25% of the applicant pool on the UKCAT to be considered for interview, but UKCAT scores alone do not give applicants an interview automatically, unlike some other medical schools. The admissions committee also looks at the UCAS applications of those students before selecting applicants for interviews. After the interview, the admission decision is based on the applicant's performance at the interview and on all aspects of the UCAS application. If a student is selected for interview when applying to the 4 year program but is not offered a place, he or she will be considered automatically for the 5 year program [1]. After students are interviewed they are ranked according to their scores, with the top ranking group of candidates gaining admission to the 4 year program, and the second highest ranking group of candidates being offered a place in the 5 year program, along with those who applied directly for the 5 year program.

4 year selection formula (cont'd)

Since only 4 schools can be chosen on the UCAS form, the university recommends that qualified graduates choose to apply only to the 4 year program, as they can be considered for the 5 year program as well this way. If students want to maximize their chances of getting into King's College, they can apply for both programs.

5 year program selection formula

Before the interview, academic achievement, personal statements, reference letters and UKCAT scores are taken into account. Note that there is no UKCAT cutoff score. Students who have done very well at GCSE (10-11A*) have a chance of gaining an interview, even with a mediocre UKCAT score [1], provided their personal statement and reference letter are also evaluated favorably. After the interview, the admissions decision is based primarily on interview performance [1].

4 year program interview

There is a mandatory interview which is MMI format, with one or two interviewers at each station.

5 year program interview

There is a panel style interview lasting 15-20 minutes with at least 2 interviewers, usually senior members of the clinical staff. Interviewees complete a short questionnaire, usually on topics that are relevant to their career choices and experience such as "why do you want to become a physician?", "what other career choices have you considered?", or "what accomplishments are you most proud of and why?" [1]. Note that the interviewers will have the applicant's personal statement and reference letter with them, but not their grades or UKCAT scores. After the interview, the admissions decision is based almost entirely on the interview performance [1].

Cost of studies 2012-2013

£9,000 per year for UK/E.U students [2]. Non-E.U: £16,800 - 31,150 per year in 2011

4 year program statistics

The program is very competitive - the admissions office reports approximately 45 applicants per 1 position offered (approximately 1600 applicants each year for 24 places). However, of the roughly 100-160 applicants interviewed [1], approximately 32 offers are made to attend the 4 year program each year, and additional offers are made for the 5 year program to those who applied for the 4 year program (approximately 50 in the 2010-2011 application cycle). In the 2011-2012 application cycle, there were 24 places for entry to the 4 year program with 2 places for international applicants.

5 year program statistics

A total of roughly 3400 UK/E.U students and 500 non-E.U students apply each year, of which approximately 1000 are interviewed. Roughly 550 acceptances are offered each year for the 330 places available, including approximately 30 places for non-E.U applicants. Graduate students make up approximately 20% of 5 year program matriculants each year.

Contact

King's College London
Guy's Campus
London, UK. SE1 1UL
Tel: +44 (0) 20 7848 6501/6502
ug-healthadmissions@kcl.ac.uk

Ref: 141. *King's College London - Medicine Graduate Entry Programme.* Available from: http://www.kcl.ac.uk/ugp09/programme/649.
142. *King's College London - Medicine 5 year course.* Available from: http://www.kcl.ac.uk/ugp09/programme/85.

Imperial College London

Programs

Graduates can apply to a 4 year or a 6 year program.

Nationality restrictions

None.

4 year program degree requirements

The minimum requirement is an upper second class honours degree in a biological subject or a Ph.D in a biological subject. Applicants' degrees are expected to fulfill criteria available from:http://www1.imperial.ac.uk/medicine/teaching/undergraduate/ge/admission/chklist.

6 year program degree requirements

The minimum requirement is an upper second class honours degree in any discipline. Only applicants who do not fulfill the criteria for the 4 year program can apply to the 6 year program.

4 year program course requirements

There are no other A-level or GCSE requirements [1].

6 year program course requirements

Applicants require BBB at A-level including biology and chemistry [1].

Admissions exams

The UKCAT is required for all 4 year program applicants. The BMAT is required for all 6 year program applicants. Both tests are only valid for one year.

4 year program selection formula

Applicants are selected for interview based on their UCAS applications and UKCAT scores. After the interview, the admissions decision is based almost entirely on the interview performance [1].

6 year program selection formula

Applicants fulfilling the minimum criteria and ranking well in all three sections of the BMAT have their UCAS applications and academic credentials reviewed by panel members. After this stage, having a high BMAT score does not give applicants a significant advantage [1]. After the interview, the admissions decision is based primarily on the interview performance [1].

4 year program interview

There is a panel style interview lasting approximately 25-30 minutes [1]. The panel usually consists of a chairperson, 2 members of the admissions committee, a senior medical student and frequently a lay observer.

4 year program interview (cont'd)

Interviewees are assessed on motivation and realistic approach to medicine as a career, capacity to deal with stressful situations, evidence of leadership and teamwork, ability to multitask, contribution to school, communication skills, maturity, understanding of mammalian cell biology and ability to think logically and draw conclusions from data.

6 year program interview

There is a mandatory interview lasting approximately 10-15 minutes. The interview panel consists of a chairperson, 2 members of the admissions committee, a senior medical student and frequently a lay observer. Interviewees are assessed on motivation and realistic approach to medicine as a career, capacity to deal with stressful situations, evidence of leadership and teamwork, ability to multitask, contribution to school, communication skills and maturity.

Cost of studies 2012-2013

£9,000 per year for UK/E.U students [2]. Non-E.U: £26,250 - 39,150 per year in 2011.

4 year program statistics

In the 2010-2011 application cycle, approximately 120 students were interviewed for 50 places. 10 places are available for non-E.U students.

6 year program statistics

In the 2010-2011 application cycle, there were approximately 2000 applicants, of which approximately 650 were interviewed. Roughly 500 offers were made for the 286 places available. 21 places are available for non-E.U students.

Contact

Registry, Imperial College London
South Kensington Campus
London SW7 2AZ
Tel: +44 (0)20 7594 7259
medicine.ug.admissions@imperial.ac.uk

Refs: 143. *Imperial College London, 4-year program.* Available from: http://www1.imperial.ac.uk/medicine/teaching/undergraduate/ge/. 144. *Imperial College London, 6-year program.* Available from: http://www1.imperial.ac.uk/medicine/teaching/undergraduate/medicine/.

St George's, University of London

Programs
Graduates can apply to the 4 year program.

Nationality restrictions
Non-E.U applicants are **not** eligible to apply.

Degree requirement
The minimum requirement is a lower second class honours degree in any discipline. Applicants with a third class honours degree but with a master's degree or other higher degree can also apply.

Course requirements
No GCSE or A-level requirements.

Admissions exam
The GAMSAT is required of all applicants. The test is only valid for two years.

Selection formula
Once applicants meet the degree requirements, selection for interview is based solely on the GAMSAT results. The GAMSAT cutoffs have been 56, 60 and 60 for 2009, 2010 and 2011 entry, respectively, and have varied from as low as 55 to as high as 64. The high score of 64 was in 2003, and the scores in recent years have been slightly lower than average [1]. Note that students must also have a minimum score of 55 in section II, 55 in section I or III and no less than 50 on the remaining section. The personal statement and reference letter submitted through UCAS play no part in getting the applicant an interview. If two students have the same interview score and are on the borderline for gaining admission, the one with the higher GAMSAT score will receive an admission offer. If two students have the same interview score and the same GAMSAT score, then the admissions committee will look at their UCAS application to decide who will get an admission offer [1].

Interview
There is a mandatory interview which is MMI format with eight 5 minute tasks to complete. Tasks can include role plays with an actor, answering questions or discussing your reasoning on scenarios like "packing a suitcase for a trip, where the case can only contain half of the items available". Other examples are available from: http://www.sgul.ac.uk/undergraduate/MBBS%20Graduate%20Stream/interviews At each station, one or more of the following competencies is being assessed:
1. Academic ability and intellect
2. Empathy
3. Initiative and resilience
4. Communication skills
5. Organisation and problem solving

Interview (cont'd)

6. Team work
7. Insight and integrity
8. Effective learning style

Note that the applicants' work and volunteer experience are assessed at the interview, usually through one station devoted to the topic, and also through other stations that may bring up applicants' healthcare experience in their reflections [1]. A rough guide of how points are assigned is available from: http://www.sgul.ac.uk/undergraduate/ MBBS%20Graduate%20Stream/work-experience-scores.pdf

Cost of studies 2012-2013

£9,000 per year for UK/E.U students [2].

Statistics

In the 2011-2012 application cycle, there were approximately 980 applicants for the 119 places available in the 4 year program [1].

Contact

St George's University of London
Cranmer Terrace
London, UK. SW17 0RE
Tel: +44 (0)20 8725 233
enquiries@sgul.ac.uk

Refs: 145.   *St George's Hospital Medical School - Graduate Stream entry requirements*. Available from: http://www.sgul.ac.uk/students/ undergraduate/medicine/mbbs-gep.cfm.

University College London

Programs

Graduates can apply to the 6 year program, which they will complete in 5 years.

Nationality restrictions

None. Note, however, that students must usually have some academic qualifications in the UK (either A-levels or higher education). Note also that the university gives preference to non-E.U applicants from countries where there are no medical schools, or where discrimination reduces their access to medical school.

Degree requirement

The minimum requirement is an upper second class honours degree in any discipline. An MSc with merit, a PhD or an MPhil may allow some students to apply even if they did not achieve upper second class honours in their first degree. These cases are considered on an individual basis.

Course requirements

Graduates should have at least BBB at A-levels. A-levels taken after the degree are expected to be at grades of A. Students must offer A-level chemistry and biology, or, if these courses were not taken, full details of any biology or chemistry courses taken at undergraduate level should be submitted to the admissions office before the application deadline. Graduates with unusual backgrounds should consult the admissions office prior to applying.

Admissions exam

The BMAT is required for all applicants. The test is only valid for one year.

Selection formula

Candidates are selected for interview based on their GCSEs, previous experience including work experience and volunteer experience (particularly related to healthcare, laboratory work or work in a caring capacity), motivation to study medicine, outside interests, personal qualities and their reference letter. Note that high BMAT scores can strengthen the application. Those whose BMAT scores are significantly below average are unlikely to be admitted. After the interview, the entire application is taken into consideration in selecting applicants for admission [1].

Interview

There is a mandatory interview which lasts 15-20 minutes and consists of a panel of 2 or 3 interviewers who are selected from the university, the hospital, the medical student body and the local (lay) community [1].

Interview (cont'd)

Interviewers are given a copy of the written response to section III of the BMAT before the interview, as this is used to form part of the interview. Interviewers then score the applicant on several parameters listed below:

1. Intellectual ability (intellectual curiosity and robustness)
2. Motivation for (and understanding of) a career in medicine
3. Awareness of scientific and medical issues
4. Ability to express and defend opinions, including discussion of the BMAT essay topic
5. Attitude, including flexibility and integrity
6. Individual strengths (e.g. social, musical, sporting interests or activities)
7. Communication skills (verbal and listening)

Cost of studies 2012-2013

£9,000 per year for UK/E.U students [2]. Non-E.U: £24,940 per year in 2011.

Statistics

In the 2011-2012 application cycle, there were approximately 2500 applicants for 330 places, including 24 places for non-E.U students. The university expects to send approximately 750 interview invitations for the 2012-2013 admission cycle [1].

Contact

Medical Admissions Office
UCL Medical School
Gower Street, London, UK. WC1E 6BT
Tel: +44 (0) 20 7679 0841
medicaladmissions@ucl.ac.uk

Ref: 146. *University College London.* Available from: http://www.ucl.ac.uk/medicalschool/index.shtml.

England - Midlands

University of Birmingham

Programs
Graduates can apply to a 4 year and a 5 year program.

Nationality restrictions
Non-E.U applicants can only apply to the 5 year program. Note that the medical school is particularly interested in students from countries without medical schools or with insufficient training facilities.

4 year program degree requirement
The minimum requirement is an upper second class honours degree in a life sciences discipline. The competition to date has been such that the university has only considered candidates with first class degrees.

5 year program degree requirement
The minimum requirement is an upper second class honours degree in any discipline.

4 year program course requirements
A-level chemistry (or equivalent) is required at grade C or higher. Students can also fulfill this requirement by doing chemistry in a pre-university examination, or as part of their degree. Note that A-level grades are used to discriminate between applicants, and in recent years the cutoff has been approximately BBB.

5 year program course requirements
Applicants are expected to have completed chemistry at A-level or equivalent. Students are also expected to have either biology at A-level, or another science at A-level with biology at AS level with a grade of A [1].

Admissions exam
No admission exam is required. The medical school is considering requiring applicants to write an admissions exam in the future.

4 year program selection formula
Students are selected for interview based on their entire UCAS application form. After the interview, the admissions decision is based mainly on the interview, but other academic and non-academic factors may also be considered [1].

5 year program selection formula
See 4 year program selection formula.

Interview

There is a panel style interview with 2 or 3 interviewers, usually at least one physician and one faculty lecturer [1].

Cost of studies 2012-2013

£9,000 per year for UK/E.U students [2]. Non-E.U: £14,650 - 26,590 per year in 2011.

4 year program statistics

In the 2011-2012 application cycle, the university received approximately 580 applications. Roughly 80 to 100 applicants are interviewed for the 40 places available each year.

5 year program statistics

In the 2011-2012 application cycle, there were approximately 2200 applicants. Roughly 800-1000 candidates are interviewed each year for the roughly 330 places available.

Contact

Admissions Tutor
Medical School
The University of Birmingham
Edgbaston
Birmingham B15 2TT
Tel: +44 (0) 121 414 3858
A.E.Spruce@bham.ac.uk and
C.J.Lote@bham.ac.uk

Ref: 147. *University of Birmingham, 4-year program.* Available from: http://www.medicine.bham.ac.uk/ug/gec/guidance.shtml.
148. *University of Birmingham, 5-year program.* available from: http://www.medicine.bham.ac.uk/ug/mbchb/.

Keele University

Programs
Graduates can apply to a 4 year, 5 year and 6 year program.

Nationality restrictions
Non-E.U applicants can only apply to the 5 year and 6 year programs.

4 year program degree requirements
An upper second class honours degree in any discipline is required. A degree in biological sciences is preferred but other degrees can be considered. Applicants should have experience in a caring role from work experience or a family setting.

5 year program degree requirements
There are three ways to meet the minimum requirements for the 5 year program.
1. An upper second class honours degree in a scientific subject with significant coursework in chemistry and biology.
2. Those with a scientific honours degree with less than second class honours or those with a non-science degree can qualify with the appropriate science A-levels (see course requirements).
3. Those with non-science degrees and non-science A-levels can qualify by scoring well on the GAMSAT (note that they must also write the UKCAT as all other applicants do). The GAMSAT cutoff for this route is the same as for the 4 year program [1].

Applicants should have experience in a caring role from work experience or in a family setting.

6 year program degree requirements
Applicants cannot apply to the 6 year program if they qualify for the 5 year program. This means applicants should usually have an upper second class honours degree in a non-science subject, with non-science A-levels. Note that students can apply to the 4 year and the 6 year program simultaneously. Applicants should also have experience in a caring role from work experience or in a family setting.

4 year program course requirements
Graduate applicants must have minimum grades of C in GCSE English and math.

5 year program course requirements
For those qualifying through method 2 in the 5 year program degree requirements, students will need AAA at at A-level to qualify, including biology or chemistry plus another science subject or math, as well as a third rigorous subject [1]. Subjects like "general studies, key skills and critical thinking" are not accepted. If only two sciences were taken, the science subject not offered at AS or A-level must be taken at GCSE level with a grade of B or above.

5 year program course requirements (cont'd)

Students must have GCSE chemistry, physics and biology (dual award science is an acceptable alternative with BB minimum), or a core science subject with an additional science course. Students must also have grades of B in English and math. They must have a total of at least four grade A passes in full GCSEs (with a broad range of courses).

6 year program course requirements

No GCSE or A-level requirements. Graduates are usually exempt from the standard A-level requirements for the program.

Admissions exams

The GAMSAT is required for all 4 year program applicants. The exam is valid for 2 years. The UKCAT is required for all 5 and 6 year applicants. The exam is only valid for one year.

4 year program selection formula

Applicants must meet the minimum academic criteria and the yearly GAMSAT cutoff. Those who meet these requirements will have their entire application assessed (personal statement, academic achievement, reference letter, etc.) before being granted an interview. In 2009, the GAMSAT cutoff was an overall score of 60, with a score of 55 on section III and scores of 50 or more on the other sections.

A scores of 55 or more with a section II score of 60 and other section scores of 50 or more were also accepted [1]. The minimum overall score in 2010 was 58, with 55 or more required on section III and 50 or more required in the other two sections. The "minimum scores do not vary much from year to year" [1]. After an applicant has been granted an interview, the admission decision is solely based on the interview performance [1].

5 year program selection formula

There is **no** UKCAT cutoff. The UKCAT is only used when there is a tie between applicants [1]. Applicants are selected for interview based on academic achievement and their entire UCAS application. After the interview, applicants are selected for admission primarily based on interview performance [1].

6 year program selection formula

See 5 year program selection formula.

Interview

There is a mandatory interview for each program which lasts 20 minutes and consists of a panel of 3 interviewers who are selected from the university, the hospital and the local (lay) community.

Cost of studies 2012-2013

£9,000 per year for UK/E.U students [2].

Cost of studies (cont'd)

Non-E.U: Foundation year £8,500, years 2-6 £19,570 - 22,500 per year in 2011.

Additional information

Applying to the 4 year program does not prevent applicants from applying simultaneously to the 5 year or 6 year program, but students cannot apply to the 5 year and 6 year programs simultaneously. Those who apply unsuccessfully for the 5 year program will not be considered for the 6 year program [1]. Students may be eligible to apply for more than one program, however, if they do apply for more than one, they must be separate choices on the UCAS application.

4 year program statistics

In the 2011-2012 application year, there were approximately 240 applications for the approximately 10 places available.

5 year program statistics

In the 2011-2012 application year, there were approximately 2700 applications for approximately 130 places, roughly 10 of which were for non-E.U applicants. Approximately 400 applicants are granted an interview each year [1].

6 year program statistics

In the 2011-2012 application year, there were approximately 190 applications for the approximately 10 places available to UK, E.U and non-E.U applicants.

Contact

School of Medicine
Keele University
Staffordshire, UK. ST5 5BG
Tel: +44 (0) 1782 734 651
Questions: www.keelemedicalschool.org.uk/keele_medical_school/contact_us.htm

Refs: 149. *Keele University, applicant brochure.* Available from: http://www.keelemedicalschool.org.uk/keele_medical_school/resources/MedSch_Brochure.pdf.
150. *Keele University - Medical School - Admissions and Entry Criteria.* Available from: http://www.keele.ac.uk/depts/ms/undergrad/courseinfo/entryrequirements.htm.

University of Leicester

Programs
Graduates can apply to a 4 year and a 5 year program.

Nationality restrictions
Non-E.U applicants can only apply to the 5 year program.

4 year program degree requirements
The minimum requirement is an upper second class honours degree in any discipline. To be eligible, all applicants also need to have at least one full year of paid experience in a caring role by the time of admission. Applicants are therefore expected to have approximately 6 months of paid healthcare experience at the time of application.

5 year program degree requirements
The minimum requirement is an upper second class honours degree with a background in biology and chemistry. Those who have not worked in a caring role for one year should apply to the 5 year program.

4 year program course requirements
No GCSE or A-level requirements.

5 year program course requirements
Applicants are generally expected to have a good background in biology and chemistry.

Admissions exam
The UKCAT is required for all applicants. The test is only valid for one year.

4 year program selection formula
Last year the UKCAT was assigned a point score as follows: >700 = 5 ; >600 = 4 ; >500 = 3 ; >400 = 2 ; all others = 1. The UKCAT, the UCAS application and the amount of experience the student had in a caring role were used to determine whether the student was selected for interview [1].

5 year program selection formula
Last year the UCAS application was scored on academic ability, UKCAT score, personal statement and reference. Each element received a score out of 10. For graduates, achieving a first with A-levels as low as BBB would earn 10 points. Upper second degrees with AAA at A-levels would earn 8 points. An upper second with less than DDD earned 5 points. For the UKCAT, 10 points were awarded for >700, and a point was deducted for every 50 points below this score (for example, 612 would earn 8 points). In the past, after the interview, the admission decision was based solely on the interview performance [1].

Interview

The interview is a panel style interview lasting approximately 15 minutes. The panel consists of a senior faculty member or physician and a 5th year medical student, each scoring the student on motivation, teamwork, professional issues, career progression and personal qualities. Previously, each attribute was scored out of 10, for a maximum of 50 points per interviewer. There was also a 30 minute written assignment, which was graded on a set of criteria worth 30 points.

Cost of studies 2012-2013

£9,000 per year for UK/E.U students [2]. Non-E.U: £13,750 - 24,895 per year in 2011.

4 year program statistics

In the 2010-2011 application cycle, 619 students applied for 64 places. This was nearly double the number of applicants compared to the previous year (327). In the 2011-2012 application cycle, there were approximately 366 applicants, of which 100 were interviewed for the 64 places available.

5 year program statistics

In the 2010-2011 application cycle, there were approximately 2400 applicants for 162 UK/E.U places. There were also 19 places non-E.U applicants. They invited approximately 950 students for interview, and made offers to approximately 350 students.

Contact

University of Leicester Medical School
Maurice Shock Building
PO Box 138, University Road.
Leicester, UK. LE1 9HN
Tel: +44 (0) 116 252 2969/2985/2966
med-admis@le.ac.uk

Ref: 151. *University of Leicester - Graduate Entry Program*. Available from: http://www.le.ac.uk/ugprospectus/courses/medicine/main.html.

University of Nottingham

Programs
Graduates can apply to a 4 year and 5 year program.

Nationality restrictions
None.

4 year program degree requirement
The minimum requirement is a lower second class honours degree in any discipline. Higher degrees such as master's degrees or PhDs can be accepted as well. Applicants are expected to have gained healthcare work-experience prior to their interview [1].

5 year program degree requirement
The minimum requirement is an upper second class honours degree in a scientific discipline.

4 year program course requirements
No GCSE or A-level requirements.

5 year program course requirements
Graduate applicants must have achieved AAA at A-level with grades of A in biology and chemistry. General studies and critical thinking cannot be used toward this requirement.

Admissions exam
The GAMSAT is required for all applicants to the 4 year program. The test is valid for 2 years. The UKCAT is required for all applicants to the 5 year program. The test is only valid for one year.

4 year program additional documents
Once an applicant has submitted the UCAS form, he or she will receive an email from the Graduate Entry Program school office asking them to fill in an online questionnaire, or "record of work experience." Relevant experience could include volunteering in a care home or working as a healthcare assistant within a hospital.

5 year program additional documents
Once an applicant has submitted the UCAS form, he or she will receive an email from the admissions office asking them to fill in an online questionnaire.

4 year program selection formula
The university sets a minimum GAMSAT cutoff each year, as well as minimum requirements for each section. Although the full application is considered, the one main factor determining whether or not an applicant is invited for interview is meeting the GAMSAT cutoff [1]. The GAMSAT cutoffs in 2009, 2010, and 2011 were 58, 60 and 61, respectively. Applicants also needed to achieve a minimum score of 55 in section 2, 55 in either section 1 or section 3 and at least 50 in the remaining section.

4 year program selection formula (cont'd)

Applicants are asked in the online questionnaire about their previous relevant work experience, as well as experience they expect to gain in the coming months. Thus, applicants who do not have relevant work experience at the time of application may still be interviewed if they have concrete plans of gaining experience in the coming months [1]. After the interview, if two students have the same interview score and are on the borderline for gaining admission, the one with the higher GAMSAT score will receive an admission offer [1]. If two students have the same interview score and the same GAMSAT score, then the admissions committee will look at their UCAS applications to decide who will get an admission offer [1].

5 year program selection formula

There is **no** minimum UKCAT score. Each application is scored based on the UKCAT results, personal statement, highest 8 GCSEs and answers to the online questionnaire. The 800 highest ranking applicants are granted an interview. After the interview, the two interviewers submit an interview report to the admissions sub-dean, who makes the final decision on whether or not the applicant is offered a place.

4 year program interview

There is a mandatory interview held at the university. The interview will likely be MMI format for the 2012-2013 admissions cycle [1].

5 year program interview

There is a mandatory interview held at the university. The interview is a panel style interview with two interviewers, one of which is a senior member of the admissions committee.

Cost of studies 2012-2013

£9,000 per year for UK/E.U students [2]. Non-E.U: £15,780 - 27,430 per year in 2011

4 year program statistics

In the 2010-2011 application cycle, there were over 1000 applicants for approximately 93 places, including 2 places for non-E.U applicants.

5 year program statistics

In the 2010-2011 application cycle, approximately 2400 students applied. Roughly 800 candidates were interviewed for the approximately 249 places available, 28 of which were for non-E.U applicants. Since not all accepted students enroll, approximately 55% of interviewees each year are offered a place in the program.

4 year program contact
School of Graduate Entry Medicine and
Health
Royal Derby Hospital
Uttoxeter Road
Derby, UK. DE22 3DT
Tel: +44 (0)1332 724622
gem@nottingham.ac.uk

5 year program contact
University of Nottingham
Medical School
Queen's Medical Centre
Nottingham, UK. NG7 2UH
Tel: +44 (0) 115 823 0000
medschool@nottingham.ac.uk

Refs: 152. *University of Nottingham - Graduate Entry Medicine webpage.* Available from: http://www.nottingham.ac.uk/mhs/gem/
students/index.php.
153. *University of Nottingham - Facutly of medicine and health science webpage.* Available from: http://www.nottingham.ac.uk/mhs/.

University of Warwick

Programs
Graduates can apply to a 4 year program.

Nationality restrictions
None.

Degree requirement
The minimum requirement is an upper second class honours degree in a biological, natural, physical or health science. A list of accepted degrees is available from: http://www2.warwick.ac.uk/fac/med/study/ugr/degrees Applicants whose degrees may qualify but are not listed here should send a copy of their syllabus to the admissions office to determine if it is acceptable. Students with a Ph.D and a lower second class honours in their undergraduate degree may also be considered.

Course requirements
No GCSE or A-level requirements.

Admissions exam
The UKCAT is required for all applicants. The test is only valid for one year.

Selection formula
Students are selected for interview based on their UKCAT scores and UCAS applications. Those meeting the UKCAT cutoff set each year have their applications assessed by two reviewers, usually clinicians and professors [1]. The reviews are submitted to the Director and Deputy Director of admissions, who then decide who is invited for interview. Based on previous years, those with UKCAT scores below 2600 are unlikely to be granted an interview. After the interviews, the Director and Deputy Director of admissions receive applicants' interview scores and select students for admission.

Interview
There is a mandatory interview held at the university's selection center. The interview lasts approximately half a day. Trained assessors observe applicants completing several tasks and grade them on criteria that assess their aptitude for studying medicine. In the past these tasks have included a group exercise, a written exercise, and watching a video of a medical consultation [1].

Cost of studies 2012-2013
£9,000 per year for UK/E.U students [2]. Non-E.U: £23,268 per year in 2011.

Statistics
In the 2011-2012 application cycle, approximately 1818 students applied for the 178 places available [1], including approximately 14 places for non-E.U students.

Statistics (cont'd)

Roughly 384 candidates were interviewed on site. In addition, the medical school partners with Barts and the London School of Medicine to be able to interview more candidates. Applicants who have applied to both medical schools and are selected for interview at both programs are sometimes interviewed only at Barts and the London School of Medicine, and the interview performance reports are used by both medical schools to make their final selections [1]. In the 2011-2012 application cycle approximately 75 more candidates were considered this way, for a total of roughly 450 students moving to the interview stage at the University of Warwick [1].

Contact

Warwick Medical School
The University of Warwick
Coventry, UK. CV4 7AL
Tel: +44 (0) 24 7657 4394
wmsinfo@warwick.ac.uk

Ref: 154. *University of Warwick - Graduate Entry Medicine*. Available from: http://www2.warwick.ac.uk/fac/med/study/ugr/.

England - North East

Hull York Medical School

Programs
Graduates can apply to a 5 year program.

Nationality restrictions
None.

Degree requirements
The minimum requirement is an upper second class honours degree. Specific undergraduate requirements for different countries are available from http://www.hyms.ac.uk/undergraduate/entry-requirements.aspx. Graduates from North America need an undergraduate degree with a minimum gpa of 3.3 each year, and a cumulative gpa of 3.5 out of 4.0.

Course requirements
Applicants must have grades of ABB at A-levels and must show evidence of recent study in biology or chemistry, either through A-levels with grades of A, Open University, Access to Medicine courses or by completing relevant courses in at least the first year of their degree. Applicants must also have 6 GCSEs and grade C or above, including GCSE English and math at grades of A. If grades of B are obtained in either subject, the applicant can contact the admissions office to provide evidence that they have subsequently used English or math skills at AS, A-level or higher qualification, or have achieved a score of 600 or higher on the corresponding section of the UKCAT.

Admissions exam
The UKCAT is required for all applicants. The test is only valid for one year.

Selection formula
The entire application including reference letter and personal statement is reviewed before inviting applicants for interview. A standard form is used to score the personal statement and reference letter based on the following criteria:
1. Academic ability
2. Motivation for medicine
3. A realistic understanding of medicine, including hands-on experience of caring and observing healthcare in hospital and community settings
4. Self-motivation and responsibility
5. Communication skills
6. Ability to work with others
7. Other unusual qualities or life-experience

The UCAS application has been scored out of 50 points in previous years. This score is combined with the UKCAT, which is given a score out of 10 based on the formula in table 45.

Selection formula (cont'd)

Note that applicants who score below 2000 on the UKCAT or who scored below 450 on any section are unlikely to be considered. Those whose UKCAT score is in the top 25%, but whose initial score is below the interview threshold will have their UCAS application re-reviewed and may be invited for an interview. Those whose initial scores are just below the threshold for interview are also re-evaluated, with the two readings averaged to determine a final working score. After the interview, the interview, the UKCAT and the UCAS application are used to rank applicants for admission. The weighting in previous years has been: 50 points for the UCAS application, 10 points for the UKCAT, and 50 points for the interview.

Interview

There is a mandatory interview with a panel of 2 interviewers, one of whom is usually a clinician. The interview lasts roughly 20 minutes. The interviewers do not see the UCAS form beforehand. One question is based on a non-technical article the interviewee reads before the interview (like a newspaper article). The other questions evaluate the following criteria:

1. Knowledge and understanding of problem-based learning
2. Motivation for medicine
3. Depth and breadth of interests, knowledge and reflection about medicine and the wider world
4. Teamwork and work experience
5. Personal insight -- knowledge of own strengths and weaknesses
6. Understanding of the role of medicine in society
7. Tolerance of uncertainty and ambiguity

UKCAT score	Points awarded
2000-2099	0
2100-2199	1
2200-2299	2
2300-2399	3
2400-2499	4
2500-2599	5
2600-2699	6
2700-2799	7
2800-2899	8
2900-2999	9
3000+	10

Table 45. Number of points awarded based on applicants' UKCAT scores at Hull York Medical School

Interview (cont'd)

At the end, each interviewer gives an independent grade. The university may interview overseas applicants in Toronto, Canada as it did two years ago [1].

Cost of studies 2012-2013

£9,000 per year for UK/E.U students [2].
Non-E.U: £23,268 per year in 2011.

Statistics

In the 2011-2012 application cycle, there were approximately 1200 applicants for 140 places. This included 90 non-E.U applicants for the 10 places available to non-E.U students [1]. Each year, roughly 550 applicants are interviewed and approximately 340 offers are extended [1]. Approximately one third of students have been graduates or mature students, but this is expected to decrease in the 2012-2013 application cycle due to the expected increase in fees. Since graduates receive tuition fee grants from the NHS for graduate entry programs but not for 5 and 6 year programs (although they are eligible for other funding as detailed in the "costs of studying medicine" section on page 468), the number of graduate applicants is expected to decrease [1].

Contact

Hertford Building, University of Hull
Hull, UK. HU6 7RX
Tel: +44 (0) 1904 321762
admissions@hyms.ac.uk

___

Ref: 155. *Hull York Medical School.* Available from: http://www.hyms.ac.uk/.

University of Leeds

Programs
Graduates can apply to a 5 year program.

Nationality restrictions
None.

Degree requirements
The minimum requirement is an upper second class honours degree in a scientific discipline. Those with non-science degrees can qualify with A-levels or an Access to Medicine course, and can contact the admissions office with any concerns.

Course requirements
Students need 6 GCSEs at grade B including English, math, and either dual award science or chemistry and biology.

Admissions exam
The UKCAT is required for all applicants. The test is only valid for one year.

Selection formula
Applicants have their UCAS application form assessed independently by two senior medical staff. They are then assigned a point score and ranked for interview. After the interview, the interview performance is the main factor determining which applicants are offered admission [1].

Interview
There is a mandatory interview which lasts approximately 20 minutes. It consists of a panel of 3 interviewers: 2 interviewers are either senior faculty, hospital staff, or local GPs, and the third interviewer is a third year medical student or junior doctor. Students are assessed on their interpersonal skills, insight into a career in medicine, social and cultural awareness, responsibility and non-academic achievements.

Cost of studies 2012-2013
£9,000 per year for UK/E.U students [2].
Non-E.U: £15,600 - 29,750 per year in 2011

Statistics
In the 2011-2012 application cycle, there were approximately 3600 applicants for 223 places, including approximately 20 places for international students. Approximately 600 students are interviewed each year [1]. The university tries to take approximately 10% of its UK/E.U intake from graduates, mature students and those from a dental background.

Contact
Room 7.09 Worsley Building, University of Leeds. Leeds, UK. LS2 9JT
Tel: +44 (0) 113 343 7194
ugmadmissions@leeds.ac.uk

Ref: 156. *University of Leeds, School of Medicine.* Available from: http://www.leeds.ac.uk/medicine/mbchb/.

University of Newcastle

Programs
Graduates can apply to a 4 year and a 5 year program.

Nationality restrictions
Non-E.U applicants can only apply to the 5 year program.

4 year program degree requirements
The minimum requirement is an upper second class honours degree in any discipline, or an integrated masters degree. Healthcare professionals can also apply if they have gained a substantial amount of experience in patient care with the NHS or a similar health care service.

5 year program degree requirements
The minimum requirement is an upper second class honours degree in any discipline or an integrated master's degree.

4 year program course requirements
No GCSE or A-level requirements.

5 year program course requirements
Applicants must show evidence of academic endeavor in the last 3 years. Examples include postgraduate A-levels, taking the GAMSAT, or taking an Access to Medicine course.

Admissions exam
The UKCAT is required for all applicants. The test is only valid for one year. The University of Newcastle's 4 year program also considers GAMSAT scores in addition to UKCAT scores if the applicant believes that this may strengthen his or her application.

4 year program selection formula
Last year, applicants were granted an interview if they met the academic requirements and met the UKCAT cutoff set each year. Once selected for interview, applicants were judged on their personal statement, reference letter and interview performance based on the following criteria:
1. Choice of Newcastle
2. Commitment to care and the role of a physician
3. Personal attributes
4. Overall impression including communication skills

More details on what each of these attribute assessments comprises is available in the admissions policy document at: http://mbbs.ncl.ac.uk/public/admissions/

5 year program selection formula
See 4 year program selection formula.

Interview

There is a mandatory interview held at the university. The interview lasts 30 minutes and consists of a panel of 2 interviewers. See "Selection Criteria" for the qualities being assessed during the interview. Note that those interviewing at Durham University for their 5 year program may have slightly different criteria which are available from: http://www.dur.ac.uk/school.health/phase1.medicine/entrancerequirements/

Cost of studies 2012-2013

£9,000 per year for UK/E.U students [2]. Non-E.U: £13,905 - 25,735 per year.

4 year program statistics

In the 2011-2012 application cycle, there were roughly 880 applicants, of which 135 were interviewed and 39 were offered a place [1]. A total of 25 students matriculated into the program that year.

5 year program statistics

In the 2011-2012 application cycle, there were roughly 2057 applicants, of which 928 were interviewed and roughly 400 were offered a place [1]. Approximately 102 students (including 7 non-E.U students) enrolled in Durham University's medical program, while 225 (including 19 non-E.U applicants) began their training

at Newcastle University (students select their preference at the time of application).

Contact

Newcastle University Medical School
Framlington Place
Newcastle upon Tyne, UK.
NE2 4HH
Tel: +44 191 222 7005
Questions: http://www.ncl.ac.uk/enquiries/

Refs: 157. *Newcastle University, medicine admissions brochure.* Available from: http://mbbs.ncl.ac.uk/public/admissions/.
158. *Newcastle University, 5-year program.* Available from: http://www.ncl.ac.uk/undergraduate/course/A100/Medicine_and_Surgery.

University of Sheffield

Programs
Graduates can apply to a 5 year and a 6 year program.

Nationality restrictions
None.

5 year program degree requirement
The minimum requirement is an upper second class honours degree in a scientific discipline. PhDs and other higher degrees can also be considered.

6 year program degree requirement
The minimum requirement is an upper second class honours degree in any discipline. Nursing, PhD and other higher degrees can also be considered.

5 year program course requirements
Those who have upper second class honours science degrees will also need to have BBB at A-level. Those with first class honours science degrees have no GCSE or A-level requirements.

6 year program course requirements
See 5 year program course requirements.

Admissions exam
The UKCAT is required for all applicants. The test is only valid for one year.

5 year program selection formula
First, applicants who meet the minimum academic qualifications are given a personal qualities score based on their personal statement and reference letters, as well as an academic achievement score. These scores are combined and the highest scoring applicants move to the second stage. In the second stage, applicants are ranked based on their UKCAT scores and selected for interview. Note that in 2011, only candidates with 2870 and above were invited for interview. After the interview, students are selected for admission solely based on their interview performance [1]. In 2011, interviewers graded each applicant from 1-5 on several dimensions and gave a final overall score. Candidates scoring 9-10 at the interview were offered admission, those with scores of 11-15 were offered a place or waitlisted depending on the interviewers' comments, and those with scores of 15 or more were not offered a place.

6 year program selection formula
See 5 year program selection formula.

Interview
There is a mandatory interview held at the university, or in the applicant's home country if an international representative is available.

Interview (cont'd)

The interview at the university is held between November and March and lasts 20 minutes. It consists of a panel of 3 interviewers who are selected from among the faculty, physicians, senior nurses, senior medical students and lay people. The interviewers have viewed the applicants UCAS application beforehand. Applicants are assessed based on the following criteria:

1. Knowledge of and interest in studying at Sheffield
2. Motivation for medicine
3. Evidence of commitment for caring
4. Depth of interests (achievements in specific fields)
5. Communication skills
6. Understanding the nature of medicine
7. Medical work experience

Cost of studies 2012-2013

£9,000 per year for UK/E.U students [2]. Non-E.U: £15,100 - 27,290 per year in 2011. There are few merit based scholarships available for exceptional international candidates.

5 year program statistics

In the 2011-2012 application cycle, there were approximately 2500 applicants for the 232 places available, including approximately 20 places for non-E.U applicants in the 5 year and 6 year programs combined [1]. The medical school interviews approximately 650 candidates for the 5 year program each year.

6 year program statistics

In the 2011-2012 application cycle, there were approximately 200 applications for the roughly 20 places available in the 6 year program [1].

Contact

Medical Admissions Office
School of Medicine and Biomedical Sciences,
Beech Hill Road
Sheffield, UK. S10 2RX
Tel: +44 (0)114 271 3727
medadmissions@sheffield.ac.uk

Ref: 159. *University of Sheffield*. Available from: www.shef.ac.uk/medicine/prospective_ug/applying.

England - North West

University of Liverpool

Programs

Graduates can apply to a 4 year and a 5 year program at the University of Liverpool, as well as a second 5 year program offered by the University of Liverpool, Cumbria and Lancashire Medical and Dental Consortium.

Nationality restrictions

Non-E.U applicants can only apply to the University of Liverpool 5 year program.

4 year program degree requirements

An upper second class honours degree in biology or health sciences is required. Healthcare experience is also a prerequisite.

5 year University of Liverpool program degree requirements

The minimum requirement is an upper second class honours degree in biology or health sciences. Graduates must hold their degree at the time of application to be considered graduate applicants. Evidence of healthcare experience or experience in a caring role is required.

5 year Medical and Dental Consortium degree requirements

See 5 year University of Liverpool program degree requirements.

4 year program course requirements

The A-level requirement is likely to drop to BBB in the 2012-2013 application cycle, compared to ABB last year [1]. Applicants must have taken biology and chemistry at A-level, and obtained a grade of A in at least one of the two subjects. General studies and critical thinking are not accepted at A-level. A grade of B in a fourth AS level subject is also expected. Applicants must also have a minimum of 5 GCSEs including English, math and dual or single sciences at minimum grades of B.

5 year University of Liverpool program course requirements

Those with an upper second class honours degree in biomedical or health sciences require a minimum of BBB at A-level including biology and chemistry. Those with an upper second class honours degree in any other subject require AAB at A-level including biology and chemistry (grades of A) and an AS level subject (grade of B). GCSEs in English and math (grades A or B) are also required for all applicants.

5 year Medical and Dental Consortium course requirements

See 5 year University of Liverpool program course requirements.

Admissions exam
No admissions exam is required.

Selection formula for all 3 programs
The UCAS application is used in combination with academic achievement to select applicants for interview. Applicants are expected to show evidence of insight into medicine as a career, experience in a caring role and strong interpersonal skills. They are also evaluated on their contribution to the local community and quality of communication in their personal statement. After the interview, the entire application is taken into consideration in selecting applicants for admission [1].

Interview
Interviews are required for each program. For the 5 year program, the interview lasts approximately 15-20 minutes and consists of a panel of 2 interviewers [1]. The 4 year program interview is identical except that applicants are given an extra 5 minutes [1].

Cost of studies 2012-2013
£9,000 per year for UK/E.U students [2]. Non-E.U: £20,500 per year in 2011. Small scholarships are available for international students.

Additional Information
Students in the Medical and Dental Consortium program follow the same curriculum as the normal 5 year program.

4 year program statistics
In the 2009-2010 application year, there were roughly 300 applicants for 32 places [1].

5 year University of Liverpool program statistics
In the 2009-2010 application year, there were approximately 2500 applicants for 292 places [1].

5 year Medical and Dental Consortium statistics
There are approximately 50 places available for the 2012-2013 application cycle.

Contact
Student Recruitment and Admissions Office. The University of Liverpool, Foundation Building. Brownlow Hill,
Liverpool, UK. L69 7ZX
Tel: +44 (0)151 795 4370
Questions: http://ask.liv.ac.uk/
University of Liverpool programs: mbchb@liv.ac.uk
5 year Consortium program: cme@lancaster.ac.uk

Refs: 160.   *University of Liverpool, 4 year program.* Available from: http://www.liv.ac.uk/study/undergraduate/courses/A101.htm.

University of Manchester

Programs

Graduates can apply to a 5 year and a 6 year program.

Nationality restrictions

None. Note that the medical school is particularly interested in students from countries without medical schools or insufficient training facilities.

5 year program degree requirement

The minimum requirement is an upper second class honours degree in any discipline, however, a background in chemistry is normally required, either by taking a chemistry related degree or by having chemistry at A-level or equivalent [1]. Voluntary work in a caring capacity is also required, and the medical school may verify this experience.

6 year program degree requirement

The minimum requirement is an upper second class honours degree in any discipline. Voluntary work in a caring capacity is also required, and the medical school may verify this experience.

5 year program course requirements

Applicants require a minimum of BBB at A2 level, including chemistry. Physics and math are required at AS or GCSE with grades of C. Dual award science or core and additional science, if offered, must be at grade BB. GCSE English at grade B (or equivalent) is also required.

6 year program course requirements

See 5 year program course requirements.

Admissions exam

The UKCAT is required for all applicants. The test is only valid for one year.

5 year program selection formula

Applicants are first screened based on meeting the minimum academic requirements. Those who meet the requirements undergo a second screening to ensure that there is evidence of the necessary work experience, motivation for medicine, teamwork and other non-academic factors in their UCAS applications. Most students pass the above two screenings. Applicants are then ranked for interview based on their UKCAT scores [1]. After the interview, the admissions decision is based solely on the interview performance [1].

6 year program selection formula

See 5 year program selection formula.

Interview

There is a mandatory interview held at the university, as well as in Singapore, Malaysia and Mauritius each year. Video-linked interviews can also be requested but are not the preferred option for the admissions committee. In the 2011-2012 application cycle all international students chose to interview on campus. At the university, the interview has two steps, each taking 30 minutes. The first 30 minutes are spent with other applicants doing a group task. For example, applicants might be asked "which five of the following ten patients in renal failure would you select for a kidney transplant?" The first ten minutes are for individual reflection, then the rest of the time is spent coming to a consensus as a group, with three observers watching. The second 30 minutes are spent at three one-on-one stations:

1. Reflection on the group discussion
2. What led you to apply to medicine
3. Other issues

Note that interviewers have a copy of your personal statement.

Cost of studies 2012-2013

£9,000 per year for UK/E.U students [2]. Non-E.U: £14,700 - 26,800 per year in 2011.

Additional information

The first year of the 6 year program is open to both medical and dental school applicants. Students who pass the first year gain automatic entry to the 5 year course.

5 year program statistics

In the 2011-2012 application cycle, there were 2500 applicants for the 380 places available, including approximately 29 places for non-E.U students. Roughly 900 applicants were granted an interview [1].

6 year program statistics

In the 2011-2012 application cycle, there were approximately 200-300 applicants, of which approximately 70 were interviewed for the 20 places available to E.U and non-E.U students [1].

Contact

School of Medicine
The University of Manchester, Oxford Road, Manchester
Tel: +44 (0)161 275 5025/5774
ug.medicine@manchester.ac.uk

Ref: 161. *University of Manchester School of Medicine.* Available from: http://www.medicine.manchester.ac.uk/.

England - South

Brighton and Sussex Medical School

Programs

Graduates can apply to the 5 year program.

Nationality restrictions

None.

Degree requirement

An upper second class honours degree in any discipline is required.

Course requirements

Adequate knowledge in biology and chemistry is required. This can be achieved with grades of A in A-levels or by taking these subjects in university.

Admissions exam

The UKCAT is required for all applicants. The test is only valid for one year.

Selection formula

Applicants are recommended for interview based on academic and non-academic criteria (multiple selectors assess each application). The admissions board then decides who is offered an interview. Good UKCAT scores or grades of A* at A2 level can give students an advantage, but poor UKCAT or no A* grades can still be overcome by other factors. After the interview, panel members make recommendations to the admissions board, which makes the final selections.

Interview

There is a mandatory interview which lasts 20 minutes and is a panel style interview with 3 interviewers. They are given a copy of the applicant's UCAS application beforehand [1]. International applicants are encouraged to attend an interview at the medical school, however, a videoconference is also an option.

Cost of studies 2012-2013

£9,000 per year for UK/E.U students [2]. Non-E.U: £23,678 per year in 2011. A £3000 fee reduction can be earned by non-E.U applicants based on merit and need.

Statistics

In the 2011-2012 application cycle, there were approximately 2170 applicants for approximately 144 places available, including 10 places for non-E.U applicants. Roughly 400 applicants were invited for interview [1].

Contact

BSMS Admissions, Registry, Checkland Building, Falmer Campus, University of Brighton, Brighton, East Sussex, BNP 9PH
Tel: +44 (0)1273 643528
medadmissions@bsms.ac.uk

Ref: 162. *Brighton and Sussex medical school.* Available from: http://www.bsms.ac.uk/undergraduate/index.php.

University of Oxford

Programs
Graduates can apply to a 4 year or a 6 year program. Graduates may be exempt from the first year of the 6 year course and thus complete the course in 5 years.

Nationality restrictions
None.

4 year program degree requirement
The minimum requirement is an undergraduate degree in an "experimental or applied science". Several undergraduate disciplines meet this criteria, and a list of options is available from: http://bmra.pharm.ox.ac.uk/FTQuals.html If you are unsure about your degree, contact undergraduate.admissions@admin.ox.ac.uk. An upper second class honours degree or a gpa above 3.5 is expected, but this is not a rigid rule. "In practice, we very seldom admit candidates with lower-second (2:2) class degrees; usually about half of our successful candidates have first-class degrees, and about half have research degrees of some kind; about a third have upper-second (2:1) class degrees with no research history".

6 year program degree requirement
The minimum requirement is an undergraduate degree in any discipline.

4 year program course requirements
Candidates are expected to have A-level chemistry or equivalent, unless their first degree has a substantial chemistry or biochemistry component. Another science A-level and GCSE level biology (or equivalent), or dual-award science is usually expected.

6 year program course requirements
The typical offer is AAA at A-levels. Applicants must have A-level chemistry, as well as one of biology, math or physics. Biology, math and physics must be taken at at least GCSE level with grades of C.

Admissions exams
The UKCAT is required for all 4 year program applicants. It is only valid for one year. The BMAT is required for all 6 year program applicants, and is only valid for one year.

4 year program selection formula
Applicants scoring roughly in the top 25% of the applicant pool on the UKCAT are usually invited for interview. Applicants in roughly the top 40% and who have a particularly strong academic background are often also interviewed. Those scoring in the bottom 50% on the UKCAT are usually not granted an interview. Note that the UCAS and Oxford applications may be taken into account as well.

4 year program selection formula (cont'd)

Applicants can choose a college they prefer, however, each application is considered by at least two of the Oxford colleges, and sometimes offers are made from a college that was not an initial preference. After the interview, the full file is reviewed in combination with the interview performance to select applicants for admission [1].

6 year program selection formula

Applicants are first selected for interview mainly based on BMAT and GCSE scores. Sections are weighted differently each year, but in the 2010-2011 application cycle, the section weightings for the BMAT were:

Section 1: 40%

Section 2: 40%

Section 3: 20%

Note that there are no cutoffs for GCSE or BMAT scores. Candidates are also judged on the proportion of A* grades across GCSE subjects, excluding short courses. Those who have not taken GCSEs are assessed even more heavily on BMAT scores. Mature students' experience is given weight as well. After the interview, the full file is reviewed in combination with the interview performance to select applicants for admission [1].

4 year program application documents

In order to apply, applicants are required to submit an Oxford application which is available from their undergraduate office. It should be completed and returned to the Undergraduate Admission Office, University Offices, Wellington Square, Oxford OX12JD, together with the supporting materials, by the closing date of October 15th. It requires applicants to submit personal information, high school and higher education information, employment and relevant occupational or volunteer work information, a personal statement explaining why they wish to study medicine at the University of Oxford and why they think they are suited to medicine as well as 3 reference letters. Note that all of this is in addition to the normal UCAS application.

Interview

All candidates selected for interview will be interviewed at two colleges, on two consecutive days. Candidates must be available for interview on both dates. The interviews are panel interviews that last about 20 minutes [1]. A report from a previous interviewee is available on the university's website at: http://www.medsci.ox.ac.uk/study/medicine/courses/sixyearsatoxford/3 The student's interviews lasted 30-40 minutes and included questions on his extracurriculars, academics and some public health initiatives in the UK.

Interview (cont'd)

Videos of staged interviews with tips to prepare for undergraduate admission at Oxford are available from the university at: http://www.ox.ac.uk/admissions/ undergraduate_courses/how_to_apply/ interviews/interview_videos.html

Cost of studies 2012-2013

£9,000 per year for UK/E.U students [2]. There may also be an additional £5,920 college fee. This fee is not applied for full-time undergraduates from the UK/E.U enrolling in this program as their first publicly funded higher education course. Non-E.U: Approximately £20,470 - 32,420 per year (including college fees) in 2011.

Additional information

Note that applicants who qualify for the graduate entry course are expected to apply for that course, and not to the 6 year course. Unsuccessful 4 year course applications are not passed to the 6 year course admissions committee for consideration. The 6 year course has two stages: a three year course studying medical sciences leading to a BA in medical science, and a three year clinical course. It is worth noting that the UCAS regulation limiting application to Oxford and Cambridge only applies to school leavers and thus if you are a graduate student, you can apply to both these medical schools at the same time.

4 year program statistics

There is a government imposed quota of 7 non-E.U students at oxford each year (including the 6 year program), however, this quota has never been a limiting factor for the graduate entry course at Oxford. "In practice students from overseas are considered alongside UK students, and selection is made according to the same criteria for everyone". In 2007, when the UKCAT had only 3 subsections, no candidate with lower than 1950 total (average subtest score of 650) was interviewed. All candidates with average subsection scores of 760 or over were interviewed. The 2008 figures were roughly the same. It is estimated that those with lower than 600 per section (2400 total) on the UKCAT this year are unlikely to be invited for interview.

6 year program statistics

In the 2010-2011 application cycle, 1490 applications were received. The mean weighted BMAT score of all applicants was 55%, and the mean proportion of GCSE's at A* was 73%. For those short-listed, the average BMAT score was 66% and the average proportion of A* grades was 89%. Roughly 30% were interviewed, and roughly 155 offers were made.

6 year program statistics (cont'd)

21% of applicants had qualifications other than A-levels, and 14% of offers were given to such applicants. Of the 198 international applicants that applied, 3 candidates received an offer. Additional statistics are available from: http://www.medsci.ox.ac.uk/study/medicine/courses/preclin/statistics

4 year program contact

The Graduate Admissions Office
PO Box 738
University of Oxford
Wellington Square
Oxford OX1 9FB
Tel: +44 (0) 1865 228975
lesley.maitland@medsci.ox.ac.uk

6 year program contact

Medical Sciences Office
John Radcliffe Hospital, Headington
Oxford, UK. OX3 9DU
Tel: +44 (0) 1865 221689
admissions@medschool.ox.ac.uk

Refs: 163. *Oxford University, 4-year program.* available from: http://www.medsci.ox.ac.uk/study/medicine/courses/accelerated.
164. *University of Oxford - Graduate Entry Medicine - prospectus.* Available from: http://www.medsci.ox.ac.uk/study/medicine/courses/prospectus.pdf/at_download/file.
165. *Oxford University, 6 year program.* Available from: http://www.medsci.ox.ac.uk/study/medicine/courses/preclin.

University of Southampton

Programs
Graduates can apply to a 4 year and a 5 year program.

Nationality restrictions
None.

4 year program degree requirement
The minimum requirement is an upper second class honours degree in any discipline.

5 year program degree requirement
See 4 year program degree requirement.

4 year program course requirements
A passing grade is required in A-level chemistry or in AS level chemistry and biology. Minimum grades of C are required in GCSE mathematics, English and double award science. Evidence of fairly recent study and non-academic requirements such as health care exposure are also important for all applicants.

5 year program course requirements
See 4 year program course requirements.

Admissions exam
The UKCAT is required for all applicants. The test is only valid for one year.

4 year program selection formula
The UCAS application is used alongside the UKCAT to select students for admission. UK and E.U graduates are **not** normally interviewed and are thus offered a place solely based on their UCAS application and their UKCAT score. Non-E.U graduates are interviewed before being offered a place. After the interview, non-E.U applicants are selected based on their interview performance and their UCAS applications [1].

5 year program selection formula
See 4 year program selection formula.

Interview
For non-E.U applicants to the 5 year program and all applicants to the 6 year program, there is a mandatory interview which lasts 20 minutes and consists of a panel of at least 2 interviewers. The interviewers each complete a sheet rating several non-academic criteria on a scale of 1 - 5. They also make individual comments about the applicant.

Cost of studies 2012-2013
£9,000 per year for UK/E.U students [2]. Non-E.U: £13,840 - 25,500 per year in 2011.

4 year program statistics

In the 2011-2012 application cycle, there were approximately 1415 applicants for the 40 places available, with one or two places available for non-E.U applicants [1].

5 year program statistics

In the 2011-2012 application cycle, there were roughly 2675 applicants for the 260 places available, including 18 places available for non-E.U applicants [1].

Contact

University of Southampton
University Road
Southampton UK. SO17 1BJ
Tel: +44 (0)23 8059 4408
bmadmissions@soton.ac.uk

Ref: 166. *University of Southampton.* Available from: http://www.som.soton.ac.uk/undergrad/course/.
167. *University of Southampton - School of Medicine Brochure.* Available from: http://www.som.soton.ac.uk/undergraduates/pdf/BM-programmes.pdf.

England - South West

University of Bristol

Programs
Graduates can apply to a 4 year, a 5 year and a 6 year program.

Nationality restrictions
Non-E.U applicants can only apply to the 5 and 6 year programs.

4 year program degree requirements
The minimum requirement is an upper second class honours degree in a biomedical sciences discipline. The degree should include at least one year equivalent of credits in topics related to human or mammalian biology such as anatomy, biochemistry, cell biology and physiology.

5 year program degree requirements
The minimum requirement is an upper second class honours degree.

6 year program degree requirements
The minimum requirement is an upper second class honours degree in a non-science discipline. Applicants with science degrees or science A2 levels must apply to the 4 year or the 5 year programs and are not eligible to apply to the 6 year program. If a student has an upper second honours degree in an arts discipline and A2 levels in arts, they must apply to the 6 year program.

4 year program course requirements
Students are expected to need BBB or ABC at A-level including a grade of B or higher in chemistry in the 2012-2013 application cycle [1]. Applicants must have a minimum of 4 subjects at AS level and minimum grades of B in GSCE math, English and science.

5 year program course requirements
Those with upper second class honours degrees in scientific disciplines are expected to require BBB or ABC at A2 level in the 2012-2013 application cycle [1]. Those with upper second class honours degrees in arts disciplines require two laboratory based science subjects at A2 level (including B in A2 level chemistry).

6 year program course requirements
Students are expected to need AAA in A-levels (including no more than one laboratory based science subject) in the 2012-2013 application cycle [1]. Applicants must have a minimum of 4 subjects at AS level and a minimum of 5 GCSEs at grades of A/A* including English, math, and two sciences.

Admissions exam
No admissions exams are required.

4 year program selection formula

Applicants are selected for interview based solely on their UCAS applications. The personal statement is scored according to six criteria, each given a score out of 4:

1. Realistic interest in medicine
2. Informed about a career in medicine
3. Demonstrated commitment to helping others
4. Demonstrate a wide range of interests
5. Contribution to school, university and community activities.
6. Range of non-academic personal achievements.

After the interview, the admissions decision is solely based on the interview.

5 year program selection formula

See 4 year program selection formula.

6 year program selection formula

See 4 year program selection formula.

Interview

There is a mandatory interview which lasts 15-20 minutes and is conducted by two interviewers. Applicants are asked questions related to why they want to go into medicine, what they know about the related courses, the career, and the recent developments in medicine. An information video on the interview process is available from: http://www.bristol.ac.uk/prospectus/undergraduate/2011/interviews/medical-applicants.html.

Cost of studies 2012-2013

£9,000 per year for UK/E.U students [2]. Non-E.U: £15,550 - 28,700 per year in 2011.

4 year program statistics

In the 2011-2012 application cycle, there were roughly 513 applicants for 19 places.

5 year program statistics

In the 2011-2012 application cycle, there were approximately 3,200 applications for the 235 places available, including 19 places for non-E.U applicants.

6 year program statistics

In the 2010-2011 application cycle, there were 309 applicants for 10 places.

Contact

University of Bristol
Faculty of Medicine and Dentistry
69 St Michael's Hill,
Bristol, UK. BS2 8DZ
T: +44 (0) 117 928 7679
med-admissions@bristol.ac.uk

Refs: 168. *University of Bristol School of Medicine*. Available from: http://www.bris.ac.uk/medical-school/.
169. *University of Bristol, 2011 prospectus*. Available from: http://www.bristol.ac.uk/prospectus/undergraduate/2011/sections/MDYF/dept_intro.

Peninsula Medical School

Programs
Graduates can apply to a 5 year program.

Nationality restrictions
None.

Degree requirements
There is no minimum degree requirement.

Course requirements
No A-level or GCSE requirements.

Admissions exam
The GAMSAT exam is required for all graduate applicants. The test is valid for two application cycles.

Selection formula
Applicants who meet the GAMSAT cutoff that is set every year are granted an automatic interview. Normally, the cutoff ranges between 62 and 65 depending on the applicant pool. In addition, applicants must meet minimum grades on each subtest (2 subtests including the written subtest with scores of 55 or higher, and no less than 50 on the last subtest). For entry in 2010 and 2011, the admissions cutoff was 64 each year [1]. This was higher than usual (the two previous years had cutoffs of 62). After the interview, the admissions decision is based solely on the interview performance [1].

Interview
There is a mandatory interview which has two parts. In the first part, students are asked to fill in a questionnaire aimed at investigating their motivation to study medicine. This section lasts approximately 20 minutes. Students are given 3 ethical scenarios related to medicine, one of which they will select as the basis of their interview. The second part of the interview process is the interview itself, which also lasts approximately 20 minutes. After the interview, the admissions decision is based on the applicant's interview performance [1].

Cost of studies 2012-2013
Tuition for UK/E.U students could be up to £9,000 per year. Non-E.U: £14,000 - 21,500 per year in 2011.

Statistics
In the 2011-2012 application cycle, approximately 1809 students applied for the 215 places available, including 15 places for non-E.U applicants. Roughly 700 applicants are interviewed each year [1]. Although there are no places reserved for graduate applicants, it has been the case that over the last few years, approximately 20% of places have been consistently offered to graduate students, which can be estimated to about 43 places.

Statistics (cont'd)

Note, however, that only about 10% of places have been filled by graduate students in recent years because UK and EU graduate students would need to pay tuition for 4 out of 5 years of study, as opposed to paying for 1 out of 4 years with 4 year programs, and thus admitted graduates usually choose 4 year programs over this program [1]. This does not apply to international students.

Contact

Peninsula College of Medicine & Dentistry
John Bull Building
Plymouth UK. PL6 8BU
Tel: +44 (0) 1752 437444
info@pcmd.ac.uk

Ref: 170. *Peninsula medical School - Admissions*. Available from: http://wdbdev.pcmd.ac.uk/pms/undergraduate/apply.php.

Scotland

University of Aberdeen

Programs
Graduates can apply to a 5 year program.

Nationality restrictions
None.

Degree requirement
The minimum requirement is an upper second class honours degree in any discipline.

Course requirements
It is expected that students will need chemistry at grade A or higher in A-level, Scottish Higher or another equivalent qualification [1]. If the chemistry requirement is not met, an offer may be made on the condition that the applicant obtains a score of 18 in chemistry at the university's summer school.

Admissions exam
The UKCAT is required for all applicants. The test is only valid for one year.

Selection formula
Applicants are ranked for interview based on their UKCAT scores, their academic scores and their UCAS application, which is given a score by the admissions committee. In 2008, the lowest average

UKCAT section score of an interviewed applicant was 513, and the highest was 776. After an applicant has been granted an interview, the admission decision is based on the entire application according to the following breakdown:

1. Academic score - up to 25% of the total score
2. UCAS application - up to 26% of the total score
3. UKCAT score, ranked in quartiles for up to 4% of the total score
4. Interview score - up to 45% of the total score.

Interview
There is a mandatory interview which lasts 20 minutes and consists of a panel of 2 or more interviewers. Applicants are given a score at the end of the interview based on several criteria including understanding of issues, problem solving and commitment to medicine. More details on the categories assessed are available from:
http://www.abdn.ac.uk/medicine/prospective/leaflets/selection/

Cost of studies 2012-2013

Tuition for UK/E.U students will be decided by the Scottish Government around February or March, 2012 [1]. Non-E.U: £13,200 - 24,000 per year in 2011.

Statistics

In the 2011-2012 application cycle, there were approximately 2400 applicants, of whom roughly 600 were interviewed for the 175 places available [1]. Each year, there are roughly 13 places for non-E.U applicants.

Contact

Medical Admissions, University of Aberdeen, Polwarth Building
Foresterhill, Aberdeen AB25 2ZD
Tel: +44 (0) 1224 554975
medadm@abdn.ac.uk

Ref: 42. *University of Aberdeen.* Available from: http://www.abdn.ac.uk/medicine/prospective/.

University of Dundee

Programs
Graduates can apply to a 5 year program and a 6 year program.

Nationality restrictions
None.

5 year program degree requirements
The minimum requirement is an upper second class honours degree in a scientific discipline.

6 year program degree requirements
The minimum requirement is an upper second class honours degree in a non-scientific discipline.

5 year program course requirements
No GCSE or A-level requirements.

6 year program course requirements
No GCSE or A-level requirements.

Admissions exam
The UKCAT is required for all applicants. The test is only valid for one year.

5 year program selection formula
Applications are given scores for their academic achievement, their reference letter and their medically related experience. The personal statement are also scored for non-academic achievement and evidence of diversity. The UKCAT score is then taken into account to produce a final score that ranks applicants for interview. After the interview, the interview performance along with the pre-interview scores are used to rank candidates for admission [1].

6 year program selection formula
See 5 year program selection formula.

Interview
There is a mandatory interview which is MMI format consisting of ten 7-minute stations. Each station assesses the applicant based on three criteria:
1. Content and substance of the interviewee's response
2. Communication
3. Global assessment of suitability for medicine.

The domains covered by the station are:
1. Communication and empathy
2. Teamwork
3. Preparation for medical school and a career in medicine
4. Critical thinking
5. Ethics, fairness, respect
6. Personal statement, integrity check and community involvement

Cost of studies 2012-2013
Tuition for UK/E.U students will be decided by the Scottish Government around February or March, 2012 [1]. Foundation year non-E.U: £12,000 in 2011. Years 2-6 non-E.U: £16,750 - 25,500 per year in 2011.

5 year program statistics
In the 2011-2012 application cycle there were approximately 1680 applicants, of whom 576 were interviewed for the roughly 140 places available [1]. There are roughly 12 places for non-E.U applicants each year in the 5 and 6 year programs [1], and each year approximately 20 places are allocated for graduate applicants from the UK.

6 year program statistics
In the 2011-2012 application cycle, there were approximately 124 applicants, of whom roughly 20 were interviewed for the roughly 15 places available [1].

Contact
Admissions and Student Recruitment
University of Dundee
Nethergate, Dundee, Scotland.
DD1 4HN
Tel: +44 (0)1382 384 697
srs-medicine@dundee.ac.uk

Ref: 171. *University of Dundee, medicine admissions.* Available from: http://www.dundee.ac.uk/medschool/undergraduate/admissions.

University of Edinburgh

Programs
Graduates can apply to a 5 year program.

Nationality restrictions
None.

Degree requirements
The minimum requirement is an upper second class honours degree in any discipline. Applicants are expected to have a strong foundation in chemistry (A2 level or equivalent) and biology (AS level or equivalent). Those who have non-science degrees but have met these requirements should speak with the admissions office to see if their qualifications will allow them to apply [1].

Course requirements
For students who took A-levels, minimum grades of BBB in the upper sixth are required. Those who took Scottish Highers must have achieved BBBB in S5.

Admissions exam
The UKCAT is required for all applicants. The test is only valid for one year.

Selection formula
Each student is assessed by two independent reviewers based on academic criteria and the UCAS application. Non-academic entry criteria include evidence in the personal statement of commitment and motivation for a career in medicine, and a clear understanding of what a career in medicine entails. These scores are combined with the UKCAT score to rank graduate applicants for interview. Note that the academic and non-academic criteria carry roughly equal weight before the interview [1]. After the interview, applicants' entire files are reviewed to select candidates for admission [1].

Additional documents
In addition to the standard UCAS form, graduates and mature applicants are advised by the medical school to submit additional information, additional reference letters and a short CV (1-2 pages) at the time of application. Graduates must also submit a financial guarantee letter showing that they can finance their education.

Interview
There is a mandatory interview which lasts 30 minutes and is made up of 3 eight minute stations with two interviewers. Students are assessed on career exploration, ethical reasoning and communication skills. Students are given 20 minutes to prepare for the ethical and communication skills questions.

Cost of studies 2012-2013

Tuition for UK/E.U students will be decided by the Scottish Government around February or March, 2012 [1]. Non-E.U: £19,600 - 33,200 per year in 2011.

Statistics

In the 2010-2011 application cycle, there were roughly 2350 applications for the approximately 202 places available to UK/E.U students, and there were approximately 400 non-E.U applicants for the 16 places available to non-E.U students. Graduates and mature students comprised approximately 10-15% of the applicant pool in the 2011-2012 application cycle [1].

Contact

University of Edinburgh
The Chancellor's Building,
49 Little France Crescent
Edinburgh, Scotland. EH16 4SB
+44 (0)131 242 6407
medug@ed.ac.uk

Ref: 172. *University of Edinburgh, medical school admissions.* Available from: http://www.ed.ac.uk/schools-departments/medicine-vet-medicine/undergraduate/medicine/applying/how-to-apply.

University of Glasgow

Programs
Graduates can apply to a 5 year program.

Nationality restrictions
None.

Degree requirements
The minimum requirement is an upper second class honours degree, which must be granted less than 5 years before entry.

Course requirements
Applicants who have not completed a science degree with sufficient chemistry and biology courses must have completed either A-level chemistry and GCSE or AS level biology (both at grades of B or higher), or Scottish Highers in Chemistry and Biology (both at grades of B or higher). These courses must have been taken no more than 5 years before the entry date. GCSE English at grade B, Standard Grade 2 English or an Intermediate 2 pass in English is also required.

Admissions exam
The UKCAT is required for all applicants. The test is only valid for one year.

Selection formula
Last year, applicants were ranked for interview according to their UKCAT scores. Applicants who fell below the national UKCAT average (roughly 2400-2500) were unlikely to be interviewed.

Interview
There is a mandatory interview with a panel of 2 interviewers, usually faculty or physicians. The interview is usually recorded, but is deleted at the end of the admissions cycle. Applicants are assessed on their commitment to medicine, understanding of the qualities needed to be a physician, team-work capabilities, other interests and knowledge of the Glasgow curriculum.

Cost of studies 2012-2013
Tuition for UK/E.U students will be decided by the Scottish Government around February or March, 2012 [1]. Non-E.U: £15,000 - 27,000 per year in 2011.

Statistics
In the 2011-2012 application cycle, there were roughly 2000 applicants, of whom roughly 800 were interviewed for the 223 places for UK/E.U students and the 18 places available for non-E.U students [1].

Contact
Medical School Office, University of Glasgow Glasgow, UK. G12 8QQ
Tel: +44 (0)141 330 6216
admissions@clinmed.gla.ac.uk

Ref: 173. *University of Glasgow*. Available from: www.gla.ac.uk/faculties/medicine/undergraduatestudy/medicine/mbchbdegreeprogramme.

University of St Andrews

Programs

Graduates can apply to a 6 year program. There is also a special 6 year program for North American applicants.

Nationality restrictions

None. Note that the medical school may add a second program for North American students this year (see "Program for North Americans" section for more details).

Degree requirements

The minimum requirement is an upper second class honours degree. Students with work experience as healthcare professionals and a lower second class honours degree should contact the admissions office to find out if their experience makes them eligible to apply [1]. At St. Andrews, a GPA of approximately 3.5 is considered equivalent to an upper second class honours degree, but note that this is not the case at all UK universities. First year undergraduates can be considered on their high school credentials, but second year university students will not be considered.

Course requirements

Applicants must have taken chemistry at university level, or achieved a grade of B in A-level chemistry. GCSE biology and English are also expected with grades of B as well as a passing grade in GCSE math. If undergraduate level biology and chemistry are used to satisfy the above prerequisites, these courses must generally have been taken in the last 5 years.

Admissions exam

The UKCAT is required for all applicants. The test is only valid for one year.

Selection formula

First, students must meet the UKCAT cutoff set by the medical school. Once this is met, applicants are selected for interview based on their personal statement, reference letter, academic qualifications and UKCAT score [1]. The UKCAT cutoff in the 2011-2012 application cycle was quoted to be 2457, but the true cutoff score is often higher than quoted because of the strength of the applicant pool [1]. Academic performance is given the highest weighting in the pre-interview and post-interview stages. After the interview, applicants are ranked for admission based on the pre-interview criteria and the interview performance. The rough weighting of each factor in the 2011-2012 application cycle was: 50% academic performance, 15% UKCAT, 15% UCAS application, 20% interview [1].

Selection formula (cont'd)

Note that because academic and UKCAT performance as well as UCAS application reviews are generally high for the applicants invited for interview, the interview is often what determines which candidates are offered admission [1].

Application documents

Applicants graduating from university must supply a reference letter from their university tutor commenting on their academic ability and suitability for medicine. Applicants who have already graduated must generally submit a reference letter from their university tutor and from someone they are currently working with (one in UCAS, the other directly to the university). This is particularly helpful for the admissions committee if it has been a long time since the applicant graduated [1]. In addition, graduate applicants must send transcripts to the admissions office directly. International students are generally expected to send recommendations from two professors who have taught or supervised them (one in UCAS, the other directly to the university).

Interview

There is a mandatory interview which is held at the university for UK/E.U students. Non-E.U students are interviewed by phone, skype or video conference, but they can also request to be interviewed at the university. The interview at the university lasts 20 minutes and consists of a panel of 2-3 interviewers, many of whom are practicing clinicians. Applicants are assessed on their communication skills, a general understanding of the course and their previous experiences that have prepared them for a career in medicine.

Cost of studies 2012-2013

Tuition for UK/E.U students will be decided by the Scottish Government around February or March, 2012 [1]. Non-E.U: £20,550 for years 1-3 in 2011. Year 4-6 tuition depends on which school the student chooses to attend for their clinical years (see the "Additional information" section below for more details).

Additional information

Students can obtain a BSc honours degree in medicine after the first 3 years. They then move to one of the University of St. Andrews' partner universities, or apply independently to other medical schools, to complete their MB ChB training. Applicants must indicate whether they would like to complete the clinical phase of their education in Manchester or Scotland at the time of application. Non-E.U applicants usually go to Manchester for their clinical years, although 10 places are now available at the University of Edinburgh for non-E.U students.

Additional information (cont'd)

Students who want to pursue this route are selected for these 10 places based on their performance in the first semester of Year 2. Students can also apply independently to other non-partner medical schools such as Cambridge for their clinical years. Note that space is limited in these programs and there is no formal arrangement established as there is for the University of Manchester and the University of Edinburgh.

Program for North Americans

The University of St. Andrews is working on starting a second program for North American students (mainly Canadians). The 2011-2012 year is the first year the program is running, but it is still in the development stage. The medical school will be working with Canadian universities to provide preparation for the Canadian medical licensing exams (MCCQE and MCCEE). They are also working on partnerships with a provincial government (possibly Alberta) to establish opportunities for clinical electives and possibly residency placements. Students will be asked to write the UKCAT to gain admission. There are expected to be approximately 20 places in the program [1]. The requirements will be exactly the same as those of the standard program, but the selection process will differ in two ways. First, more emphasis will be placed on academics and UKCAT scores. Second, the medical school will not use a points formula. For example, rather than assigning a score for the UKCAT and for academics, if a student has a GPA that just meets the 3.5 cutoff, but has very strong UKCAT scores, the university may still review their UCAS application and invite them for interview [1].

Statistics

In the 2011-2012 application cycle, there were roughly 1000 applicants for the approximately 160 places available, including 40 places for non-E.U applicants [1].

Contact

University of St Andrews
Admissions Application Centre
St Katherine's West, The Scores
St Andrews, Fife, Scotland. KY16 9AX
+44 (0)1334 462150
medadmiss@st-andrews.ac.uk.

Ref: 174. *University of St. Andrews*. Available from: http://medicine.st-andrews.ac.uk/prospectus/index.aspx.

Wales

Cardiff University

Programs
Graduates can apply to a 5 year and a 6 year program.

Nationality restrictions
None.

5 year program degree requirements
Applicants are usually expected to have an upper second class honours degree in any discipline. North American and Pakistani applicants are expected to hold a BSc. with a GPA above 3.5. It may also be possible to qualify based on high school credentials.

6 year program degree requirements
Applicants are usually expected to have an upper second class honours degree in any discipline.

5 year program course requirements
Previous academic qualifications for graduate applicants are considered in addition to their undergraduate degree performance. Generally, applicants should have completed at least two of biology, chemistry and physics. If applicants have completed none or only one of these courses, they are usually expected to apply to the 6 year program. Applicants are expected to have at least a grade of B at GCSE English (or equivalent).

6 year program course requirements
See 5 year program course requirements. Note that applicants to the 6 year program must have completed no more than one science course.

Admissions exam
The UKCAT is required for all applicants. The test is only valid for one year.

5 year program selection formula
Applicants are first ranked for file assessment based on their GCSEs and A-levels. For the GCSEs, only the top 9 are taken into account, and they are given 3 points for A*, 2 points for A, and 1 point for B [1]. The UKCAT is typically only used when applicants are on the borderline for qualifying for file assessment [1]. Applicants who qualify for file assessment at this stage will have their UCAS applications evaluated based on the following criteria:
1. Motivation for and awareness of a career in medicine
2. Caring nature and social awareness
3. Sense of responsibility
4. Non-academic interests and personal achievements

5 year program selection formula (cont'd)

5. Study skills
6. Reference letter

Applicants are then ranked for interview according to their academic and non-academic scores. After the interview, the interview panel agrees on an overall recommendation and passes this on to the admissions committee. A final decision is then made based on all aspects of the applicant's file.

6 year program selection formula

See 5 year program selection formula.

Interview

There is a mandatory interview held at the university between November and March. It lasts approximately 20 minutes and is conducted by a panel of 2-3 interviewers. Normally at least one of the interviewers is a physician, and sometimes a senior medical student will be on the panel as well.

Cost of studies 2012-2013

Tuition for UK/E.U students could be up to £9,000 per year. Non-E.U: £13,750 - 24,500 per year in 2011.

Statistics

In the 2011-2012 application cycle, there were over 3200 applications for the 280 places available in the 5 year program, and roughly 250 applicants for the approximately 16 places available in the 6 year program [1]. There are approximately 24 places for non-E.U applicants in both programs combined.

Contact

Admissions Deanery
Cardiff University School of Medicine
UHW Main Building, Heath Park
Cardiff, Wales. CF14 4XN
Tel: +44 (0)29 2074 4740
medicaladmissions@cardiff.ac.uk

Refs: 175.   *Cardiff University.* Available from: http://medicine.cf.ac.uk/en/degree-programmes/undergraduate/.
176.   *Cardiff University, 2011 undergraduate prospectus.* Available from: http://www.cardiff.ac.uk/for/prospective/ug/prospectus/.

Swansea University

Programs
Graduates can apply to a 4 year program.

Nationality restrictions
Currently, only UK and E.U applicants are eligible to apply, although non-E.U applicants may be allowed to apply in the coming years.

Degree requirement
The minimum requirement is an upper second class honours degree in any discipline.

Course requirements
Applicants are required to have GCSE math at grade C or above, and ideally should have experience in biology and chemistry at a level higher than GCSE.

Admissions exam
The GAMSAT is required of all applicants. The test is only valid for two years.

Selection formula
Selection for interview is based on the UCAS application form (academic achievement, personal statement and reference letter) and university grades. The GAMSAT score is not used to select applicants for interview. After the interview, the interview performance, the GAMSAT score and the other aspects of the applicant's file are used to make the admissions decision [1].

Interview
There is a mandatory interview held at the university. The interview consists of a panel of 2-3 interviewers selected from the admissions staff, consultants and clinical tutors.

Cost of studies 2012-2013
Tuition for UK/E.U students could be up to £9,000 per year.

Statistics
In the 2011-2012 application cycle, there were approximately 680 applications received. 245 applicants were selected to interview for the approximately 70 places available [1].

Contact
Swansea University
Singleton Park
Swansea, Wales. UK SA2 8PP
Tel: +44 (0)1792 602618
medicine@swansea.ac.uk

Ref: 177. *University of Wales, Swansea*. Available from: http://www.swansea.ac.uk/medicine/GraduateEntryMedicineProgramme/.

Northern Ireland

Queen's University Belfast

Programs
Graduates can apply to a 5 year program.

Nationality restrictions
None.

Degree requirement
The minimum requirement is an upper second class honours degree in any discipline.

Course requirements
Applicants must have a minimum of BBB at A-level. Higher degrees, such as a PhD, may allow students to apply with slightly lower A-level performance [1].

Admissions exam
The UKCAT is required for all applicants. The test is only valid for one year.

Selection formula
To select applicants for interview, the medical school awards all applicants up to 36 points for academics and up to 6 points for the UKCAT. Graduates meeting the minimum criteria are automatically given the full 36 points for academics, which is why they are routinely interviewed. The UKCAT scores are given up to 6 points according to the formula in table 46. Applicants are expected to show evidence of commitment and motivation toward medicine in their personal statement and must have a satisfactory reference letter. After the interview, applicants are ranked for admission based solely on their interview performance [1].

Interview
There is a mandatory interview held at the university. Occasionally, an interview can be scheduled in the applicant's home country. Otherwise, the interview is MMI format with 9 stations. Sample interviews are available from:
www.qub.ac.uk/schools/mdbs/medicine/Prospectivestudents/MultipleMiniInterviews

Cost of studies 2012-2013
Tuition for UK/E.U students is expected to be posted by April, 2012 [1]. Non-E.U: £11,576 - 21,830 per year in 2007.

Statistics
There are 750-850 applicants each year for approximately 250-260 places, including 12 places for non-E.U applicants [1].

Contact
Admissions and Access Service, Queen's University Belfast, University Road, Belfast, Northern Ireland. BT7 1NN
Tel: +44 (0) 28 9097 2757
admissions@qub.ac.uk

UKCAT score	Points awarded
1200-1899	0
1900-2099	1
2100-2299	2
2300-2499	3
2500-2699	4
2700-2899	5
2900-3600	6

Table 46. Number of points awarded based on applicants' UKCAT scores at Queen's University Belfast.

Ref: 178. *Queen's University Belfast.* Available from: http://www.qub.ac.uk/schools/mdbs/ProspectiveStudents/.

USA

Rolling admissions

The importance of early application cannot be overemphasized [43, 44]. Most schools in the US have rolling admission, including Johns Hopkins, Mayo Medical School, the University of California, San Francisco and many others. Schools with rolling admission only accept students until the class is full; as such, your target date for submission of the primary application should be around the third week of June [44] or as early as possible during the summer. "**There is a sharp decline in the number of interviews and, consequently, possible acceptances that students receive with late summer or fall applications**. Some students are still waiting for interviews months after schools have accepted their first students." *Yale University, Applying to Medical School.*

Medical Programs

There are 133 accredited 4 year medical programs in the US, of which approximately 60% are public and 40% are private. Public medical schools are usually funded in part by the state in which they teach, and as such they usually favor in-state applicants and offer subsidized tuition for them. They also generally have less places for international students. Private medical schools often do not favor in state applicants (although some colleges may have an agreement with a specific state, such as the agreement between Dartmouth Medical School and the state of Maine through which a few students apply), and tend to have places allocated for international applicants.

A listing of all the medical schools by name and by state is available from the AAMC at http://services.aamc.org/memberlistings/index.cfm?fuseaction=home.search&search_type=MS

A range of statistics on US medical schools is available from https://www.aamc.org/data/facts/

In addition, the Medical School Application Requirements (MSAR) guide and online database provides information relevant to applicants on each school from the US and Canada such as entrance statistics and financial information, as well as the number of applicants and places available at most schools, including international student entrance statistics, which can save students a lot of time combing through websites. The resource is available from https://www.aamc.org/students/applying/requirements/msar/

GPA and MCAT requirements in the US

Private Medical Schools	Average GPA*	Average MCAT*
Creighton University School of Medicine [111]	3.78	30P
Dartmouth Medical School [120]	3.83	34
George Washington University School of Medicine [112]	3.71	30Q
Harvard Medical School [63]	3.88	36
Jefferson Medical College [117]	3.72	32Q
Loma Linda University	3.8	30P
Rosalind Franklin, Chicago Medical School	3.75	31Q
University of Pennsylvania [116]	3.87	37R
Yale University	3.86	37R
Public Medical Schools	Average GPA*	Average MCAT*
University of Hawaii, John A. Burns School of Medicine [113]	3.68	32Q
University of Kentucky College of Medicine [114]	3.79	31Q
University of Minnesota Medical School – Twin Cities [121]	3.76	33Q
State University of New York (SUNY) Upstate University	3.74	23Q
University of Texas Medical School at Southwestern [45]	3.86	35Q

Table 47: Average GPA and MCAT requirements at private and public US medical schools in 2010.

Although the averages may give some insight, there is a large range of accepted scores. For example, the University of Texas Medical School at Southwestern reported an average entering GPA of 3.81 and MCAT of 33.1, however, the MCAT scores of accepted students ranged from 25-40, and the GPAs of accepted students ranged from 3.1 to 4.0 [45]. The reason for this range in MCAT and GPA is the importance that admissions committees place on the personal attributes necessary to make a good physician. Good grades will earn you points, but medical schools are looking for well-rounded applicants. Your essays, your extracurricular activities and the way that your references describe your character will have a significant impact on your overall pre-interview assessment.

Entrance statistics

The selection ratios for the US medical schools with high international acceptance covered in detail in this guide, as well as some additional randomly selected medical schools, are listed below. Note that the number of students offered admission usually exceeds the number of students who actually enroll, so the calculated selection ratios are higher than the true admissions ratio.

University	Entering Class Statistics	Selection Ratio
Harvard University	457 in state applicants for 15 places 5355 out of state applicants for 141 places 416 international applicants for 9 places	IS*: 30:1 OS: 38:1 Int'l: 46:1
Yale University	225 in state applicants for 8 places 4570 out of state applicants for 82 places 437 international applicants for 10 places	IS: 28:1 OS: 56:1 Int'l: 44:1
Loma Linda University	2093 in state applicants for 79 places 2581 out of state applicants for 71 places 303 international applicants for 15 places	IS: 26:1 OS: 36:1 Int'l: 20:1
SUNY Upstate	1941 in state applicants for 131 places 2523 out of state applicants for 22 places 439 international applicants for 8 places	IS: 15:1 OS: 115:1 Int'l: 55:1
Rosalind Franklin University, Chicago medical school	1160 in state applicants for 79 places 8238 out of state applicants for 96 places 668 international applicants for 15 places	IS: 15:1 OS: 86:1 Int'l: 45:1
Pennsylvania State University	1057 in state applicants for 72 places 6045 out of state applicants for 70 places 460 international applicants for 3 places	IS: 15:1 OS: 86:1 Int'l: 153:1
University of Hawaii	234 in state applicants for 58 places 1318 out of state applicants for 3 places 116 international applicants for 3 places	IS: 4:1 OS: 439:1 Int'l: 39:1
University of Kentucky	427 in state applicants for 81 places 1419 out of state applicants for 28 places 153 international applicants for 4 places	IS: 5:1 OS: 51:1 Int'l: 38:1
University of Minnesota - Twin Cities	800 in state applicants for 195 places 2764 out of state applicants for 30 places 286 international applicants for 4 places	IS: 4:1 OS: 92:1 Int'l: 72:1
University of Texas Medical School at Southwestern	2672 in state applicants for 199 places 676 out of state applicants for 26 places 137 international applicants for 5 places	IS: 13:1 OS: 26:1 Int'l: 27:1

Table 48. Selection ratios at medical schools in the United States in 2010 [46]

Again, these selection ratios can be helpful, but just as the University of Saskatchewan accepted 39 out-of-province students for the 5 places they needed to fill, some of the universities above may have much better true selection ratios than what the calculated ratios above suggest.

University Rankings

A few agencies rank US medical schools each year using different criteria.

US News and World Report 2011 - Medical Research

This ranking gives each medical school an overall score out of 100 depending on:

1. MCAT average of entering class (13%)
2. GPA average of entering class (6%)
3. Acceptance rate (1%)
4. Faculty-to-student ratio (10%)
5. Peer assessment (20%)
6. Residency Director assessment (20%)
7. Total research activity (15%)
8. Research activity per faculty member (15%)

The top 11 medical schools in this ranking are:

1. Harvard University	5. University of California - San Francisco
2. University of Pennsylvania	5. Yale University
3. Johns Hopkins University	9. University of Washington
4. Washington University in St. Louis	10. Columbia University
5. Duke University	10. University of Michigan - Ann Arbor
5. Stanford University	

The full ranking is available at: http://grad-schools.usnews.rankingsandreviews.com/best-graduate-schools/top-medical-schools/research-rankings

US News and World Report 2011 - Primary Care

This ranking gives each medical school an overall score out of 100 depending on:

1. MCAT average of entering class (9.75%)
2. GPA average of entering class (4.5%)
3. Acceptance rate (0.75%)
4. Faculty-to-student ratio (15%)
5. Peer assessment (25%)
6. Residency Director assessment (15%)
7. Rate of entry into primary care fields (30%)

The top 13 medical schools in this ranking are:

1. University of Washington	8. University of Massachusetts - Worcester
2. University of North Carolina - Chapel Hill	9. University of Pennsylvania
3. Oregon Health and Science University	10. East Carolina University (Brody)
4. University of California - San Francisco	10. University of Alabama - Birmingham
5. University of Colorado - Denver	10. University of Iowa (Carver)
6. University of Minnesota	10. University of Wisconsin - Madison
7. University of Nebraska Medical Center	

The full ranking is available at: http://grad-schools.usnews.rankingsandreviews.com/best-graduate-schools/top-medical-schools/primary-care-rankings

For a critique of the US News and World Report medical school rankings published in the AAMC journal, please see https://www.aamc.org/about/medicalschools/ at the bottom of the page under "America's Best Medical Schools: A Critique of the U.S. News & World Report Rankings"

QS Top Universities - World University Rankings 2010/2011 - Overall

This ranking gives each university an overall score based on several factors including academic peer review, employer review, research and faculty. More details are available on page 118.

The top 10 US universities with medical schools in this ranking are given below:

2. Harvard University	13. Stanford University
3. Yale University	14. Duke University
8. University of Chicago	15. University of Michigan
11. Columbia University	16. Cornell University
12. University of Pennsylvania	17. Johns Hopkins University

The full world ranking is available at: www.topuniversities.com/world-university-rankings

QS Top Universities - World University Rankings 2010/2011 - Medicine

This ranking gives each medical school a ranking based on similar criteria to the QS Top Universities overall ranking outlined above.

The top 10 US universities with medical schools in this ranking are given below:

1. Harvard University	10. University of California, San Diego
5. Stanford University	14. Duke University
6. Yale University	16. Columbia University
7. University of California, Los Angeles	17. University of California, San Francisco
8. Johns Hopkins University	19. University of Chicago

The full world ranking is available at: www.topuniversities.com/university-rankings/world-university-rankings/2010/subject-rankings/life-science-biomedicine

Shanghai Consultancy World University Rankings 2010 - overall

This ranking also gives universities an overall ranking, not a medical school ranking, based on Nobel Prizes, Fields Medals and research. More details are available on page 119.

The top 10 US universities with medical schools in this ranking are given below:

1. Harvard University	12. Cornell University
3. Stanford University	13. University of California, Los Angeles
8. Columbia University	14. University of California, San Diego
9. University of Chicago	15. University of Pennsylvania
11. Yale University	16. University of Washington

The full ranking is available at: www.arwu.org/ARWU2010.jsp

Shanghai Consultancy World University Rankings 2010 - Clinical Medicine and Pharmacy

This ranking gives universities worldwide a ranking for their medical and life science related faculties, based on research, as well ass alumni and faculty awards in medicine. More details are available on page 120.

The top 10 US universities with medical schools in this ranking are given below:

1. Harvard University	6. University of California, Los Angeles
2. University of California, San Francisco	7. University of Texas Southwestern Medical Ctr. Dallas
3. Johns Hopkins University	8. University of Michigan - Ann Arbor
4. University of Washington	9. University of Pittsburgh
5. Columbia University	12. Stanford University

The full ranking is available at: www.arwu.org/FieldMED2010.jsp

International and out-of-state statistics

If you are an international or an out-of-state student, one of the most important considerations when applying to a school is how many international students or out-of-state students this school accepts. In 2010, 8 schools had more than 10 international students who matriculated, and 13 schools had 5-9 international matriculants (see table 49 below). In recent years, over 60 schools have accepted zero international applicants (rejecting approximately 3000 applications from international students each year). There are many schools accepting only 1 or 2 international students as well.

10 or more international matriculants	5 to 9 international matriculants
Case Western Reserve University (10)	Columbia University (8)
Dartmouth College (15)	Harvard University (9)
Loma Linda University (15)	Howard University (8)
Northwestern University (13)	Indiana University (6)
Rosalind Franklin University, Chicago medical school (15)	Jefferson University (7)
Wayne State University (15)	Mt Sinai School of Medicine (6)
Yale University (10)	Saint Louis University (9)
	State University of New York (SUNY) Upstate (8)
	Texas A&M Health Science Center (5)
	Tulane University (5)
	University of Texas Dallas Southwestern Medical Center at Dallas Southwestern Medical School (7)
	University of Texas Medical Branch (7)
	University of Virginia (6)

Table 49: Schools who accepted high numbers of international students in 2010 [46]

It is really important to consider these statistics because if a school accepts very few international students or has not accepted any in the past, it may be better to apply to another school instead. The most authoritative, up-to-date source for this information is the MSAR book [31].

Other websites exist such as the Duke health professionals advisory committee website for international students: www.fiu.edu/~preprofc/International_Students_School_Policies.htm which gives schools' policies from 2005, but will not give specific statistics about interviews and number of applicants for most schools.

Note that many US schools require that at least part of an applicant's undergraduate degree was completed at a US or Canadian university, making it easier in some cases for Canadians to apply than for other internationals.

The AMCAS application

Outline

The AMCAS application is the primary application used by almost all MD programs, as well as several MD-Ph.D programs. The application has several sections: personal information, grades and coursework, choice of schools, 15 activity/award/experience entries and one or more personal statements.

Personal information: Contact information, previous education, history of criminal activity or institutional action, financial information.

Grades and coursework: This section requires you to outline all courses taken in the past as well as the courses you are currently taking or planning to take. Note that AMCAS will review this section and mark any corrections they have had to make. It is thus useful to read your grades section over several times to avoid mistakes as much as possible. The current/future course entries are not binding. They are simply intended to give medical schools an indication of what you are planning to complete before entering medical school. If you change your course plans after your AMCAS application has been submitted, you can notify the medical schools directly of the change [47].

Programs you are applying to: Note that the list of schools you are sending your application to will not be sent to any admissions committees.

Personal Statement: 5,300 characters (including spaces), or roughly one full page. Hard returns ('enter' key) counts as 2 spaces [48]. The topic usually relates directly to why the applicant wishes to attend medical school. For those applying to an MD-Ph.D program through AMCAS, an additional essay explaining the applicant's reasons for wanting to enrol in the MD-Ph.D program (3,000 characters) and a research experience Essay (10,000 character limit) will also be required with the AMCAS application.

Experience entries: This section asks students to list and describe 15 experience entries. These can include:

Paid Employment - Not Military	Conference Attended
Paid Employment - Military	Presentations/Posters
Community Service/Volunteer - Not Medical/Clinical	Publications
Community Service/Volunteer - Medical/Clinical	Extracurricular/Hobbies/Avocations
Research/Lab	Leadership - Not Listed Elsewhere
Teaching/Tutoring	Other
Honors/Awards/Recognition	

Table 50. Categories for AMCAS experience entries [48]

Note that the AAMC is considering making significant changes to the AMCAS application in the 2012-2013 application cycle for the first time since 2001 [49].

Also, keep in mind that using point form in your descriptions will be difficult or impossible since pressing the 'enter' key produces a 'tab' rather than a new line in the final printable copy of the application.

Common errors

There are two mistakes commonly made on the AMCAS application which were mentioned in the 'Application Tips' document supplied by the AAMC in 2010.

Common error 1: Applicants creating multiple entries for related experiences or awards. For example, if you have been on the dean's honour list more than once, create one entry for this and use the description to clarify that you received it on more than one occasion.

Common error 2: Applicants failing to follow application case instructions. For experience titles, enter the information the way you would write it normally, instead of using all capital letters or all lower case. Use normal writing practices as medical schools have indicated that they prefer this format [50].

Dual degree programs

MD/Ph.D and MSTP

As is the case in Canada, the Ph.D portion of this degree can be completed in just about any field. The cost of tuition is covered for most students, and in general, the medical school and other sources of funding will be able to provide a stipend for the student during their degree. Just like in Canada, the program usually requires 7-8 years, although some students take 6 years, while others may take 10 or more [26].

MSTP (Medical Scientist Training Program) is a title given to about one-third of US MD/ Ph.D programs which are given funding by the National Institute of Health. Two examples are Stanford University and the University of Chicago. Other than the source of funding, MSTP programs are no different from MD-Ph.D programs [26].

International students are eligible to apply to most MD-Ph.D programs in the US, however, schools with MSTP programs usually have more difficulty funding international students since NIH/federal funding is only available to U.S. citizens and sometimes permanent residents [51, 52]. These schools can sometimes accept international students by obtaining funds from other sources.

Other dual degree programs

MD/MPH: MD and Master's in Public Health. Available at approximately 70 universities in 2010 [53]. Usually requires 1 additional year. Some schools like Tufts University and Boston University allow students to complete the dual degree in the same time that a normal MD program would require (4 years) [54, 55]. A good website comparing MD/MPH programs is www.amsa.org/AMSA/Homepage/About/Committees/CEH/MDMPHPrograms.aspx

MD/JD: Combined MD and Doctor of Jurisprudence. Offered by 23 schools in 2010 [53]. At most universities including Vanderbilt and the University of Pennsylvania, students accepted to both the law school and medical school can complete the degree in 6 years [56, 57]. Details on how to apply to these programs and the length of study are available on the schools' websites.

MD/MEd: MD and Master's degree in Education. Available only at a few universities (Vanderbilt and University of Pennsylvania in 2009) [53].

MD/MBA: MD and Master's degree in Business Administration. Offered by approximately 50 schools in 2010 [58]. The program usually requires 1 extra year.

MD/MS: MD and Master's degree in Science. Offered by most schools. Usually requires 1 additional year.

Other degrees such as a Master's degree in Arts, a Master's degree in Health Administration or a Master's degree in Biomedical Engineering can also be combined with an MD degree. Details on these programs are available on the schools' websites.

Additional Examinations/prerequisites

Aside from MD/Ph.D programs, most dual degree programs require applicants to apply to the medical school and the other faculty (business school, graduate school etc.) separately, although the degree will still be a joint degree and will take less time than the two degrees separately. This usually means taking any additional examinations (GMAT, LSAT), but in most cases not the GRE. MD-Ph.D applicants can often submit one application which includes essays for both programs. This is the case for Boston University, Harvard and many others. Prerequisite courses usually need to be satisfied for both programs as well.

Course requirements

General course requirements

One very important thing to consider is schools' policies regarding the completion of prerequisite courses. Most schools require you to have completed or have signed up for all prerequisite courses at the time of application. A few schools, like Harvard and Columbia in 2010, required students to have completed their course requirements only before matriculation, meaning that candidates were allowed to apply without having registered for or completed all of the prerequisites [59, 60]. However, at Harvard, the admissions committee states that most successful applicants completed most of the required courses prior to application, and at Columbia, the number of incomplete prerequisite courses at the time of application is limited to one or two [59, 60].

There are several prerequisites common to many schools. These include biology, organic chemistry, inorganic chemistry and physics which are required at almost all schools. English, college mathematics and humanities are also common requirements. It is a good idea to look at prerequisites for the school you want to apply to early as some of them require quite a few courses that many students may not normally take. For example, Johns Hopkins requires 24 credit hours of humanities or social and behavioural sciences [61].

AP and IB credit

Some schools allow you to use AP credits to satisfy prerequisites if certain conditions are met. For example, universities like Penn State require you to have received earned credit toward your degree for the AP courses from your undergraduate institution [62], while some universities like Harvard require only that the credits allowed you to take upper level courses at your university [63]. Several schools including Loma Linda, the University of Nebraska and many other schools either don't accept AP credit toward prerequisite courses or strongly recommend that all AP credit be supplemented with higher level subjects [64, 65]. A free listing of US medical schools that do not accept AP/IB credit and that accept AP/IB credit only if supplemented is available from www.colorado.edu/aac/noapib.htm, although the listing is a few years old. It is important that you double check the policies from the admissions offices or the schools' website for the programs you wish to apply to.

Several of the schools that accept AP credit still set strict limitations on how much AP credit you can use and what subjects you can use it for. Two examples are Harvard and Johns Hopkins [63, 66]. In 2010, both schools allowed a maximum of half the inorganic chemistry requirement to be satisfied by AP credit. All applicants were required to take an additional semester of inorganic chemistry at university. Another example is Cornell Medical School, which only allows students to use AP credit toward the physics requirement [67].

If you have received credit for prerequisites, you need to check the policies regarding AP credit for the schools you wish to apply to. Doing this early in your undergraduate degree will allow you to take any additional courses you need to take.

Essay requirements

In addition to one personal statement and the mini-essays/activity descriptions on the AMCAS application, many schools will ask for an essay or a few essays in their secondary applications. Below is a table outlining the secondary application requirements of a few schools in the

2008-2009 admission cycle. Note that essay questions change each year and this is just to give you an idea of the type off essays you may be asked to write for your application. The information was obtained from students who completed the secondary applications in the 2008-2009 admissions cycle:

School	# of essays	Summarized topics	Length
Boston University	1 required, 1 optional	1.Asked to provide a narrative or timeline to describe features of educational history that may be particularly relevant to the admissions committee. 2.Optional essay on anything else that may be relevant to the admissions committee	1. 2000 characters 2. 500 words
Case Western	1 required, 1 optional	1.What have you found most challenging to this point in your life and how has it helped shaped you as a person 2.Optional essay on anything else that may be relevant to the admissions committee	1. 1 page 2. 1 page
Columbia	5	1.What satisfaction do you expect to receive from your activities as a physician 2.In what collegiate extracurricular activities did you engage 3.Please list collegiate honors, awards, and memberships in honorary societies 4. About how many hours per week, if any, did you spend in work for which you were recompensed during the college year 5.What sort of work did you do (include summer employment)	1. 2475 characters 2. 760 characters 3. 345 characters 4. 200 characters 5. 1100 characters
Cornell	1	Brief statement giving your reasons for applying to Weill Cornell Medical College	200 words
Dartmouth	2	1.Indicate your plans for the current academic year. If in school, list courses. If working, let us know something about the nature of your job. 2.Share something about yourself not addressed elsewhere in the application that could be helpful to the Admissions committee when reviewing your file	1. No length restriction 2. No length restriction

Emory	2	1.Briefly describe any health related experience and/or research experience including time and frequency of your involvement	1. Approximately 100 words
		2.Briefly describe your interest in Emory	2. Approximately 100 words
Georgetown	1	Why you chose to apply to Georgetown and how you think your education at Georgetown will prepare you to become a physician for the future	5000 Characters
Mt. Sinai	2	1.What makes you special, someone who will add to the Mount Sinai community	1. 250 words
		2.Indicate the reasons for your specific interest in Mount Sinai	2. 200 words
Penn State	3	1.Explain the negative aspects of medicine that you consider in making this career decision	1. 50 words
		2.Is there a unique aspect of your application that should be considered by the admissions committee	2. 50 words
		3.Explain why you decided to apply to Penn State College of Medicine	3. 50 words
University of Chicago	2	1. Describe yourself as a great fit for the University of Chicago Pritzker School of Medicine, including examples of past service, community, clinical, educational, and research purposes. Also discuss your future goals	1. 3500 characters
		2. Tell us about a difficult or challenging situation that you have encountered and how you dealt with it. Identify both the coping skills that you called upon to resolve the dilemma, and the support person(s) from whom you sought advice.	2. 2400 characters

Table 51. Secondary application essay requirements at US medical schools in the 2008-2009 admissions cycle

Although unofficial, one of the best places to find secondary application questions from current and previous years is the student doctor network [68]. Almost all previous and current application questions and requirements are posted by other applicants.

Reference letter requirements

Most schools in the US encourage students to send a pre-health advisory committee letter if this exists at their school. At some schools like Boston University and Creighton University, this letter fulfils the minimum letter requirement, while other schools like Harvard will only count it as one letter toward their maximum [69-71]. Many schools like the Florida International University require 1 or 2 letters from science faculty [72], while others like Harvard require at least one non-science faculty letter as well [71]. For students having done extensive research or having spent time outside of school, additional letters from employers or research supervisors may be appropriate depending on the school, particularly for MD/Ph.D programs.

Details on individual schools' requirements are listed on their websites and for those schools that accept reference letters through AMCAS, details are available in the applicant instruction manual [47].

Note that although some schools have a high maximum number of letters or say that there is no limit, these schools often have specific letters they are looking for and do not encourage students to send too many additional letters. These recommendations vary widely. One example is the University of Washington: "Letters of reference from current employers may be advantageous; however, too many additional letters are discouraged." [73]. Because of the variability in guidelines, it is a good idea to see the school's website or sometimes even contact the school if unsure.

Timeline of the application process

AMCAS release date, processing time and deadline

The AMCAS application is released on or around May 5th each year, and AMCAS will begin accepting transcripts at letters of recommendation at this time. AMCAS begins accepting and processing completed applications the first week of June. Since it takes 4-6 weeks to process [47], your target date for submitting the application should be no later than the third week of June [44] (or as early as possible in the summer). If you are applying to the Early Decision Program (EDP), the deadline for sending your completed application and your transcripts is on or around August 1st each year. If you are applying through the standard route, the application deadline differs from one school to another. You should receive an email from AMCAS confirming reception of your application. You can also call +1 (202) 828 0600 which is an automated system where you can check the status of your application at any time.

Transcripts timeline

Your transcripts need to be submitted directly to AMCAS. Problems with transcripts are the number one reason for processing delays, and it has happened in the past that AMCAS has lost student transcripts. To avoid having something like this delay your application, your transcripts should be sent to AMCAS along with the AMCAS transcript request form, which is available once you have created an account with AMCAS. When you request transcripts from your undergraduate university's registrar office, it is important that you insist that they attach the AMCAS transcript request form along with your transcripts. AMCAS starts accepting transcripts on or around May 5th [74] and although some students may need to wait for their term grades to be released, it is always a good idea to send your transcripts early to avoid any delay in the processing of your application. The deadline for sending your transcripts to AMCAS is on or around August 1st if you are applying to the EDP and 14 days after the school's application deadline if you are applying through the standard application process. You can check the receipt of transcripts online when you log into your AMCAS application. It is important that you follow up regularly with your application after you have sent all the required documents. It is the applicant who is responsible for notifying AMCAS if their designated schools have not received application material within two to four weeks from the date their AMCAS application was processed [75].

Reference letter timeline

Some schools require reference letters to be submitted through AMCAS while others require reference letters to be submitted directly to their admissions office. Schools participating in the AMCAS reference letter system are listed at www.aamc.org/students/amcas/faq/amcasletters.htm. There are three key things to consider when asking your referees for your reference letters:

1. Getting your application complete as soon as possible
2. Giving your referees enough time and informing them of why you want to go into medicine
3. Meeting with your referees in person before leaving school if you will not be able to meet with them in the summer

Let us bear in mind that the AMCAS application takes 4-6 weeks to process, that reference letters submitted through AMCAS take at most 3 weeks to process and that your reference letters will not be forwarded to the schools before your AMCAS application has finished processing.

We thus think that in many cases, it makes the most sense to focus on your AMCAS application first and submit it as soon as possible. Then, during the 4-6 week processing period, you should give your personal statement and activity descriptions to your referees. If your referees take 3-4 weeks to write the letters, they will arrive within 4-5 weeks at schools not using the AMCAS reference letter system, and will arrive within 4-7 weeks at schools using the AMCAS system.

For professors however, you will want to set up a meeting with them before leaving school if you are going away for the summer. In most cases this is much more effective than sending them an email during the summer. You can then begin working on your application and forward your personal statement and 15 activity/award descriptions to your referees once completed as well as any material you did not provide them with during the first meeting.

Most schools consider your application complete once they have received their minimum reference letter requirement even if you plan on sending more letters.

Note about pre-health advisory committees

Some undergraduate institutions like Yale University provide health professional evaluations, premedical committee letters or other similar letters of evaluation for students [44]. If this is the case, you may need to submit a personal statement and reference letters to these offices well before the targets listed above so they can complete their evaluations and send them to the schools you apply to. See your undergraduate institution's career office to find out if this is the case.

Early Decision Program

Students participating in EDP are initially allowed to select only one school to apply to. If accepted at this school, they must accept the offer and cannot apply to any other schools. If not accepted, applicants may join the normal pool of applicants after they have been notified by the

EDP school. The deadline for EDP application is on or around August 1st, although some schools have set different deadlines in the past. Approximately 80 schools participate in EDP. Information regarding which schools have EDP programs and how many students were accepted through EDP the previous year are available in the MSAR book [31]. More information is also available on the AAMC website [76]. Medical schools are required to notify you of their decision on or around October 1st each year. If unsuccessful, most schools like Penn State and Baylor College keep your application on file and consider you for regular admission as well. **If you are a very strong applicant and wish to save yourself the trouble and cost of applying to several schools, you might want to consider applying through early decision.** The program carries its risks, since applicants who are not selected do not join the normal pool of applicants until they are notified of their negative decision by October 1st - **carrying the disadvantage of a very late application at rolling admission schools.**

Sample timeline

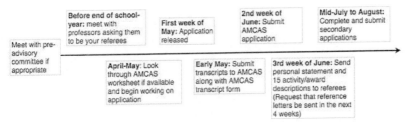

Figure 2. Timeline of the U.S. Application process

Deferring entry

It is possible at many schools to defer entry for a year or more once accepted. Information on which schools allow deferment is included in the MSAR book [31]. Some schools ask students to sign an agreement stating that they will not apply to other medical schools during their deferment, while others permit you to submit more applications during the deferment period [31]. Specific information on deferment policies can be obtained directly from the schools.

School by school (high international acceptance)

Harvard University

Programs

Students can apply to the New Pathway Program and the Health Sciences and Technology program (HST) offered by Harvard University and the Massachusetts Institute of Technology (MIT). The New Pathway Program has a strong focus on small group tutorial sessions, problem based learning and the patient-doctor relationship. The HST program is in some ways more academically rigorous, and is oriented more toward students who want to pursue a career in biomedical research.

Degree requirement

Applicants must have at least three years of undergraduate work and a bachelor's degree before matriculation. No preference is given to a specific major.

Course requirements

One year of biology with lab experience, two years of chemistry with lab experience (which may include biochemistry and/or organic chemistry), one year of physics, one year of calculus and some non science courses with expository writing. Students applying to the HST program are required to have a calculus course that includes differential equations, and linear algebra. A year of calculus based physics is also required. Harvard has also just launched a new list of course requirements that students can use now if they wish, but will become mandatory in 2016. In the new requirements, the laboratory components of the science courses are not obligatory. Also, computational skills/mathematics, analytical and writing skills, as well as language (foreign language not required but beneficial) are all considered important. Also, courses in literature, languages, the arts, humanities, and the social sciences (e.g., psychology, sociology, anthropology, and ethics) are encouraged. At least 16 hours should be completed in these areas. In addition, familiarity with computers is necessary. Honors courses and research are encouraged, because they permit a student to explore an area of knowledge in depth and provide a scholarly experience that will facilitate a lifelong habit of self-education.

GPA requirement

There is no minimum GPA requirement. The average GPA for the 2010 entering class was 3.8.

Based on Medical School Admissions Requirements 2009-2010, published by the AAMC and the university websites.

MCAT requirement

All applicants must write the MCAT. There is no minimum MCAT requirement. The average MCAT score for the 2010 entering was 35.6. VR - 10.78; PS - 12.48; BS - 12.36.

Application fee

The secondary application fee is USD85. The fee is waived for students who received an AMCAS fee waiver.

Selection Formula

Harvard is one of the handful of schools in the US that does not use a rolling admissions policy. All aspects of the file are reviewed prior to inviting students for interview including grades, MCAT scores, applicant's essay, the letters of recommendation, employment, life experiences and experience in the health field, including research and community work. The HST program is particularly interested in students who show potential for research in their career.

Application documents

All applicants receive the Harvard supplemental application after submitting their AMCAS application. In the past, students who are re-applying, students who have already graduated and students applying to the HST or dual-degree programs have been required to submit additional essays. In the 2010-2011 application cycle, applicants to the HST program were asked to write the following:

The HST Division represents a unique environment that draws on the combined resources of Harvard University and MIT to provide a distinct preclinical education tailored to preparing students for a career as a physician-scientist, with an emphasis on quantitative and analytic approaches to areas of critical importance to medicine. Please explain your interest in HST, including how your prior experiences, including research, have prepared you for this challenging opportunity. In lieu of identifying specific HST faculty or research opportunities, please focus on your particular experiences, interests and aspirations. Please limit your comments to the equivalent of one page of single spaced text with a font size of 10 or 12." Students can also submit up to 6 letters of recommendation, including at least two letters from science professors with whom they have taken classes, and one from a non-science professor. Students also need to submit letters from all of their research supervisors. Those who have graduated and worked are advised to submit a letter from their place of employment. Premedical advisory committee packets count as one letter toward the 6 letter maximum.

Interview

There is a mandatory interview held at the medical school for both programs. Applicants invited to interview for the NP or HST program meet one-on-one with members of the admissions committee.

Interview (Cont'd)

HST applicants also interview with a faculty member and student together. Students applying for the MD/PhD program have additional interviews. The interviewers usually have access to the applicant's AMCAS essay and HST essay prior to the interview.

Application deadline

Supplemental applications must be submitted by November 1st, 2011. AMCAS must also receive letters of recommendation by this date.

Cost of studies 2011-2012

Approximately USD47,500 per year in tuition fees. Approximately 70% of students receive financial assistance every year.

Additional information

Students can only apply to the medical school twice.

Statistics

For the August 2010 entry class, there were 5,324 completed applications received. Every year, there are approximately 800-1000 students interviewed for the 135 places in the New Pathway Program and the 30 places available in the HST program. Note that students who do not have a baccalaureate or advanced degree from an institution in the United States or Canada are rarely accepted for admission. Students who have studied outside North America are encouraged to supplement their education with at least one year of college or university level training in North America. In the class entering in August 2010, students were selected from 74 undergraduate institutions, 32 states and 10 foreign countries. 73% had majored in the sciences and 6% held advanced degrees. 21% of students are from groups that are traditionally underrepresented in medicine and the class ranges in age from 20-33.

Contact

Office of the Committee on Admissions
Harvard Medical School
25 Shattuck Street
Boston, Massachusetts, USA 02115-6092
Tel: +1 617 432 1550
Admissions_Office@hms.harvard.edu

Loma Linda University

Degree requirement

The university recommends that students complete an undergraduate degree prior to matriculation, however, exceptional students may be eligible to apply after completion of a minimum of 90 semester hours (135 quarter hours). Students from schools outside the US and Canada must complete at least one year of study at an accredited school in the US. No preference is given to science or non-science majors. Applicants from schools outside the United States and Canada are required to present a minimum of one year of study at an accredited United States or Canadian college or university prior to applying for admission.

Course requirements

One year of biology or zoology, one year of general chemistry, one year of organic chemistry and one year of physics. Students are also advised to study English, Religion and/or ethics as required to satisfy their degree requirements. Biochemistry is strongly recommended, and introductory statistics is also recommended. Students are also encouraged to include humanities and social science courses that prepare them for their role as a physician. The prerequisites must be completed prior to matriculation.

GPA requirement

For the 2010 entering class, the average GPA was 3.78.

MCAT requirement

All applicants must write the MCAT. MCAT scores more than three years old (prior to 2009 for the 2012-2013 application cycle) are not accepted. The average MCAT score for the 2010 entering class cycle was 31, with an average of 10 in each subsection.

Application fee

The secondary application fee is approximately USD75. The fee is waived for students who received an AMCAS fee waiver.

Selection Formula

Students are selected for interview based on their entire application including grades, MCAT scores, letters of reference, AMCAS applications and supplementary applications. Students are strongly encouraged to gain experience where they are directly involved in providing health care. The school is owned and operated by the Seventh-day Adventist Church, thus, preference is given to members of the church. However, each year applicants not affiliated with the church are admitted provided they demonstrate a commitment to Christian principles and are well suited for medicine. There is a mandatory interview.

Application documents

Students receive instructions on how to complete the secondary application after they apply to the school. In the past, the supplementary application has included seven 750 character essays and two 250 character response. In the 2010-2011 and the 2011-2012 application cycle, the questions in the supplementary application were the following:

1. Describe the extent and source of your knowledge of Loma Linda University School of Medicine (LLUSM). (750 characters max)

2. What makes LLUSM particularly attractive to you? (750 characters max)

3. What qualities make you a desirable candidate for admission to LLUSM? (750 characters max)

4. Discuss how your spiritual experience has influenced your life and how you integrate it into your daily life. (750 characters max)

5. What experiences in your life would illustrate your perspective on service to others? (750 characters max)

6. As a Christian educational institution the medical curriculum integrates spiritual, ethical, and relational issues from a Christian perspective into the practice of medicine. Weekly chapel services and religion courses are part of this program. Please respond to the above as it relates to your personal educational and career goals. (750 characters max)

7. Loma Linda University is a Seventh-day Adventist institution that has lifestyle expectations that include abstinence from alcohol, tobacco and illicit drugs/ substances in all forms. In the past year, have you used any of these substances? If so, which one(s)? (250 characters max)

8. If accepted to LLUSM, are you willing to abide by the lifestyle policies of Loma Linda University School of Medicine? (250 characters max)

9. Describe your involvement with your religious group (750 characters max)

Regarding reference letters, if the student's school provides a pre-health advisory committee recommendation or packet of recommendations, this must be submitted as part of the application and no other letters need to be submitted. If this is not available, the school requires a minimum of three letters of recommendation from individuals who know the applicant well. The school requires that one letter come from a science professor who has taught the applicant, and recommends that the other letters come from "a physician, employer, pastor (or other clergy), or other persons who know the applicant." The supplementary application form includes a reference form that referees can choose to use, or they can choose to write the letter in their own style.

Interview
There is a mandatory interview held at the university. The interviews are usually one on one interviews lasting approximately 45 minutes. The interviewers usually have access to the applicant's file beforehand.

Application deadline
Students applying through the Early Decision Program must submit their AMCAS applications by August 1st, and their supplementary applications by September 1st. Applicants will hear the final decision by October 1st. For students applying through the standard route, the supplementary application deadline is November 15th.

Cost of studies 2011-2012
Approximately USD45,600 per year.

Additional information
Weekly chapel services are part of the program. Students have also been asked in previous years if they have used any alcohol, tobacco or drugs/substances in the past year as part of the supplementary application.

Statistics
In the 2010-2011 application cycle, there were approximately 4977 applicants, with a total of 375 students interviewed for the 165 places available. 303 international applicants applied, 33 were interviewed, and 15 matriculated into the program.

Contact

Tel: +1 909 558 4467 or +1 800 422 4558
admissions.sm@llu.edu

Rosalind Franklin University, Chicago Medical School

Degree requirement

Applicants must have completed 90 hours of undergraduate study to apply.

Course requirements

One year of the following are required: biology with lab experience, inorganic chemistry with lab experience, organic chemistry with lab experience and physics with lab experience. One year course in calculus and a semester course in statistics are advised, but not required. A one semester in organic chemistry supplemented by a semester course in biochemistry can substitute the normal organic chemistry requirement.

GPA requirement

For the 2010 entry class, the average GPA was 3.75. The lowest 10% of accepted students had a GPA of approximately 3.38 or lower, and the highest 10% of students had GPA of 3.96 or higher [133].

MCAT requirement

All applicants must write the MCAT. For the 2012 entering class, the oldest scores accepted are from 2009. The average MCAT score for the 2010 entering class was 31Q [133].

Application fee

The secondary application fee is USD105. The fee is waived for students who received an AMCAS fee waiver.

Selection Formula

Students are strongly encouraged to submit their application early. In selecting students for admission, all aspects of the application are considered including grades, MCAT scores, essays, references and interviews.

Application documents

Students receive a link to a secondary application after they apply to the school. In the 2008-2009 application cycle, the questions in the supplementary application were the following:

1. Future physicians and research scientists are expected to work in an inter-professional environment, and Rosalind Franklin University allows students to learn in such an environment. Describe what you envision to be your greatest challenge in working on an inter-professional team.

2. What do you believe will be your greatest strength as a physician? What will be your greatest weakness?

3. Chicago Medical School promotes a diverse learning environment, including diversity in the student body. Keeping a broad definition of diversity in mind, how would you contribute to student diversity?

Application documents (Cont'd)

4. Why do you feel Rosalind Franklin University is the "best fit" for your learning style and personality?

In the 2009-2010 application cycle and the 2010-2011 application cycle, the questions in the supplementary application were the following:

1. At Rosalind Franklin University, we celebrate and support a Life in Discovery. Briefly describe what a Life in Discovery means to you.

2. Future physicians, research scientists, and other healthcare professionals are expected to work in an inter-professional environment, and Rosalind Franklin University allows students to learn in such an environment. Describe what you envision to be your greatest challenge in working on an inter-professional team.

3. How did you hear of Rosalind Franklin University?

Applicants must also submit either a composite/committee letter from their school or three individual letters of evaluation. The university suggests submitting two letters from professors under whom the applicant has studied, and a third letter from a person who have supervised in their work experiences or who are uniquely qualified to comment on their potential for the study of medicine.

Interview

There is a mandatory interview held at the university. Most interviews in the past have been on one interviews, although some students have had group interviews. Interviews usually last between 30 - 45 minutes. In previous years, most interviewers have had access to the applicants' files beforehand.

Application deadline

The supplementary application, including all additional documents must be received by December 1st, 2011.

Cost of studies 2011-2012

Approximately USD46,873 per year.

Statistics

For entry in 2010, there were approximately 10,066 applications received. Approximately 684 students were interviewed for the roughly 190 places available. This included roughly 668 international applicants, of which 54 were interviewed and 15 matriculated into the program [133].

Contact

Tel: +1 847 578 3204
cms.admissions@rosalindfranklin.edu

State University of New York (SUNY) Upstate University

Credit requirement

Applicants must have at least 90 semester credits of undergraduate work at an institution in the US or Canada.

Course requirements

One year of biology, general chemistry, organic chemistry, physics and English are required. They must be completed with a grade of "B" or higher prior to enrolling. The university also recommends several courses that are not required: physiology, genetics, cell biology and biochemistry, microbiology and immunology. For non science courses, the university recommends psychology, statistics and experimental design courses as well as courses related to public health, ethics and communication skills. Advanced placement credits can be used to fulfill prerequisite requirements provided they are listed on the official transcript of the student's primary undergraduate application. Note that the university recommends that applicants complete higher level science courses to be competitive for admission.

GPA requirement

The average GPA for the class of 2012 was 3.59.

MCAT requirement

All applicants must write the MCAT. MCAT scores from tests written more than 3 years prior to the application date are not accepted. The average MCAT score for the class of 2012 was 30.08.

Application fee

The secondary application fee is approximately USD100. The fee is waived for students who received an AMCAS fee waiver.

Selection Formula

Grades and MCAT scores are the two most heavily weighted factors in the initial interview selection. Non-academic factors including clinical experience, volunteer work, the AMCAS application and the letters of recommendation are also taken into account. Note that slight preference is given to students from New York state, but the school accepts many out of state applicants each year. There is a mandatory interview as well. After the interview, the applicant's file qualifications and the interview performance are used to make a final admissions decision.

Application documents

Students receive a link to a secondary application after they apply to the school. There have not been any additional essays required in previous years. Students currently completing their undergraduate studies should submit a Pre-health advisor letter, or if none exists at their university, they should submit two letters of recommendation from faculty in different departments. At least one must be from a science faculty member.

Application documents (cont'd)

Graduate students must also submit a letter of recommendation from a graduate advisor or department chairperson. Students who graduated from an undergraduate program more than 5 years ago and are employed full-time can submit one letter from a science faculty and one letter from a current supervisor.

Interview

Each applicant is interviewed independently by an MD or a faculty member and a current student, usually in their 2nd, 3rd or 4th year of medical school. Most interviews last between 30 and 45 minutes. Interviewers usually have access to the applicant's file before the interview.

Application deadline

For those applying for early decision, the AMCAS application is due August 1st, and all the materials must be submitted by August 15th. For those applying through the standard route, the full AMCAS application must be received by October 15th. The secondary application must be submitted by December 1st.

Cost of studies 2011-2012

For New York State residents = approximately USD27,090 per year, and for non-New York State residents = approximately USD53,650 per year. Students can apply for some merit based scholarships during their spring semester.

International students are not eligible for financial aid from the university.

Additional information

At the start of the third year, approximately 25% of the class moves to the Binghamton Clinical Campus one hour south of Syracuse. Most students who go decide to stay there for their fourth year. Application counseling is available through the school. Sessions are offered once a month and can be scheduled online or by calling the office of admissions.

Statistics

For the 2010 entering class, 4903 applied and 746 were interviewed for the 161 places available. There were 439 international applicants, of whom 19 were interviewed and 8 matriculated [133].

Contact

Office of Student Admissions
1215 Weiskotten Hall
766 Irving Avenue
Syracuse, NY 13210
Tel: +1 315 464 4570 or +1 800 736 2171
admiss@upstate.edu

Yale University

Degree requirement

Applicants must have at least 3 academic years of undergraduate coursework prior to matriculation. The undergraduate work must have been completed in the US or Canada. No preference is given to any field of undergraduate study.

Course requirements

One year of general biology or zoology, one year of general chemistry, one year of organic chemistry and one year of physics. The courses should have a laboratory component. Acceptable courses extend over 1 year and are given 6 to 8 semester hours credit. Community college coursework may be accepted in fulfillment of prerequisites on a case by case basis.

GPA requirement

In 2010, the average GPA was 3.86. The lowest 10% of accepted students had a GPA of 3.62 or lower, and the highest 10% of students had a GPA of 3.99. There is no minimum GPA requirement.

MCAT requirement

All applicants must write the MCAT. For entry in August 2012, the earliest test date accepted in January 2008 and the latest date is September 2011. The average MCAT for the 2010 entering class was 37R. There is no minimum MCAT score requirement.

Application fee

The school does **not** use a rolling admissions policy. The secondary application fee is USD85. The fee is waived for students who received an AMCAS fee waiver.

Selection Formula

All aspects of the applicant's file are taken into consideration when selecting candidates for interview. After the interview, all aspects of the students file including grades, MCAT scores, essays, extra-curricular achievements, letters of reference and the interview are taken into account to make a final decision.

Application documents

The supplemental application can be found online and can submitted before or after the AMCAS application. The supplemental application deadline is August 31, 2011 for EDP applicants and November 15, 2011 for all other applicants. In the 2010-2011 and 2011-2012 application cycles, the supplemental application has included a 500 word essay discussing the applicant's interest in Yale Medical School, and a second optional 500 word essay on any information not previously discussed. Applicants must also submit a letter from their pre-medical advisory committee, or, if none exists at their university, they should submit at least three letters (maximum of five letters) of recommendation, including two individuals in the sciences who are familiar with the applicant.

Interview

In-person interviews are required, and invitations are sent out by email from August to February. Applicants who are invited for an interview will meet with two members of Committee on Admissions. Most interviews last between 30 and 45 minutes.

Application deadline

For those applying for early decision, the AMCAS application is due August 1st, and the all materials must be submitted by August 31st. Applicants receive a final decision by October 1st. For those applying through the standard route, the full AMCAS application must be received by October 15th. The secondary application must be submitted by November 15th. Note that for students who apply before receiving their MCAT scores, the admissions office encourages them **not** to wait to submit their application. The school will wait to process their application until their new scores arrive, but students should submit their application as soon as it is ready.

Cost of studies 2010-2011

Approximately USD41,100 per year for tuition fees. Living expenses and health insurance adds approximately USD20,000 per year. International students are eligible for financial aid.

Additional information

Students can choose to do a fifth year in the program, tuition free. Students can spend the extra year at Yale doing research, or can work at another university, or can choose to do clinical work at home or abroad.

Statistics

Last year, there were approximately 5,232 applications received. Approximately 794 students were interviewed for the roughly 100 places available. This included roughly 437 international applicants, of which 52 were interviewed and 10 matriculated into the program. 225 applicants were in state and 4,570 applicants were out of state. 43 in state applicants were interviewed and 8 matriculated. 699 out of state applicants were interviewed and 82 matriculated.

Contact

Yale School of Medicine
Office of Admissions
367 Cedar Street
New Haven, CT 06510
Tel: +1 203 785 2643
medical.admissions@yale.edu

Australia

Graduate Entry medical programs

The 12 English taught graduate entry medical programs are listed below:

1. Australian National University
2. Deakin University
3. Flinders University
4. Griffith University
5. Monash University, Gippsland
6. The University of Melbourne
7. The University of Notre Dame Australia, Fremantle
8. The University of Notre Dame Australia, Sydney
9. The University of Queensland
10. The University of Sydney (not using GEMSAS)
11. The University of Western Australia
12. The University of Wollongong

New admissions process

The GAMSAT Consortium is introducing an on-line application and matching system for applicants to Australian graduate-entry medical schools. GEMSAS will increase the number of preferences available for applicants to medical schools and provide an equitable and transparent allocation process.

Applicants for a medical school place starting in 2012 need to apply through the Graduate Medical Admissions Centre (GMAC) at http://gmac.acer.edu.au/register. Once applications are complete, GEMSAS takes over the processing of applications, including calculation of GPAs and application of school selection rules.

Features of GEMSAS are:

1. Applicants will submit an on-line application to ACER, which is then forwarded to GEMSAS.
2. Applicants will be offered up to six preferences.

3. Applicants who completed an undergraduate degree at most Australian universities will have their results retrieved automatically. This will significantly reduce number of applicants required to obtain original transcripts of results.

4. GPAs will be calculated using all available results, including 2011 first semester results for applicants completing the final year of a qualifying degree.

5. Individual medical schools' selection rules will be applied to each preference listed by applicants.

6. Institutions will allocate applicants to interview at one of their preferred medical schools.

7. Interview scores will be standardised for use by all medical schools so that the interview score can be incorporated into the selection methods of all preferred medical schools.

8. Following interviews, institutions will use GEMSAS to allocate successful applicants to offers of a place according to their preferences and the selection rules of preferred medical schools. Applicants completing the final year of their qualifying degree will receive provisional offers.

9. GEMSAS will notify applicants if they are unsuccessful in gaining an offer.

10. Following the release of final semester results, provisional offers will be confirmed for applicants with satisfactory GPAs.

11. An applicant who has not achieved a satisfactory GPA will be informed that the offer has been withdrawn. The place will be offered to the highest ranked unsuccessful applicant at that medical school.

Please note that at the time of publication of this guidebook, GEMSAS is not yet certain if they will manage international student applications through GEMSAS next year but they are in discussion with the schools about that. If this does happen, then international applicants would have the choice of applying directly to the universities or through GEMSAS. If they apply through GEMSAS they would be offered up to six preferences. This information comes directly from the GEMSAS office.

Places of international applicants

There are 12 graduate entry programs in Australia offered by 11 universities. The estimated number of places available for international students in the 2012-2013 application cycle at each Australian medical school is:

- Up to 20 places at the Australian National University
- 16 places at Deakin University
- 25 places at Flinders University

- Up to 60 at Melbourne Medical School
- 20 at Monash University
- 170 at the University of Queensland
- 80 at the University of Sydney
- 5 at the University of Western Australia
- 12 at the University of Wollongong

University Rankings

QS Top Universities - World University Rankings 2010/2011 - Overall

This ranking gives each university an overall score based on several factors including academic peer review, employer review, research and faculty. More details are available on page 118.

The top 10 Australian universities with graduate entry medical schools in this ranking are given below:

20. Australian National University	89. University of Western Australia
37. University of Sydney	251. Flinders University
38. University of Melbourne	267. University of Wollongong
43. University of Queensland	323. Griffith University
61. Monash University	362. Deakin University

The full world ranking is available at: www.topuniversities.com/world-university-rankings

QS Top Universities - World University Rankings 2010/2011 - Medicine

This ranking gives each medical school a ranking based on similar criteria to the QS Top Universities overall ranking outlined above.

The top 7 Australian universities with graduate entry medical schools in this ranking are given below:

15. University of Melbourne	51. University of Western Australia
29. University of Sydney	151. Flinders University
33. University of Queensland	
36. Monash University	
46. Australian National University	

The full world ranking is available at: www.topuniversities.com/university-rankings/world-university-rankings/2010/subject-rankings/life-science-biomedicine

Deakin University, Griffith University, the University of Notre Dame and the University of Wollongong were not ranked in the top 200 schools overall in 2011 according to this ranking.

Shanghai Consultancy World University Rankings 2010 - overall

This ranking also gives universities an overall ranking, not a medical school ranking, based on Nobel Prizes, Fields Medals and research. More details are available on page 119.

The top 8 Australian universities with graduate entry medical schools in this ranking are given below:

59. Australian National University	151. Monash University
62. University of Melbourne	301. Flinders University
92. University of Sydney	301. University of Wollongong
101. University of Queensland	
101. University of Western Australia	

Deakin University, Griffith University and the University of Notre Dame were not ranked in the top 500 schools overall in 2010 according to this ranking.

The full ranking is available at: www.arwu.org/ARWU2010.jsp

Shanghai Consultancy World University Rankings 2010 - Clinical Medicine and Pharmacy

This ranking gives universities worldwide a ranking for their medical and life science related faculties, based on research, as well ass alumni and faculty awards in medicine. More details are available on page 120.

The top 3 Australian universities with graduate entry medical schools in this ranking are given below:

> 41. University of Melbourne
> 51. University of Queensland
> 51. University of Western Australia

The other Australian medical schools were not ranked in the top 100 in 2010 according to this ranking.

The full ranking is available at: www.arwu.org/FieldMED2010.jsp

School by School

Australian National University

Degree requirement
Successful completion of a bachelor's degree in any subject at the time of matriculation.

Course requirements
None.

GPA requirement
The minimum weighted GPA cutoff is normally 34 out of 42. The weighted GPA is calculated by assigning each course a grade between 0 and 7. Only courses counting toward the undergraduate degree are considered. Although the exact grading depends on each students' university, a rough guide on how percentage scores are converted to scores from 0 to 7 is provided in table 52. An average score from 0 to 7 is calculated for the most recent 3 years, and students finishing a three year undergraduate program will have their third year average score (from 0 to 7) multiplied by 3, the second year score multiplied by two and the first year score multiplied by one. The scores are then added to give a total out of 42. Students in four or five year undergraduate programs will only have the most recent three full-time years counted in the calculation, with the final year score tripled and the second last year doubled. For students who have completed two undergraduate degrees, the most recent degree will be used to calculate the GPA.

Examination requirements
Students with less than 55 on the GAMSAT are unlikely to be interviewed. International students can take the GAMSAT or the MCAT. For the GAMSAT, students require 55 overall with no less than 50 on any section. For the MCAT, scores are only valid for two years. Thus, students applying for entry in 2012 can write the exam between January 2009 and May 2011, inclusive. Students writing the MCAT must obtain minimum scores of 8 on each multiple choice section and M on the writing section.

Selection Formula
Students must first meet the minimum weighted GPA and minimum examination cutoffs. Applicants are then ranked for interview with a weighting of approximately 50% weighted GPA and 50% GAMSAT/MCAT score. Students can also be granted a small improvement in their ranking for completing honours or graduate degrees. The highest ranking applicants are invited for interview.

Information obtained from the school's websites and by contacting the admissions offices directly.

Selection formula (cont'd)

After the interview, those who perform satisfactorily are offered places in the program according to their rank. Those who performed satisfactorily but were not ranked high enough to be offered a place may be placed on a waiting list.

Application documents

Brief application form.

Interview

There is a mandatory interview conducted by telephone. For applicants who live in Australia or can come to the university, they can choose to interview with the Australian nationals, usually at the end of September. Telephone interviews are usually conducted in July and August. At the school, the interview includes observation in a group setting as well as MMI stations.

Cost of studies 20011-2012

Approximately AUD54,048 per year for international students.

Statistics

There are approximately 20 places available each year for international students, and 90 places available for local students.

Contact

Admissions Officer
Medical School
Frank Fenner Building #42
The Australian National University
Canberra ACT 0200
Tel: +61 2 6125 1304
medadmissions@anu.edu.au

Number of Credit hours the applicant has completed	Credit hours that the admissions committee will drop
>80	7
75-79	6.5
70-74	6
65-69	5.5
60-64	5
55-59	4.5
50-54	4
<50	0

Table 52. Weighted GPA conversion guideline at the Australian National University.

Deakin University

Degree requirement
Successful completion of a bachelor's degree in any subject at the time of matriculation.

Course requirements
None.

GPA requirement
Students must have a GPA of 5.0 on a 7.0 scale (which the university estimates to be an average of approximately 70% for international students). The median GPA in the 2010-2011 application cycle was 6.2, with a range of 5.0 to 7.0.

Examination requirements
Local applicants have to write the GAMSAT. International applicants can write the GAMSAT or the MCAT. For the GAMSAT, a minimum average score of 50 and minimum scores of 50 on all three sections are required. Students writing the MCAT must have minimum scores of 8/8/8/M to be eligible to apply.

Selection Formula
Students are selected for interview based on their GAMSAT/MCAT scores and GPA. Each of these carries roughly 50% of the pre-interview weighting. Additional points (up to 2%) are allocated for students who completed a major component of biomedical sciences or health sciences as part of their undergraduate degree. Applicants with one year of clinical practice as a health professional (nursing, dentistry, pharmacy etc.) also receive a 2% bonus. After the interview, applicants are given a score which is calculated from the GAMSAT/MCAT score, the weighted GPA and the interview. Each of the 3 elements count equally.

Application documents
Brief application form and a copy of the applicant's CV.

Interview
For local applicants, interviews at the university are MMI format with ten 5 minutes stations. Interviews for international applicants are either conducted in person in the applicant's home country or the country in which they are studying, or are conducted by videoconference. The interview is either one-on-one or a panel style interview with up to three interviewers. The questions are generally determined before the interview starts and focus on the medical school's course outcomes which include:
1. Communication skills
2. Commitment to rural practice
3. Evidence-based practice
4. Self-directed learning
5. Teamwork
6. Motivation for a career in Medicine
7. Social Justice
8. Professionalism
9. Effective use of resources

Cost of studies 2011-2012
Approximately AUD52,290 per year for international students.

Statistics
In the 2011-2012 application cycle, there were re approximately 16 places available for international students and approximately 163 places available for local applicants.

Contact
Deakin University, School of Health, Medicine, Nursing, and Behavioral Science
Geelong Campus at Waurn Ponds
Building ka, Level 3, Room 205
Tel: +61 3 522 72929
hmnbs-support@deakin.edu.au

Flinders University

Minimum credit requirement

Successful completion of a bachelor's degree in any subject at the time of matriculation.

Course requirements

None.

GPA requirement

Students who have completed a degree requiring more than three years only have the final three years counted in their weighted GPA calculation. The final year is weighted times 3, and the second last year is weighted times two. Higher degree grades are not included in the calculation. A GPA of around 3.3 out of 4.0 is suggested as a guideline for the minimum requirement, but students with higher MCAT scores or higher grades at the end of their degree (since these are weighted double and triple the first year grades) may be interviewed with lower GPAs.

Examination requirements

All local applicants must write the GAMSAT exam. International applicants can write the GAMSAT or the MCAT. GAMSAT scores are valid for two years, and if the exam is written more than once, applicants can choose which of the two scores the admissions committee will use. A minimum score is set each year for every section of the test based on the applicant pool. MCAT scores must be no more than three years old

(for the June 17, 2011 application deadline, the earliest MCAT scores can be from August 2008). An MCAT score of 30P is suggested as a cutoff guideline, but students with a good GPA may be interviewed with a lower MCAT score. As a guideline for international applicants, the GAMSAT scores required for interview have been a little lower than those for the Australian applicant pool. The GAMSAT cutoffs have ranged from 56-62 in recent years, with a cutoff of 61 in 2011. Applicants also needed section scores of at least 50, 45 and 50. Australian students with high GPAs and slightly lower GAMSAT scores were also accepted.

Selection Formula

Local applicants are ranked for interview primarily based of their GAMSAT results. Applicants with outstanding GPAs may also be interviewed despite lower GAMSAT scores. For international applicants, students are selected for interview based on their GPA and GAMSAT or MCAT scores. After the interview, applicants are ranked by combining scores on a scale of 100 for admission based on their GPA, GAMSAT/MCAT scores and interview. These 3 components are weighted equally in determining the entry score for ranking.

Application documents

Brief application form.

Interview

There is a mandatory interview conducted at the university, at international locations determined each year (previous locations have included Los Angeles and Seattle in the US, Calgary, Toronto and Ottawa in Canada, and Singapore) or by phone. Interviews are usually held in July and August with 1-3 interviewers that assess the applicants motivation for medicine, learning style, team skills, communication skills, pro-social attitude, personal management, self-evaluation skills, and approach to decision making, among other qualities. The interview is semi-structured, meaning most questions and scenarios are determined before the interview starts.

Cost of studies 2011-2012

AUD45,000 per year for international students. There are no scholarships available for international students.

Statistics

There are up to 25 places available for international students, and approximately 111 places available for local students in the graduate entry program.

Contact

International Office, The Flinders University of South Australia, GPO Box 2100
Adelaide. South Australia. 5001
Tel: +61 8 8204 4262
Toll free USA : +1 800 686 3562
intl.office@flinders.edu.au

Griffith University

First intake
This program will take its first intake in 2013.

Degree requirement
Successful completion of a bachelor's degree in any subject at the time of matriculation.

Course requirements
None.

GPA requirement
Students must have a GPA of 5.0 on a 7.0 scale or 2.67 on a 4.0 scale. Only courses in the undergraduate degree are used to calculate the GPA. The GPA is not included in the calculation of the final score used to rank applications. However, it will be used as a tie-breaker if necessary. Applicants with a masters or PhD will be automatically deemed to have met the GPA requirement.

Examination requirements
All students must write the GAMSAT. The cutoff varies each year depending on the applicant pool performance, so no set cutoff is decided until the applications are received.

Selection Formula
As long as applicants meet the minimum GPA requirement and score a minimum of 50 in each section of the GAMSAT, they are selected for the interview based on their GAMSAT result only. After the interview, students are ranked based on the following formula: 50% GAMSAT score and 50% interview score. The top ranking applicants are offered admission.

Interview
The interview is MMI format. The assessors will have no information about the applicant prior to the interview. The total length of the interview is 2.5 hours and each applicant is rated by the individual assessors on a criterion-defined rating scale.

Cost of studies 2010-2011
AUD50,000 per year for international students.

Statistics
In the 2012-2013 application cycle, there are a maximum of 10 places available for international students [1].

Contact
Gold Coast campus, Loading Bay
Little High Street, Southport Qld 4215
Tel: +61 7 5678 0704
medicine@griffith.edu.au
A list of international agents is available from: www.griffith.edu.au/international/international-degree-students/how-to-apply/recruitment-agents

Melbourne Medical School

Degree requirement
Successful completion of a bachelor's degree in any subject at the time of matriculation.

Course requirements
Applicants must have completed second year university anatomy, physiology and biochemistry.

GPA requirement
Only the final three years are counted in the weighted GPA. The final year is weighted times 3, and the second last year is weighted times two. Applicants with a post graduate degree may be given special consideration.

Examination requirements
Local applicants must write the GAMSAT. International applicants can write the GAMSAT or the MCAT, unless they are residing in Australia at the time of the GAMSAT [1]. The GAMSAT is valid for two years (2010 and 2011 for 2012 entry), and the MCAT is valid for three years (January 2009 to May 2011 for 2012 entry).

Selection Formula
For international applicants, selection for interview is based on a combination of GPA and GAMSAT/MCAT scores. The university interviews 25% more students than they plan to accept. After the interview, the GPA, GAMSAT/MCAT scores and interview are weighted equally in ranking students for admission.

Application documents
Brief application form. Students must select two referees who may be contacted by the university.

Interview
There is a mandatory interview. Interviews at the university are held in the MMI format. International applicants located overseas are offered a modified MMI by Skype.

Cost of studies 2011-2012
AUD60,000 per year for international students. Some scholarships are available for international students.

Statistics
Of the 330 places available, 60 are available to international students and local students willing to pay the full cost of their education. Typically, more than half of these 60 places are filled by international students [1]. The other 270 places are subsidized by the government and only open to local students.

Contact
Tel: +61 3 8344 5890
sc-mdhs@unimelb.edu.au
International representatives are listed at: offshore.unimelb.edu.au/OverseasReps.aspx

Monash University, Gippsland Medical School

Degree requirement

Successful completion of a bachelor's degree in any subject at the time of matriculation.

Course requirements

None.

GPA requirement

Students who have completed a degree requiring more than three years only have the final three years counted in their weighted GPA calculation. The final year is weighted times 3, and the second last year is weighted times two. Honours year grades are included, and bonus points are given for PhD and master's degrees. A minimum weighted GPA of 5.0 out of 7.0 is required to be considered.

Examination requirements

Local applicants must write the GAMSAT. International applicants can write the GAMSAT or the MCAT. For the GAMSAT, a minimum score of 50 is required on all sections of the exam, and a total score cutoff is determined each year. The overall cutoff has been between 55 and 60 for the past three years [1]. Students writing the MCAT must have minimum scores of 8/8/8/M

Selection Formula

As long as applicants meet the minimum GPA requirement and score a minimum of 50 in each section of the GAMSAT, they are selected for the interview based on their GAMSAT results only. After the interview, students are ranked based on the following formula: 40% GAMSAT score and 60% interview score. The top ranking applicants are offered admission.

Application documents

Brief application form.

Interview

Interviews are usually held in Gippsland, Australia in September, in Singapore in August and in some previous years in Vancouver, Canada in August as well. The school may conduct interviews in Canada again in 2013 [1]. Interviews include two stations lasting 10 minute each. There is no interview by telephone or videoconference.

Cost of studies 2011-2012

AUD56,800 per year for international students.

Statistics

There are up to 65 places for Australian citizens, and up to 20 places for international students.

Contact

Monash University, Gippsland campus
Northways Road, Churchill, Victoria 3842
Tel: +61 3 9902 6445
gippslandmed@med.monash.edu.au

University of Queensland

Degree requirement
Successful completion of a bachelor's degree in any subject at the time of matriculation.

Course requirements
None.

GPA requirement
Students who have completed a degree requiring more than three years only have the final three years counted in their weighted GPA calculation. The final year is weighted times 3, and the second last year is weighted times two. A minimum weighted GPA of 5.0 out of 7.0 is required to be considered. This generally translates to approximately 2.67 on a 4.0 scale where 2.0 is a passing grade, or approximately 2.00 where 1.0 is a passing grade.

Examination requirements
Local applicants must write the GAMSAT. International applicants can write the GAMSAT or the MCAT. For the GAMSAT, a minimum score of 50 is required on all three sections of the exam. Students writing the MCAT are expected to have minimum scores of 8/8/8/M. Students may also apply if they have a score of 7 on only one section, but still have a total minimum score of 24M. Note that American students on US federal loans must submit an MCAT score. For local applicants, the GAMSAT cutoff in 2011 was between 64 and 66 depending on which applicant pool was considered. Note that cutoffs change every year.

Selection Formula
As long as applicants meet the minimum GPA requirement and score a minimum of 50 in each section of the GAMSAT, they are ranked based on their GAMSAT result only. The GPA may be used as a tie breaker for applicants with the same GAMSAT results. The top ranked applicants are then offered admission. The school uses a rolling application system, meaning that students gain an advantage by applying earlier in the application cycle.

Application documents
Brief application form. Students can apply directly to the university, via ACER, or through an international representative. For US citizens applying to the Ochsner/Queensland Program, students will need to answer three short essay questions on their educational objectives, and how they believe the program will enhance their educational goals.

Interview
None.

Cost of studies 2011-2012
Approximately AUD49,920 per year for international students. There are some scholarships available for international students.

Statistics

In the 2012-2013 application cycle, there are approximately 170 places available for international applicants, including the 40 places available to US citizens and permanent residents wishing to complete the last two years of their education in the Ochsner Health System in New Orleans, Louisiana. Most international students to date have been from Canada, but there are also international students from other countries including the US, UK, Singapore and Malaysia.

Contact

The University of Queensland
Mayne Medical Building, Herston Road, Herston QLD 4006
Telephone: +61 7 334 65206
Email: international@som.uq.edu.au
International representatives are listed at: www.uq.edu.au/international/index.html?page=18255

University of Notre Dame

Programs
Graduate entry programs are offered on both the Sydney campus and the Fremantle Campus.

Nationality restrictions
International students are NOT eligible to apply to either program.

Degree requirement
Successful completion of a bachelor's degree in any subject at the time of matriculation.

Course requirements
None.

GPA requirement
Students must have a GPA of 5.0 on a 7.0 scale. At the Fremantle campus, a bonus of up to 0.5 can be granted for masters or PhD degrees at the discretion of the admissions committee. This bonus is almost always given in full to candidates with master's degrees or PhDs [1]. At both campuses, the GPA is calculated on the most recently completed three years in the undergraduate degree.

Examination requirements
All students must write the GAMSAT. At the Fremantle campus, the minimum score to obtain an interview is 50 overall, and there may be individual section score cutoffs and higher overall cutoff scores required based on the applicant pool. At the Sydney campus, the minimum scores are 50 overall and 50 on each component of the test.

Selection Formula
Students are selected for interview based on their GAMSAT scores, GPA, and evaluation of personal qualities and motivation to study medicine from the application. After the interview at Fremantle campus, the interview comprises 60% of the post-interview score, and the rest of the application comprises 40%. At the Sydney campus, the GPA, GAMSAT, SOMAS form and interview are all weighted roughly equally to determine who is granted admission [1].

Application documents
The application form includes a list of activities related to leadership, service to the community, working with others and other extra-curricular activities. Students are also required to submit 2-3 written references, their CV, and a 750 word personal statement describing their personal qualities and motivation to study, reasons for wanting to study at Notre Dame, and reasons for wanting to study medicine.

Interview
There are mandatory interviews for both programs with a panel of interviewers. The panel usually consists of 3 interviewers, often a medical practitioner, an academic and a community representative [1]. The interviews last approximately 40 minutes.

Cost of studies 2011-2012

Approximately AUD29,230 per year for full paying domestic students and AUD9,080 for Commonwealth supported domestic students.

Statistics

In the 2011-2012 application cycle, there were approximately 800 applicants for the 100 places available at the Fremantle Campus [1] and roughly 1200 applicants for the 112 places available at the Sydney campus [1].

Contact

Admissions Office, Fremantle
The University of Notre Dame Australia, Fremantle,
21 High Street, Fremantle WA 6959
Tel: +61 8 9433 0540
admissions@nd.edu.au

Admissions Office, Sydney
The University of Notre Dame Australia, Sydney
140 Broadway, Broadway NSW 2007
Tel: +61 (2) 8204 4430
sydneyadmissions@nd.edu.au

University of Sydney

Minimum credit requirement
Successful completion of a bachelor's degree in any subject at the time of matriculation.

Course requirements
None.

GPA requirement
In previous years, students who had completed a degree requiring more than three years only had the final three years counted in their GPA calculation, and all years were weighted equally. A minimum weighted GPA of 5.5 out of 7.0 is required to be considered. This is equal to approximately 2.7 out of 4.0 for North American students and a lower second class for UK students). Postgraduate courses are not counted in the GPA calculation. Applicants from Canada can contact AustraLearn to help them calculate their effective GPA.

Examination requirements
Local applicants must write the GAMSAT. International applicants can write the GAMSAT or the MCAT. For the GAMSAT, a minimum score of 50 is required on all three sections of the exam. In 2012, the cutoff was 67 and in 2011, it was 62. The cutoffs change yearly so this is just to be used as a guide. Students can write the exam more than once and choose which test date they would like the admissions committee to use.

Students writing the MCAT must have minimum scores of 8/8/8/M to be eligible to apply. Note that GAMSAT and MCAT results are only valid for two years. Thus, for the GAMSAT, students applying for entry in 2012 must have taken the exam in 2010 or 2011. For MCAT results, students who applied for entry in January 2012 must have taken the exam between January 2009 and May 7, 2011.

Selection Formula
For local applicants who meet the minimum GPA of 5.5, the selection for interview is based in their overall GAMSAT score only. Note that candidates with a research PhD are automatically interviewed if they meet the minimum GAMSAT/MCAT qualifications, and are given 3 bonus percentage points in their total final score. No extra points are given for other degrees. Local applicants need to meet or exceed a minimum MMI score that will be set. Then, they are ranked based on a score calculated as follows: 50% GAMSAT and 50% MMI performance. The highest ranked applicants are offered a place and the highest GAMSAT score is used as a tie breaker. The exact selection formula for international applicants is not disclosed.

Application documents
Brief application form. Students can submit their application directly to the university office or to one of the university's representatives abroad.

Interview

There is a mandatory interview of MMI style conducted by video conference over Skype. It lasts 81 minutes and consists of 9 stations, each lasting 7 minutes. Interviews are conducted by panelists selected from the faculty, medical student body and lay community. Interviewers are not provided with any information about applicants.

Cost of studies 2011-2012

AUD59,280 per year for international students. Some scholarships are available for international students.

Additional information

Students rank their preferences for clinical school (where some of the first two years and most of the final two years are spent) when they apply. Note that this is the one medical programs that does not accept applications via ACER and thus all applications must be sent directly to the university or an official representative.

Statistics

For local applicants, the university interviews between 1.4 and 1.6 times the total places available and there were 228 places available in 2011. In the 2012-2013 application cycle, up to 80 international students will be accepted into the program.

Additional information

Students rank their preferences for clinical school (where some of the first two years and most of the final two years are spent) when they apply. Note that this is the one medical program that does not accept applications via ACER and all applications must thus be directly to the university or an official representative.

Contact

Sydney Medical School
Edward Ford Building, A27
The University of Sydney
NSW 2006
Australia
Tel: +61 2 9351 3132
medicine.admissions@sydney.edu.au
A list of international representatives is available from:
sydney.edu.au/internationaloffice/agents/

University of Western Australia

Degree requirement
Successful completion of a bachelor's degree in any subject at the time of matriculation.

Course requirements
None.

GPA requirement
Students must have a GPA of 5.5 on a 7.0 scale (estimated by the school to be an average of roughly 65%). All years are weighted equally, and graduate degrees are included in the average.

Examination requirements
Local applicants must write the GAMSAT. International applicants can write the GAMSAT or the MCAT. For the GAMSAT, a minimum score is set each year for each section (usually at least 50), and for the overall score. Students with a section score marginally below 50 should contact the admissions office as a high GPA or overall GAMSAT score may compensate for this. Students writing the MCAT must have minimum scores of 8/8/8/M to apply. GAMSAT scores are valid for 2 years.

Selection Formula
Students are selected for interview based on their GAMSAT/MCAT scores and GPA, which are given equal weight. After the interview, the test scores, GPA and interview scores are given equal weight to determine which applicants are selected for admission.

Application documents
Brief application form.

Interview
Interviews are held in Perth each September, as well as in Singapore and Malaysia for applicants from these countries. Interviews last 25-40 minutes and are conducted by a community member and a university representative. A moderator or an interviewer in training will sometimes join. The questions asked can focus on a variety of criteria including ability to work with others, decision making, and social responsibility. There may also be a 25 minute listening skills exercise where applicants view media clips and answer multiple choice questions.

Application documents
Brief application form.

Additional information
The 2012 entry is the last intake for graduate entry to the MBBS. UWA will be moving to a postgraduate Doctor of medicine course which will start in 2012. For this reason, there will be no option to defer a 2012 offer.

Statistics

Of the 65 places available in the 2012-2013 application cycle, approximately 5 will be granted to international applicants. In the 2011-2012 application cycle there were roughly 580 applicants, of which 380 were received after the preference system screening. 100 applicants were selected for interview.

Contact

Tel: +61 8 6488 4646 / (08) 6488 8500
meddentadmissions@uwa.edu.au
International representatives are listed at: www.studyat.uwa.edu.au/undergraduate/apply/agents

University of Wollongong

Degree requirement
Successful completion of a bachelor's degree in any subject at the time of matriculation.

Course requirements
None.

GPA requirement
Students must have a GPA of 2.8 on a 4.0 scale or 5.0 on a 7 point scale to be eligible to apply. The university may set a higher GPA cutoff to receive an interview invitation depending on the applicant pool each year. Students who have completed a degree requiring more than three years only have the final three years counted in their GPA calculation. The final year is weighted times 3, and the second last year is weighted times two. Students completing their third year of a three year of undergraduate program at the time of application will not have their third year counted in the calculation, but can still apply and will have their second year counted times two in the weighted GPA calculation.

Examination requirements
Local applicants must write the GAMSAT. International applicants can write the GAMSAT or the MCAT. For the GAMSAT, a minimum score of 50 is required on all three sections of the exam, as well as an overall score of 50. Students writing the MCAT must have minimum scores of 24M to be eligible to apply. Only tests from 2 years prior to application are accepted. Note that the university may set higher test score cutoffs for interview each year depending on the applicant pool.

Selection Formula
Students are selected for interview based on their GPA, GAMSAT/MCAT scores and their University of Wollongong portfolio score. After the interview, students are selected for admission based on their interview scores and portfolio. The University uses a rolling admission process, starting with admission for the early application cycle applicants.

Application documents
Students submit a University of Wollongong portfolio, which asks them to list their extracurricular activities and volunteer work that demonstrate experience in the following areas:
1. Leadership
2. Capacity to work with others
3. Service ethic
4. Diversity of experience
5. Higher level of performance in an area of human endeavor
6. Academic experience

Application documents (cont'd)

Note that there is also a component asking about rural residency which is **not** scored for international applicants. If the applicant has lived in a rural area or has attended school in a rural area however, this should still be included in the portfolio as this will be viewed positively by the admissions committee. The portfolio template and guidelines for completing the form are available online through the university website. International applicants can apply through ACER, directly to the school, or through AustraLearn.

Interview

There is a mandatory interview conducted using the best available technology (teleconference or videoconference). Interviews are usually held between April and September. For North American applicants, interviews are held in several locations in the USA or Canada. International interviews are done in panel format and assess several criteria including teamwork, problem solving ability, leadership and self-reflection.

Cost of studies 2011-2012

AUD43,300 per year for international students. Some scholarships are available for international students.

Additional information

There is an early application round in late March through AustraLearn or directly to the school in addition to the standard ACER application route in June. There are approximately 56 students at the Wollongong campus and 28 at the Shoalhaven campus.

Statistics

In the 2012-2013 application cycle, there were 72 places for local applicants and 12 places for international students.

Contact

Graduate School of Medicine
Building 28
University of Wollongong
NSW, 2522, Australia
Tel: +61 2 4221 4111
gsm_info@uow.edu.au
The international representative for Canadian and US applicants is AustraLearn, www.degreesoverseas.com
Canada Tel: +1 800 980 0033 ext. 140
canada@degreesoverseas.com
US Tel: +1 800 980 0033 ext. 108
info@degreesoverseas.com

Caribbean
Medical programs in English

This is not an exhaustive list. Medical schools in Cuba are not included and there may be programs missing from this list as new schools are opening every year in the Caribbean Islands.

1. All American Institute of Medical Sciences
2. American Global University School of Medicine
3. American International Medical University
4. American International School of Medicine
5. American University of the Caribbean School of Medicine
6. Atlantic University School of Medicine
7. Aureus University School of Medicine
8. Avalon University School of Medicine
9. Caribbean Medical University School of Medicine
10. Central American Health Sciences University, Belize medical college
11. Destiny University School of Medicine and Health Sciences
12. GreenHeart Medical University
13. International American University, College of Medicine
14. International University of Health Sciences School of Medicine
15. Medical University of the Americas
16. Ross University School of Medicine
17. Saba University School of Medicine
18. Spartan Health Sciences University School of Medicine
19. St George's University
20. St James School of Medicine - 2 campuses Bonaire and Anguilla
21. St Martinus University Faculty of Medicine
22. St Matthew's University School of Medicine
23. Trinity School of Medicine
24. University Autonoma de Guadalajara School of Medicine
25. University of Health Sciences Antigua
26. University of Medicine and Health Sciences - St Kitts
27. University of Sint Eustatius School of Medicine
28. University of West Indies: 3 campuses Cave Hill in Barbados, Mona in Jamaica and St Augustine in Trinidad

29. Windsor University School of Medicine
30. Xavier University School of Medicine at Aruba

University rankings

To the best of our knowledge, there is no agency ranking Caribbean medical schools officially. The Caribbean medical schools were not listed in the QS World University Rankings, or the Shanghai Consulting Group rankings.

Things to consider

Some of the most important things to consider when choosing a Caribbean school are the accreditation of the school, where you will do your clinical rotations (including the opportunities at Green Book hospitals for those that want to complete their residencies in the US), USMLE pass rates (although these are often not a fair indicator for the reasons described below) and the opportunities to complete residency in the country of your choice. You may also want to consider how long the medical school has been established for and students comments in forums such as the student doctor network forum.

Accreditation

Not all Caribbean medial schools are accredited, even if their websites say that they are accredited and that they allow you to write the USMLE. This means that not all degrees are accepted in the US, the UK and Canada. In California, Florida, New York and New Jersey, the state evaluates foreign medical schools individually, and most Caribbean medical schools are not accredited in those states. The Caribbean schools that have obtained accreditations in every American state are St George's University, American University of the Caribbean, Ross School of Medicine, University of the West Indies and SABA School of Medicine.

The state of california posts the schools which are disapproved at http://www.medbd.ca.gov/applicant/schools_ unapproved.html

The list of approved schools is available from http://www.medbd.ca.gov/applicant/schools_recognized.html

Note that in most countries, licensure is based on the year of study. This means that if a school is licensed starting in 2010, a physician who graduated from that school in 2008 will not be licensed to practice in that state or country. For this reason, even if a school says it will receive accreditation soon, it is important to note that this will not be valid if you study there before they receive approval.

Green book hospitals

Although many medical schools in the Caribbean allow students to complete their rotations in the US, not all US rotations are viewed equally by state licensing committees. Many states require that if an applicant does core rotations in the US (core rotations are mandatory, non-elective rotations such as surgery, family medicine, pediatrics, etc.) every US rotation must be completed at a hospital that satisfies two criteria: (1) the hospital must be affiliated with an accredited US medical schools and (2) the hospitals must have a residency program in the field of the core clerkship. Hospitals meeting these criteria are called "green book hospitals" because the list of these hospitals was first published in a green colored book. The list is now available using the link below.

www.acgme.org/adspublic/

This is very very important for students applying to the Caribbean. If a student from the Caribbean completes their core surgery rotation at a hospital that is not affiliated with a medical school, or that does not have a residency program in surgery, the student will not be allowed to practice as a physician in any state with a green book requirement. The law may differ from state to state, and it can be difficult to find this information online. One example of a green book law is available from the links below, however, it can be easier to contact the state medical licensing boards directly.

In Florida, the core clerkships in medicine, surgery, obstetrics-gynecology, and pediatrics need to be completed either in the country of the medical school or at Green Book hospitals as defined by the State of Florida. For more details, visit the Department of State, Library website at https://www.flrules.org/ and search "64B8-4.018".

For those wanting to complete their residency in the US or practice there, schools' affiliations with green book hospitals is an important consideration, as well as the number of green book hospital rotations compared to the number of students.

USMLE pass rates are not always a good indicator

The USMLE pass rates can be helpful to look at from school to school, since there is large variation in the passing rates from school to school. The pass rates for the USMLE step 1 varied from 19.4% in the poorest performing Caribbean country to 84.4% in the best performing Caribbean country [15]. Some Caribbean countries have students take the USMLE Step 1 an average of 2.84 times to pass, while others take just 1.19 attempts on average [15]. These are sometimes published on the schools' websites, and sometimes they can be obtained from scientific studies on Caribbean medical schools, such as the study mentioned above entitled: "Medical education in the Caribbean: a longitudinal study of United States medical licensing examination performance, 2000-2009". It is available for purchase or through university libraries. For example, the Cayman Islands, where only St. Matthews University School of Medicine is present, had a pass rate of 51% (out of 349 test takers) in 2009. The pass rate in Dominica, where there were two schools in 2009, was 88.2% (of the 901 test takers) [15].

It is important to consider, however, that some schools only allow the students who are already performing well to write the USMLE, and may even ask students who are not doing well to repeat years of medical school or leave the school. For example, a school may require students to pass the NBME Comprehensive Basic Science Exam or the Kaplan Comprehensive Exam, or both (sometimes called "Comp" exams), before taking the USMLE. It may be the case that 60% of people pass the Comp exams, and of those 60% that pass, 95% pass the USMLE. It can be helpful to look into the school's exam policies, their pass rates, and the policy on failing Comp exams and USMLE exams before choosing a Caribbean medical school. This information is usually available in the student handbook, or from the school directly. For example, the Ross University student handbook is available from http://www.rossu.edu/medical-school/shared-content/documents/RUSM_STUDENT_HANDBOOK.pdf and describes the conditions under which students can be withdrawn from the program, including how many times they can attempt the NBME Comprehensive Basic Science Examination, and how many attempts they are allowed on the USMLE steps. In this case, there are three attempts allowed for all of these exams in 2011 at Ross University.

Getting a residency position in your country

One of the most important factors in choosing a school will be the opportunity to complete a residency in the country of your choice after you graduate. Note that many Canadians who have difficulty going directly to Canada for residency decide to complete their residency in the US, then hope to move to Canada once they complete their residency training.

Some schools say that their students usually get their first or second choices for residency, but this can be a misleading statement, both for US and Caribbean schools. It is a misleading statement because in the matching process, applicants first apply to schools, then receive interviews, and then create their rank list only from the schools that interview them. For example, if an applicant applies to eight programs, and only interviews at 2 programs, he or she will only rank those two programs. This applicant would technically have received their first or second choice, although they may have wanted to go to one of the six places where they were not interviewed. Still, many students from the Caribbean match where they want to. The match lists for St. George's University, American University of the Caribbean, Ross School of Medicine, and SABA School of Medicine are provided in the school specific sections below.

When to apply

Students often assume that September is the best start date to apply for, and for some students it may be the best start date, but it is not the best date for everyone. It is often the most competitive session to apply for, and for Canadians in particular, having to start in September usually means finishing in mid-June, with residency starting in July. This can cause a compressed schedule without extra time to study for the MCCQE and possibly other international tests like the USMLE Step 2 before the start of residency.

School by School

American University of the Caribbean

Degree requirement

Successful completion of a bachelor's degree in any subject. Experience in healthcare is also strongly recommended.

Course requirements

Full year of biology, English, general chemistry, organic chemistry and physics. Also some courses are recommended but not required: mathematics, humanities and social sciences.

GPA requirement

For the 2009 entering class, the average cumulative GPA was 3.23 and the average science GPA was 3.05. There is no minimum GPA requirement, however, students are expected to have about 2.8/4.0 overall and 2.8/4.0 in their science courses to be competitive. A strong application in other areas may compensate for this.

MCAT requirement

For the 2009 entering class, the average MCAT score was 25. MCAT scores must be less than 5 years old. All students, including non-North Americans, must write the MCAT. The minimum expected MCAT score is 20, and students are rarely admitted with a lower score.

Selection Formula

The university uses rolling admissions and thus, although there is no deadline for application, applying early significantly increases the chance of admission. Applicants should plan to complete their application 4 to 5 months prior to the term they wish to apply for. The program start dates are in September, January and May. The university may request a personal interview at the discretion of the admissions committee. Selection for interview is based on the entire application. After the interview, all aspects of the application are considered in selecting students for admission.

Application documents

The application includes a list of employment and volunteer experiences. Students also submit official letters from a pre-medical advisory committee or a minimum of 2 reference letters from science professors who have taught the applicant. Finally, a personal statement summarizing the applicant's interest in medicine, their goals and personal attributes that make them suitable for a career in medicine, and the skills and values they believe a physician should possess to practice in the 21st century.

Application documents (cont'd)

The essay is limited to 750 words. Information on relevant experience should also be included in the essay. Note that the university accepts additional reference letters from professors or employers with details regarding previous medical experience. Also note that all foreign transcripts need to be evaluated by the World Education Services, Inc. (www.wes.org), or another accredited evaluation organization.

Interview

The university may request an interview at the discretion of the admissions committee. The interview is either done at a location near the applicant, or is done by phone.

Cost of studies 2010-2011

The total cost for all semesters = approximately USD162,000, for an average annual tuition of approximately USD40,500 if the degree is completed in 48 months. Some merit based scholarships are available through the university.

Additional information

The university's clinical curriculum is composed of 42 weeks of core clerkships and 30 weeks of electives. Core clerkships are completed at affiliated sites lin the United States and the United Kingdom. Core clerkship sites in Ireland may be offered again in the future but are currently on hold.

Electives can be done in the US, UK, Canada or abroad.

Statistics

In 2008, 88% of admitted students were U.S citizens or permanent residents, 9% were Canadians and 4% were from other countries [40]. There are approximately 100 students admitted in the spring, 100 students admitted in January, and 200 students admitted in September each year. There are total of approximately 1700 - 1800 applicants per year, and roughly 40% of applicants are offered a place in the program.

Residency match list

The university's match list is available from: www.aucmed.edu/alumni/residency-appointments.html

Contact

Medical Education Administrative Services
901 Ponce de Leon Blvd, Suite 700, Coral Gables, FL, USA 33134
Tel: +1 305 446 0600
North American recruiters are listed at www.aucmed.edu/prospective/contact-recruiter.html

Information obtained from the school's websites and by contacting the admissions offices directly.

Ross University

Degree requirement
Successful completion of at least 90 credits of undergraduate studies.

Course requirements
Full year of biology, English, general chemistry, organic chemistry and physics. A half semester of mathematics is also required (courses which include calculus or statistics are preferred). In addition to the prerequisite courses, the university strongly recommends that applicants complete coursework that provides a broad background in the humanities as part of their pre-medical education.

GPA requirement
Currently, the average undergraduate GPA of enrolled students is roughly 3.4. The undergraduate GPA of accepted students ranges from 2.7 to 4.0.

MCAT requirement
There is no minimum MCAT requirement, but most competitive applicants have MCAT scores of 17 or higher [1]. The average MCAT for matriculating students is approximately 27 [1]. Note that applicants who have taken the MCAT more than once must submit all test results prior to enrollment. All students, including non-North Americans, must write the MCAT.

Selection Formula
The academic year is divided into 3 semesters at Ross University starting in September, January and May, and students can apply to start the program in any of these three terms. Ross University uses a rolling admissions system. When the number of accepted students exceeds the number of students that can be accommodated in the class, a waiting list is established. Students who apply for the fall term may be put on the waiting list, in which case they are automatically accepted for the spring (January) term. Students should note that the class is usually full 6 months before the start date [1]. The application for enrollment in September usually closes the earliest [1]. Selection for interview is based on the entire application. After the interview, all aspects of the application are considered in selecting students for admission.

Application documents
The application process includes an application form and either a pre-medical advisory committee letter or at least one academic (preferably a science professor) [1] and one professional letter (which can be a previous employer, volunteer coordinator, a physician the applicant has shadowed to name a few examples) [1].

Application documents (cont'd)

The application form includes personal information, academic history, a list of academic awards, research and publications, MCAT scores, a list of extra-curricular activities since high school, a list of clinical experience in hospitals, clinics or other health professional practice as well as a personal essay. The personal essay should state in no more than 300 words why you want to become a physician and what you can bring to the world of medical health in today's multicultural society. Also note that all foreign transcripts need to be evaluated by an accredited evaluation organization in order to be accepted.

Interview

The admission process includes a mandatory interview. The interview is either done at a location near the applicant in Canada or the US, or is done by phone.

Cost of studies 2010-2011

The total cost for all semesters = approximately USD165,000, for an average annual tuition of approximately USD41,000 if the degree is completed in 48 months.

Statistics

There are approximately 350 students matriculating at the start of each trimester. Roughly 75% of students who apply are granted an interview, and roughly 50% of students who are interviewed are offered a place in the program [1]. Approximately 98% of students are Canadian or US residents.

Residency match list

The university's match list is available from: www.rossu.edu/medical-school/residencyappointments.cfm

Contact

Ross University, Administrative Office
630 US Highway 1,
North Brunswick, NJ 08902
Tel: +1 877 767 7338
admissions@RossU.edu
North American recruiters are listed at: www.rossu.edu/contact/territory.cfm

SABA University

Degree requirement
Successful completion of at least 90 credits of undergraduate studies. An undergraduate degree is recommended but not required. Students are also required to have 50 hours of direct patient care experience. This experience can be fulfilled through volunteering in a hospital setting, shadowing physicians or paid work. Students who do not meet this requirement at the time of application must fulfill it prior to matriculation.

Course requirements
Full year of biology or zoology, full year of general chemistry, and a full year of either organic chemistry or biochemistry. Exceptions for completion of the pre-requisite courses are considered on an individual basis. In addition to the pre-requisite courses, a broad background in humanities, social sciences or physical sciences and computer skills is recommended. Additional courses in biology and related subjects is also strongly recommended, and students who complete courses like "anatomy and physiology, genetics, biochemistry, molecular biology and psychology/interpersonal skills and communication" are given preference for admission.

GPA requirement
There is no minimum GPA requirement to apply. The admissions office looks at overall scores, but also places a significant emphasis on grade trends and courses chosen.

MCAT requirement
The MCAT is required for all applicants who are US citizens, nationals, or permanent residents. In addition, the MCAT is strongly recommended for all other applicants, and is required for the following 3 applicant groups:
1. Students with outdated required science coursework (>5 yrs. old)
2. Students who completed required science coursework at a community college
3. Students with 'C' grades or lower in the required science coursework

Selection Formula
There are three entering classes per year: January, May and September. Students may apply at any time during the year. Since the school uses rolling admission, applicants are encouraged to submit their documents early, between 6 to 12 months in advance, to ensure that their files are ready for consideration at least three months prior to the trimester of their first choice. Selection for interview is based on the entire application. After the interview, all aspects of the application are considered in selecting students for admission.

Selection formula (cont'd)

Note that the time of year with the most applications for roughly the same number of places is September, each year. Students tend to have significantly better chances if they apply for one of the other start dates (see page 354 for more information on this) [1].

Application documents

The application includes an application form and a minimum of 2 reference letters (or a premedical committee advisory letter). The application form includes employment history, a list of extra-curricular activities since high school, a list of clinical experience in hospitals, clinics or other health professional practices, a list of hobbies and countries visited, a list of all medical schools you have applied to in the US, Canada and elsewhere as well as a personal essay. Students can upload their CV. There is also a personal essay, which should state in no more than 500 words your purpose for considering a career in medicine, why you would be an asset to SABA University School of Medicine as well as significant activities, accomplishments, personal interests and unique aspects of your pre-medical preparation. Also note that all foreign transcripts need to be evaluated by the World Education Services, Inc. (www.wes.org), or another accredited evaluation organization.

Interview

The admission process includes an interview. An in-person interview at the main administrative office in Massachusetts is preferred, however, if this is not feasible, a telephone interview with members of the admissions committee can be scheduled. The interview is normally done with one or two members of the admissions staff.

Cost of studies 2010-2011

The total cost for all semesters = approximately USD98,500, for an average annual tuition of approximately USD24,600 if the degree is completed in 48 months.

Additional information

The basic science component of the medical curriculum is five semesters in length and may be completed in 20 months. The clinical medicine component is composed of 72 weeks of clinical rotations at hospitals in the United States, Canada and abroad. Although 95% of all SABA University students complete their clinical rotations in the United States, and Canada, rotations outside the United States are also available. SABA University graduates have participated in rotations in Great Britain, Ireland, Israel, Canada, Australia, India and the Netherlands-Antilles. SABA University students have also completed elective rotations with voluntary groups in Africa, Central America and Bosnia.

Statistics
There are approximately 90 to 95 students matriculating at the start of each trimester.

Residency match list
The university's match list is available from: www.saba.edu/saba/images/Forms/ 2010_residency.pdf

Contact
Saba University School of Medicine
C/o R3 Education Inc.
One Jackson Place
27 Jackson Road, Suite 301
Devens, MA, USA 01434
Tel: +1 978 862 9600
admissions@saba.edu

St. George's University

Degree requirement

The minimum requirement for North American applicants is a bachelor's degree from an accredited university. A candidate may apply before the completion of their bachelor's degree, however, a candidate's acceptance will be withdrawn if the degree is not obtained. The minimum requirement to apply directly to the 4-year medical programs for British applicants is an undergraduate degree with a strong science background. Applicants with passes at A levels are assessed individually and are considered for appropriate entry into the premedical sciences program. A student can be selected to enter the premedical sciences program for a period of 1 year to 3 years, meaning the full medical program will last between 5 and 7 years depending on the student's point of entry.

Course requirements

Full year of biology or zoology, one semester of English, full year of general chemistry, full year of organic chemistry and one semester of physics. One semester of mathematics is also required. In addition to the pre-requisite courses, students are required to have a basic knowledge in the use of computers. Courses in microbiology, biochemistry and physiology are also recommended.

GPA requirement

For the entering class in spring 2009, the average cumulative GPA was 3.3, the average science GPA was 3.17.

MCAT requirement

North American applicants are required to submit MCAT scores. For the entering class in 2009, the average MCAT score was 26. Non-North American students do not need to write the MCAT.

Selection Formula

The School of Medicine at St George's University begins first term classes in mid-August and again in mid-January. The school uses rolling admission and thus applicants may significantly increase their chances of admission by submitting their documents early. Prospective students may apply to SABA School of Medicine at any time during the year. Since the school uses rolling admission, applicants are encouraged to submit their documents early, between 6 to 12 months in advance, to ensure that their files are ready for consideration at least three months prior to the trimester of their first choice. Applications are assessed within one month and are selected for interview at that time.

Application documents

The application process includes an application form and a minimum of 2 reference letters. The application form includes a minimum of 2 essays as outlined below. Applicants should indicate in the application form if they are applying for the Keith B. Taylor Global Scholars Program. All applicants are required to write a personal statement providing personal information that is not included elsewhere in the application. This personal statement should be no longer than 1500 words. Applicants applying to the medical program in Grenada (not for those applying to the Keith B. Taylor Global Scholars Program) need to write a second essay discussing the most significant issue affecting the future of healthcare delivery in the country they intend to practice medicine in. This essay should be approximately 500 words. Applicants applying to the Keith B. Taylor Global Scholars Program need to write an essay describing their commitment to dedicating at least part of their professional life to practicing medicine in a developing country or underserved region. This essay should be no longer than 500 words. All applicants can also write an optional essay on the following topic: If you feel that your academic record and/or background is somewhat unusual, please state to the Board of Admissions a concise explanation of your path towards medicine. Please note that 2 additional short answers are required for those applying to the dual degree programs. The topics are as follows:

1. If you have experience in the area you wish to study, describe that experience.
2. What are the most significant issues facing your chosen area of study?

Interview

The interview can be held at the student's convenience in Grenada or in the United States, the United Kingdom, Africa, the Middle East, the Far East, the Caribbean or other locations.

Cost of studies 2010-2011

The total cost for all semesters = approximately USD205,000, for an average annual tuition of approximately USD51,300 if the degree is completed in 48 months. Note that the top 50 students are awarded a one-third tuition scholarship automatically. The minimum grades to qualify are 3.7 cumulative GPA, 3.5 science GPA and a 29 on the MCAT. There is also another scholarships for academic excellence.

Additional information

There are two medical programs offered at St George's University. One program consists of the first two years, which cover the basic sciences, spent on the True Blue campus in Grenada. The other medical program is called the Keith B. Taylor Global Scholars Program. Students entering this program spend their first year on the campus of Northumbria University in the United Kingdom. Both medical programs differ only in the location where the first year is complete. They are similar in every other aspect including courses and examinations. During the last two years of these medical programs, which cover the clinical sciences, students move on to study at the university's clinical centers and affiliated hospitals in the United States and the United Kingdom. In addition to the medical programs, St George's University offers a premedical sciences program. Applicants may enter this program for a period of 1 to 3 years depending on their previous academic achievements. Note that St George's University also offers dual degree programs: MD/MPH and MD/MSc.

Statistics

For entry in spring 2009, there were 1663 applicants. 417 students enrolled at the Grenada campus and 101 students enrolled at the campus of Northumbria University in the United Kingdom.

Residency match list

The university's match list is available from: http://www.sgu.edu/alumni/student-profile-alumni-residency-appointments.html

Contact

Office of Admission
St. George's University
c/o The North American Correspondent
University Support Services, LLC
One East Main Street
Bay Shore, NY, USA 11706-8399
US Tel: +1 800 899 6337 ext. 9 280
UK Tel: 0800 1699061 ext. 9 380
Other Tel: +1 (631) 665-8500 ext. 9 380
SGUEnrolment@sgu.edu

Croatia

Medical programs in English

1. University of Split, 6 year program
2. University of Zagreb, 4 and 6 year programs

University Rankings

In 2010, the universities in Croatia were not ranked in the top 640 universities in the world according to the QS World University rankings, or the top 500 universities according to the Shanghai Consultancy World University Rankings. They were also not ranked in either agency's top medical school rankings.

Accreditation Information

Croatia is not currently part of the European Union. This means that at the moment the medical degrees completed in Croatia do not allow students to practice in the E.U. Croatia is expected to enter the E.U in early 2013, and after that, graduates from Croatian medical schools will have their degrees recognized in the European Union.

Graduates from Croatian medical school are eligible to write the American and Canadian licensing exams. However, recognition of the individual medical schools vary by State and province.

School by school

University of Split

Programs
Students with an undergraduate degree can apply a 6 year program.

Nationality restrictions
Note that Croatian citizens living abroad are eligible to apply but Croatians living in Croatia are not eligible for the program in English.

Academic requirements
A secondary school diploma is required.

Admissions Exam
Students who have written the MCAT or SAT are given admissions priority. See "Selection formula" for more details.

Application documents
The application includes a CV and a written statement on the reasons for applying to study medicine in English in Split.

Selection formula
Applicants are given priority for admission in the following order: (1) University graduates (or final year students) who have written the MCAT (2) University students (or final year) with premedical majors in biology, chemistry or physics (3) Secondary school students who have written the SAT (4) Secondary school students with percentage grades that indicate their ranking in their country (5) Other students graduating from secondary school.

Cost of studies 2011-2012
€7,000 per year in tuition fees.

Statistics
There are approximately 30 places available each year in the English medical program.

Contact
School of Medicine in Split, Application for the study programme Medicine in English
Šoltanska 2, 21000 Split
Tel: +385 21 557 903
zoran.valic@mefst.hr

Ref: 179.   *University of Split*. Available from: http://www.mefst.hr/default.aspx?id=47.

University of Zagreb

Programs
Students with an undergraduate degree can apply to a 4 year and a 6 year program. Note that some students with some pre-medical courses may be exempt from the first year. Students can also combine the first two years of the 6 year program completing it in 5 years.

4 year program academic requirements
Applicants are usually expected to have graduated from a university pre-medical program, or to have completed a sufficient number of premedical courses at university.

6 year program academic requirements
A secondary school diploma is required.

Admissions Exam
There is a mandatory entrance examination in chemistry, physics and biology. A sample of their admission exam is available from mse.mef.hr/link1.php?grupa=01060000 Students who have written the MCAT, or earned a university degree with courses in chemistry, physics and biology may be exempt from writing the entrance examination. Students from the US are strongly encouraged to take SAT II subject tests from the required subjects. These will be considered alongside their SAT I or ACT scores for entrance exam exemption.

Application documents
The application includes a 200 word personal statement about why the applicant wants to study medicine and become a physician. Students must also submit their CV.

Selection formula
Applicants are evaluated on their secondary school grades, with additional emphasis placed on grades in biology, chemistry and physics if these courses have been taken. If required, the admissions exam will be taken into consideration as well, alongside the CV and application form.

Cost of studies 2010-2011
Approximately €7,000 per year

Contact
University Of Zagreb Medical School
Salata 3, 10000 Zagreb Croatia
Tel: +385 145 64 111
mse@mef.hr

Ref: 180. *University of Zagreb*. Available from: http://mse.mef.hr/.

Czech Republic

Medical programs in English

1. Charles University, Faculty of Medicine in Hradec Kralove
2. Charles University, Faculty of Medicine in Pilsen
3. Charles University in Prague, first faculty of Medicine
4. Charles University in Prague, second faculty of Medicine
5. Charles University in Prague, third faculty of Medicine
6. Masaryk University, Faculty of Medicine
7. Palacky University, Faculty of Medicine, Olomouc

University Rankings

The QS World University rankings have ranked two of the three universities in the Czech republic offering medical programs in English. Palacky university was not ranked in the top 640 in 2010. The Czech universities ranking in the top 640 according to this source are:

267. Charles University
551. Masaryk University

The Shanghai Universities also ranked Charles University in Prague in 201st place overall worldwide. Palacky University is not ranked in the top 500 according to this source, and none were ranked in the top medical schools worldwide by either agency. More details on these rankings are available on page 118.

School by school

Charles University, Faculty of medicine in Hradec Králové

Programs
Students with an undergraduate degree are eligible to apply to a 6 year program.

Academic requirements
Students must have a secondary school (high school) diploma. Courses in biology, chemistry and physics may be helpful for the exam but are not required [1].

Admission Exam
Most applicants must write an entrance exam, however, up to 15 applicants with course grades of AAB in A-level (or equivalent) biology, chemistry and either math or physics will be admitted without the exam. The exam is held in Hradec Králové or at other sites including Cyprus, Germany, Malasia, India, and the UK. Additional sites can be arranged with agencies. The multiple choice test covers biology, chemistry and either math or physics depending on student preference.

Selection formula
Test scores from all worldwide test centers are received by the office of admissions. Applicants are ranked for admission based on these results [1].

Application documents
Brief application form and CV.

Interview
A 5 minute interview for all applicants discussing the applicants motivation for a career in medicine, and why they want to study medicine in the Czech republic, is usually performed by the vice-dean [1].

Cost of studies 2011-2012
Approximately €11,820 per year

Statistics
In the 2012-2013 application cycle, there are 60 places. In the 2010-2011 application cycle, 8 students were admitted without an admissions exam, 100 were admitted after writing the exam, and 82 who took the exam were not granted admission. In total there were roughly 500 applicants [16]. One student was admitted from North America, and some students came from Malaysia, Botswana, Taiwan, Germany, Norway and several other countries [16].

Contact
Tel: +420495816487
students@lfhk.cuni.cz
Country representatives available from: www.lfhk.cuni.cz/article.asp?nArticleID=3742&nDepartmentID=1013&nLanguageID=2

Charles University in Prague, Faculty of Medicine in Pilsen

Programs
Students with an undergraduate degree are eligible to apply to a 6 year program.

Nationality Requirements
None [1].

Academic requirements
Students must have a secondary school (high school) diploma.

Admission Exam
All applicants must take an entrance exam in Pilsen or in their home country (organized by the application agency). The test is multiple choice and covers biology, chemistry and physics. The test is held in June at the university, and can be scheduled at another time near the applicant's home country with their admissions admissions agencies.

Selection formula
There is no interview for admission. The admissions exam is the most important component in the admissions process, but the university may look at other factors when applicants have equal exam scores [1].

Cost of studies 2010-2011
Approximately €9200 per year

Statistics
In the 2012-2013 application cycle, there were roughly 90 places available. There is no limit on the number of non-E.U students admitted, but the university does not make the number of non-E.U students or the number of applicants public [1].

Contact
Center of Studies in English, Lidická 1
301 66 PLZEN
Tel: + 420-377 593 175
medstudy@lfp.cuni.cz
Contact details for different country's partner representative are available from: www.lfp.cuni.cz/study_english.aspx

Ref: 181. *Charles University in Prague, Faculty of Medicine in Pilsen.* Available from: http://web.lfp.cuni.cz/studies/studies and http://www.lfp.cuni.cz/study_english.aspx.

Charles University in Prague, First Faculty of Medicine

Programs
Students with an undergraduate degree are eligible to apply to a 6 year program.

Nationality Requirements
None [1].

Academic requirements
E.U students must have a secondary school (high school) diploma. North American students are expected to have an undergraduate degree before enrolling. Students are expected to have taken at least one science course [1].

Admission Exam
Students take an entrance exam in Prague or at a location specified by official representatives of the university in June (locations include the US and UK). Late examinations are available in September for students with extenuating circumstances. The exam covers biology, chemistry and either physics or math (applicants choose which subject they prefer).

Selection formula
The admissions committee takes the entire application into account in deciding which applicants are granted admission, including the written exam and the interview [1].

Interview
There is a mandatory interview for those who pass the written portion of the exam. The interview is one on one and lasts approximately 15 minutes. It focuses on the student's motivation, communication skills. There may also be questions about the medical profession, the history of medicine or other miscellaneous topics [1].

Cost of studies 2012-2013
Approximately €13,000 per year [1]

Statistics
In the 2012-2013 application cycle, there are 120 places available. In previous years, there have been between 400-500 applications. There are roughly 22 US students in the school, 13 Canadian students, and 115 UK students, and an average entrance of 2 Canadians, 4-5 Americans and 25-30 British students each year [1].

Contact
Tel: +420 224968483
otomar.kittnar@lf1.cuni.cz
International representatives are listed at: www.lf1.cuni.cz/en/master-studies#Reps

Ref: 182. *Charles University in Prague, First Faculty of Medicine.* Available from: http://www.lf1.cuni.cz/en.

Charles University in Prague, Second Faculty of Medicine

Programs

Students with an undergraduate degree are eligible to apply to a 6 year program.

Nationality Requirements

None [1].

Academic requirements

Students must have a secondary school (high school) diploma.

Admission Exam

Students can either take the American SAT exam (also offered outside the US), or the university subject tests in physics, biology and chemistry.

Selection formula

For students taking the SAT, applicants who score above the cutoff set each year are admitted on a first come, first serve basis. Applicants with scores below the cutoff are evaluated after the submission deadline. In the 2012-2013 application cycle, the SAT cutoff will be 1850 [1]. Those who achieve this score are automatically admitted. Students may need to take SAT II subject tests in biology, chemistry and physics as well [1]. Those not achieving 1850 points can either wait to be considered if there are additional places, or can take the university test. The university exam comprises a written and oral exam administered by the school are given a score out of 225 for the written exam and 60 on the oral exam. The highest scoring candidates are admitted. An sample test is available from www.lf2.cuni.cz/parallel/example.htm

Interview

The university exam includes an interview. Students are evaluated based on demonstration interest in a career in medicine and ability to defend their opinion.

Cost of studies 2011-2012

Approximately €10,000 for the first year and €11,600 per year for years 2-6. International students in the top 10% of the class are eligible to pay only €10,000 per year for years 2-6.

Statistics

In the 2012-2013 application cycle, there were roughly 60-70 places available [1].

Contact

Charles University in Prague - 2nd Faculty of Medicine
V Úvalu 84, Praha 5 - Motol, 150 06
Tel: +420 22 44 3 58 33
relenata.habetinova@lfmotol.cuni.cz

Ref: 16. *Charles University, 2nd Faculty of Medicine.* Available from: http://www.lf2.cuni.cz/Studium/pr/eindex.htm.

Charles University in Prague, Third Faculty of Medicine

Programs
Students with an undergraduate degree are eligible to apply to a 6 year program.

Nationality Requirements
None [1].

Academic requirements
Students must have a secondary school (high school) diploma.

Admission Exam
There is a mandatory admission exam covering secondary school physics, biology and chemistry.

Selection formula
Students are admitted primarily based on the entrance exam. The interview normally does not play a major role in the admissions process [1].

Interview
There is a brief mandatory interview for all students held after the entrance examination [1].

Cost of studies 2011-2012
Approximately CZK290,000 (roughly €11,150) per year.

Additional information
The university offers a pre-term program in physics, biology and chemistry that prepares students for the entrance exam [1].

Statistics
There are approximately 60 places available in the program each year [1].

Contact
Charles University in Prague
Third Faculty of Medicine
Ruská 87, 100 00 Praha 10
Tel: +420-267 102 206

Ref: 183. *Charles University, 3rd Faculty of Medicine.* Available from: http://old.lf3.cuni.cz/english/.

Masaryk University

Programs
Students with an undergraduate degree are eligible to apply to a 6 year program. Note that some students with previous medically related coursework may be granted credit for up to the first 2 years of the program. The number of credits given is determined by comparing the syllabi of the courses taken by the applicant to the corresponding courses at Masaryk University.

Nationality Requirements
None [1].

Academic requirements
Students must have a secondary school (high school) diploma.

Admission Exam
Entrance examinations are administered by representatives of the medical university or at the university campus in Brno, Czech Republic. The exam is multiple choice and covers biology, chemistry and either math or physics.

Selection formula
Selection is based solely on the entrance examination scores [1]. There is no interview in the application process. A list of topics, practice examinations and recommended study materials are available from is.muni.cz/

prihlaska/info.pl?lang=en;op=n;utyp=BM;beh=646;vcskdl=1

Cost of studies 2011-2012
Approximately €9000 per year

Interview
None.

Statistics
Approximately 200 students apply each year for the 100 places available.

Contact
Masaryk University, Faculty of Medicine
Komenskeho nam. 2
662 43 Brno, Czech Republic
Tel: +420 549 498 188
admission@med.muni.cz
International representatives are listed at: www.med.muni.cz/index.php?id=9 under "Information for Applicants"

Ref: 184. *Masaryk University.* Available from: http://www.med.muni.cz/index.php?id=9.

Palacky University

Programs
Students with an undergraduate degree are eligible to apply to a 6 year program. For North American students, strong grades in the prerequisite courses coupled with good MCAT section scores may allow the applicant to receive transfer credits, however, the degree usually takes 6 years regardless of credits given since applicants must complete Czech language studies before clinical years [1].

Nationality Requirements
None [1].

Academic requirements, E.U applicants
Applicants from the UK and Ireland must have completed A-levels in chemistry, biology and one other subject (math or physics is recommended). Other applicants are expected to take biology and chemistry, usually to a level that allows them to apply to medical schools in their country [1].

Academic requirements, North American applicants
Applicants are required to hold a secondary school diploma and have university level courses in biology, general chemistry, organic chemistry and physics.

Academic requirements, other international applicants
See academic requirements, E.U applicants.

Admission Exam
Canadian and US applicants with good MCAT scores may be invited directly for interview. All other North American students and students from other countries are required to write a screening multiple choice examination. The exam covers physics, chemistry and biology. In 2011, the exam dates were set to June 20, 2011 (Olomouc) and July 7, 2011 (London), with the possibility of a late examination in August as well. Examinations may also be scheduled in North America.

Application documents
Once the application is submitted, students are asked to submit a CV, personal statement and two letters of recommendation.

Selection formula, E.U applicants
Students with AAB at A-level (or equivalent) will be invited automatically for an interview. Other students need to write the screening exam to qualify for interview, after which a final admissions decision is made.

Selection formula, North American applicants

Applicants with good MCAT scores or who pass the screening exam will be invited for interview, after which a final admissions decision is made.

Selection formula, other international applicants

Applicants may qualify for an automatic interview with very strong secondary school grades at the discretion of the admissions committee [1], however, most students need to write the entrance exam to qualify for interview, after which a final admissions decision is made.

Interview

The interview is conducted by the board of admissions and evaluates applicants on their motivation for entering a medical career, their reasons for wanting to study in the Czech Republic, and their academic history [1]. Some basic science questions in biology or chemistry may be asked as well. An important component of the interview is evaluation of English language fluency [1]. Canadian and US applicants can be interviewed in their home countries. Interviews are usually scheduled at the same time as entrance examinations. Occasionally, interviews can be held in another city if there is a large number of applicants in that city needing to be interviewed. This has happened in the past in Norway [1].

Cost of studies 2011-2012

Approximately €9500 per year

Statistics

There are roughly 100 applicants each year for the roughly 50 places available. For non-E.U applicants, the country most represented in the program is Malaysia. There are some British students, a few Taiwanese students and some North Americans as well [1].

Contact

Faculty of Medicine, Palacky University
Trida Svobody 8, 771 26
Olomouc, Czech Republic
Tel: +420-58 563 2015
coordin@tunw.upol.cz

Ref: 185. *Palacky University.* Available from: http://www.upol.cz/en/faculties/faculty-of-medicine-and-dentistry.

Hungary

Medical programs in English

1. Semmelweis University
2. University of Debrecen, Medical and Health Science Center
3. University of Pecs
4. University of Szeged, Albert Szent-Gyorgyi Medical University

University Rankings

The QS World University rankings ranked the University of Szeged in 2011 as 451st. The other Hungarian universities offering programs in English were not ranked that year. The University of Szeged also moved up to the top 300 universities worldwide on the Shanghai Consultancy World Rankings overall in 2010. It was the only university to rank in the top 500 worldwide overall according to this source. The hungarian universities were not ranked in either agency's top medical school rankings.

School by school

University of Debrecen, Medical and Health Science Center

Programs
Students with an undergraduate degree are eligible to apply to a 6 year program.

Academic requirements
Students must have a secondary school (high school) diploma.

Admissions exam
Foreign applicants have to write the entrance examination to be admitted. The exam consists of two parts: a multiple choice test covering biology, chemistry and physics and an oral exam covering biology and either physics or chemistry. Applicants who have a B.A or B.Sc degree in a biology related natural science may be exempted from the entrance examination. The deadline to submit requests for exemption from the entrance examination is May 31st. There are 3 dates to sit the entrance examination from April to July.

Application documents
Basic application form and CV.

Application Deadline
The deadline of application for the next academic year is 30th June.

Application Fee
The application fee is USD150. The entrance examination fee is USD350.

Interview
The interview covers either biology and chemistry or biology and physics. The applicant can choose the subjects he or she prefers.

Cost of studies 2011-2012
USD13,500 for the first year's tuition.

Contact
Tel: +36 52 258-051
info@edu.unideb.hu
A list of the representatives in each country is available from http://www.ud-mhsc.org/index.php?option=com_map&Itemid=81

University of Pécs

Programs

Students with an undergraduate degree are eligible to apply to a 6 year program. Students with a B.A or BSc, or studying in a medicine related field may be granted credit for the first year of the program. If courses in anatomy, histology or embryology are not completed, an intensive summer course can be completed to start in 2nd year.

Nationality restrictions

None [1].

Academic requirements

Students must have a secondary school diploma. Courses in biology and chemistry are encouraged but not required [1].

Admission Exam

There is an entrance exam either in Pécs or through one of the university's agencies in another country. In Pecs, the written exam is 3 hours and covers biology, chemistry and physics and is followed by an oral interview. Exams administered by local representatives may differ. Students with degrees may receive exemption from the exam [1].

Selection formula

Selection is based on the CV, reference letters, exam and interview. Students who do not do well at the exam but who do well in the interview can still be admitted [1].

Application documents

Applicants are required to submit a CV and 1 or 2 letters of recommendation [1].

Interview

Students taking the entrance examination in Pécs can schedule it in August, and have an oral examination with 1-2 interviewers.

Cost of studies 2011-2012

Approximately USD14,000 per year.

Statistics

In the 2010-2011 application cycle, there were approximately 600 applicants for the 200 places available [1].

Contact

Tel: +36 72 536 000 ext. 6018
studentservice.center@aok.pte.hu
A list of the representatives in each country is available from www.studyhungary.hu

---

Ref: 186. *University of Pécs*. Available from: http://www.pote.hu/index.php?&nyelv=eng.

Semmelweis University

Programs

Students with an undergraduate degree are eligible to apply to a 6 year program.

Nationality restrictions

None [1].

Academic requirements

Applicants must have a secondary school diploma with some background in biology and chemistry.

Admission Exam

Applicants must write a multiple choice entrance examination in biology, chemistry and English. The exam is held in several locations in Europe, Asia, as well as other locations like Nigeria. Students can contact their local representative to set up an exam. Exam topics are listed at www.semmelweis-english-program.org/index.php?option=com_content&task=view&id=45&Itemid=66&limit=1&limitstart=2

Application documents

Applicants are required to submit a CV and one letter of recommendation.

Selection formula

The entrance exam, the CV, the other application documents and the interview are all used to select applicants for admission [1].

Interview

There is a mandatory interview, which begins with an oral examination testing the applicant's knowledge of biology, chemistry and English, followed by a personal interview.

Cost of studies 2012-2013

Approximately USD16,400 per year. Students performing very well in the program are eligible for a 10-15% fee reduction.

Statistics

Each year, there are approximately 120 places available for international students. Among the medicine, dentistry and pharmacy programs, there are roughly 1000 applicants for the 350 places available, roughly 10% of which are filled by North Americans [1].

Contact

Tűzoltó u. 37-47.
Budapest Hungary H–1094
Tel: + 36 1413-3015
Send a message at: www.semmelweis-english-program.org/index.php?option=com_contact&Itemid=3. A list of the representatives in each country is available from www.studyhungary.hu

ReF: 187. *Semmelweis University.* Available from: http://english.sote.hu/.

University of Szeged, Albert Szent-Györgyi Medical University

Programs

Students with an undergraduate degree can apply to a 6 year program. Students can be granted credit for the first year (or rarely the first two years) if they have taken courses which have a similar curriculum to the courses at the University of Szeged. Bsc. holders may also be eligible to complete an anatomy summer course and enter into the second year of the program. The university cannot grant credit before August, so students will not know in advance if they have received credit for part of the program [1].

Nationality restrictions

None [1].

Academic requirements

Students must have a secondary school diploma.

Admission Exam

Applicants not meeting one of the following criteria are required to write the entrance exam:

1. IB graduates with grades of at least 5 in English and 2 of biology, chemistry and physics are exempt
2. A-levels graduates with B+ or higher in 3 natural science subjects, as well as A or A* at GCSE level
3. BSC holders in natural, biomedical, life sciences, chemistry or biology with good grades at university

Applicants whose first language is not English may also need to write the TOEFL to be exempt from having to write the entrance exam. Applicant's whose first language is English may need to provide supporting documentation to the admissions committee [1]. All applicants who do not qualify according to the criteria above must write the entrance exam which covers chemistry or physics, as well as biology and English. The exam is held between February and August in Hungary, and is also held in locations in Europe, Asia, Africa and the US.

Selection formula

For students who do not qualify for entry based on their secondary school or university results, the entrance exam is the main factor determining which applicants are granted admission.

Application documents

Applicants must also submit a CV and 2 reference letters. Most students submit letters from health professionals [1].

Interview

There is a mandatory interview following the written exam, and there is also an interview for students who want to receive exemption from part of the program.

Interview (cont'd)

The interview consists of biology and chemistry questions, as well as questions about the applicant's motivations to study medicine. The interview is also meant to test applicants' proficiency in English [1].

Cost of studies 2011-2012

Approximately USD13,900 for years 1-5, then approximately USD7,000 for year 6 depending on the rotations chosen [1]. The anatomy preparatory course costs approximately USD7,800 [1].

Statistics

In the 2011-2012 application cycle, there were approximately 900 applicants for the 130 places available [1].

Contact

Foreign Students Secretariat of the University of Szeged
H-6720 Szeged, Dóm tér 12
Tel: +36 62-545-836
english.program@medea.szote.u-szeged.hu
Local representative contacts for the University of Szeged are available from http://angoltit.webesmegoldas.hu/prospective_students?q=agents

Ref: 188. *University of Szeged, Albert Szent-Györgyi Medical University.* Available from: http://www.szote.u-szeged.hu/AOK/eng/.

Ireland

Medical programs

The medical schools offering 4-year programs are:

5. The Royal College of Surgeons in Ireland (RCSI)
6. University College Cork
7. University College Dublin
8. University of Limerick

The medical schools offering 5-year programs are:

1. The Royal College of Surgeons in Ireland (RCSI)
2. The National University of Ireland, Galway
3. Trinity College Dublin
4. University College Cork (this program is generally not open to North American Applicants) [18]
5. University College Dublin (this program is generally not open to North American Applicants) [18]

Three universities offer 6-year medical programs.

1. The National University of Ireland, Galway
2. The Royal College of Surgeons in Ireland (RCSI)
3. University College Dublin

University rankings

All medical schools in Ireland have a high standard of education. To our knowledge there are no rankings specifically for Irish medical schools. We have listed some of the rankings based on universities overall, recognizing of course that these may not reflect the reputation of the schools. When choosing which schools to apply to, students take in many other factors including curriculum and how much experience the school has placing students in the country they want to practice.

TIMES ONLINE - Irish university guide 2010

This ranking gives each Irish university an overall score out of 750 depending on:

1. Irish leaving certificate points
2. Research
3. Employment
4. Firsts/2:1 awarded
5. Student/staff ratio
6. Completion rate

Note that the Royal College of Surgeons Ireland (RCSI) which has a very good reputation is not ranked in this guide, as it is not a general studies university. The top Irish universities in this ranking are:

1. Trinity College Dublin
2. University College Dublin
3. University College Cork
4. National University of Ireland, Galway
7. University of Limerick

The complete ranking is available at: www.timesonline.co.uk/tol/life_and_style/education/sunday_times_university_guide/ireland/ Note that students must sign up for an online membership (£1 for 1 day trial) to access this link.

QS Top Universities - World University Rankings 2010/2011 - Overall

This ranking gives each university an overall score based on several factors including academic peer review, employer review, research and faculty. More details are available on page 118.

Again, RCSI is not ranked in this list for the reasons mentioned above. The Irish universities' rankings according to this list are:

52. Trinity College Dublin
114. University College Dublin
184. University College Cork
232. National University of Ireland, Galway
451. University of Limerick

None of the Irish schools ranked in the top 200 in the QS World University rankings for medicine. The full world ranking is available at: www.topuniversities.com/world-university-rankings

Shanghai Consultancy World University Rankings 2010 - overall

This ranking also gives universities an overall ranking, not a medical school ranking, based on Nobel Prizes, Fields Medals and research. More details are available on page 119.

Again, RCSI is not ranked in this list for the reasons mentioned above. The Irish universities' rankings according to this list are:

201. Trinity College Dublin
301. University College Dublin
401. University College Cork

The National University of Ireland, Galway and the University of Limerick did not rank in the top 500 universities worldwide in 2010 according to this source. Note that none of the Irish schools ranked in the top 100 in the Shanghai Consultancy World University Ranking for clinical medicine and pharmacy. The full ranking is available at: www.arwu.org/ARWU2010.jsp

Note that RSCI has an excellent reputation but is not part of these global rankings only because it it not a general studies university.

E.U Applicants - summary of requirements

E.U applicants applying to 4-year GEPs are required to hold an upper second class honours in their undergraduate degree, which can be in any discipline and must write the GAMSAT exam. All applications are submitted through the Central Application Office of Ireland: www.cao.ie

For GEPs, there are only 2 factors considered in the application process:

1. Applicants are expected to hold a minimum of an upper second class honours in their first undergraduate degree. The undergraduate degree must be an NFQ level 8 degree* (honours bachelor's degree, higher diploma or equivalent). Even if the applicant completes a second undergraduate degree, it is in their first undergraduate degree that they must have achieved an upper second class honours.

2. If the first criteria is met, applicants are selected solely based on their GAMSAT result. The applicant with the highest GAMSAT result will be selected first, then the applicant with the second highest GAMSAT result and so on. There are no interviews for these programs [77].

*A NFQ level 8 degree in Ireland is not the same as a level 8 degree in Wales, England or other parts of the E.U. For a guide to comparing qualifications within the UK, see www.nfq.ie/nfq/en/awards_in_the_framework.html Note that many students, particularly those from outside the UK, will be asked by the schools to have their qualifications assessed, either by the National Qualification Authority of Ireland (www.qualificationsrecognition.ie/recognition) or another similar institution.

E.U applicants with undergraduate degrees applying to the 5 or 6-year undergraduate medicine programs have different application requirements depending on whether or not they qualify as mature students. **Mature students are those that will be 23 years of age or older as of January 1st of the year of matriculation** [78].

Mature and standard applicants both need to write the HPAT-ireland exam to apply to the 5 and 6-year programs [78]. Both pools of applicants apply through the CAO of Ireland: www.cao.ie

The HPAT-Ireland is a two and a half hour multiple choice, paper based test with 3 equally weighted sections: logical reasoning and problem solving, interpersonal understanding and non-verbal reasoning. Applicants are given an overall score out of 300 points. In 2011 there was only one date to sit the exam. Applicants who could not attend on that date were not given an alternative date and were forced to wait until the following year to write the exam. If an applicant wrote the test in 2011, their scores will be valid for 2011 and 2012 only [79]. In 2011, the test centres were located in Cork, Dublin, Galway, Sligo and Waterford [80]. More information is available at: www.hpat-ireland.acer.edu.au. The deadline to register for the exam in 2011 was the January 20th, 2011. Students who missed this deadline could register until February 3rd but were required to pay a late registration fee of 50€ in addition to the standard 95€ fee [78, 80].

If an applicants does not qualify as a mature student, his or her undergraduate degree will not be taken into consideration for admission to the 5 and 6-year programs [78]. Admission will be based solely on his or her secondary school (high school) examination results and the HPAT exam as outlined below.

The standard application requirements (for those who do not qualify as mature applicants) for the 5 and 6-year medicine programs in 2011 were as follows:

1. Achieving a minimum score of 480 in the same sitting on the Irish Leaving Certificate Exam or equivalent (for example, RCSI uses the following conversion for AS and A2 Level examinations: A2 Levels - A is 150 points; B is 130 points; C is 105 points; D is 80 points and E is 40 points. AS Levels - A is 75 points; B is 65 points; C is 55 points; D is 40 points and E is 20 points)[81]. Note that recent A-level graduates have different grade conversions according to a new system incorporating A* grades [1].
2. Applicants must meet the minimum course requirements for the program they wish to apply to.
3. Applicants must write the HPAT-Ireland exam within the 2 years immediately preceding matriculation to the medicine program [78].

Once the minimum requirements above have been met, the Leaving Certificate Examination (LCE) scores (or equivalents from abroad) are combined with the applicants' HPAT-Ireland scores to give each applicant a total score. This score will be the sole factor determining which applicants are offered admission. There is no interview in for non-mature students applying to 5 and 6 year programs.

The HPAT-Ireland is given a score out of 300. The LCE scores are normally out of 600 points and thus carry twice the weight of the HPAT score in the calculation of the applicant's total score. However, above 550 points at the LCE examinations, applicants are only given 1 point for every 5 additional points they score. This means that their total LCE score cannot exceed 560 points [78]. In 2010, the minimum entry levels varied from 725 to 731. Additional details on score calculation are available from the undergraduate medical program application brochure at www.cao.ie/index.php.

Applicants rank their school choices in the CAO application form. Schools calculate cutoffs for entry based on the competition and the number of students they can accept each year. If the applicant qualifies for admission at several schools, they will be offered a place only at the school they ranked most highly that offered them admission. After admission offers have been made, the cutoffs for admission can still drop as some applicants will decline some schools' offers. Thus, if an applicant does not obtain an offer from his or her top choice, he or she might still receive an offer from that school at a later date after other students have rejected their offers. More details are available from the CAO handbook at www2.cao.ie/handbook/handbook.

For mature students, the HPAT-Ireland exam is also required for all 5 and 6-year medicine programs. In addition, there is an extra section in the CAO of Ireland application where mature applicants are required to write a personal statement with the following information, or as much of it as is relevant to their case [82]:

1. Relevance of life/educational experience. State your educational goals and objectives.
2. Final secondary level qualification awarded
3. Post-secondary level qualifications
4. Current studies
5. Non-certificate courses
6. Employment
7. Voluntary (unpaid) work
8. Hobbies or interest

Applicants can complete their personal statement on additional pages if they wish. In addition to this application form, some schools have additional application requirements that are outlined in the school specific sections on page 389. Some undergraduate programs have a separate quota for mature applicants, and will consider many factors other than grades and LCE scores to select mature applicants for admission.

The determination of E.U residency status varies from school to school. European Union citizens that are not residents in the E.U are not eligible to apply for places within the E.U quotas at some schools [18]. RCSI is one example, where students are required to not only hold an E.U passport, but also to have been residents in an E.U country for the 3 to 5 years preceding entry to medical school to be considered for the E.U quota [83]. Other schools like Trinity College Dublin consider someone for the E.U quota under a variety of conditions, including those with an E.U passport who have completed all of their full time post-primary education in the E.U [84]. Because the definition of an E.U student differs from school to school, it is a good idea to check the schools' websites if you are unsure of your status.

North American applicants - summary of requirements

Up to 200 US and Canadian applicants are admitted each year, and there are currently approximately 900 North American students studying medicine in Ireland [85].

North American applicants are required to hold an undergraduate degree in any discipline and are strongly advised to have completed at least one university level course in Biology, one in Chemistry and one in Physics or Mathematics [18]. Note, however, that most students will apply with more science courses than the three mentioned above which will strengthen their application at some of the Irish medical schools [18]. In addition, all of the 4-year GEPs require North American applicants to submit MCAT scores.

All North American applicants need to submit a personal statement, two reference letters (or one premedical advisory committee letter if such a committee exists at the student's university), a resume and their transcripts (as well as MCAT scores if applicable) to the Atlantic Bridge Program: www.atlanticbridge.com. Applicants can discuss which medical programs they should apply to with the Atlantic Bridge staff. The Atlantic Bridge Program then makes copies of their application and sends them to the admissions offices of the Irish medical schools. The next step depends on the school. Most schools do not interview North American applicants, however, the Royal College of Surgeons in Ireland and the University of Limerick will conduct interviews before accepting students [1, 18]. These interviews are conducted in North America.

Note that on rare occasion, if a student applies to the 4-year program and is not successful, the school may offer them a place in their 5 or 6-year program instead [18].

The three medical schools offering 5-year programs to North American students are:

1. The Royal College of Surgeons in Ireland (RCSI)
2. The National University of Ireland, Galway
3. Trinity College Dublin

North American students applying to one of the three 5-year programs are required to hold an undergraduate degree in any discipline and are strongly recommended to have completed at least one university level course in Biology, one in Chemistry and one in Physics or Mathematics [18]. These programs do not require North American applicants to submit MCAT scores [1, 17].

North Americans are also eligible to apply to all three 6-year programs listed on page 383.

Note that it can be more difficult for North American applicants to try to stay in the E.U as internship posts in the E.U must be offered to qualified E.U students before non-E.U students by law [86]. In addition, the Irish government has been increasing the intake of Irish/E.U medical students recently, making it even more difficult for non-E.U citizens to secure residency positions because of the increasing competition. Most American and Canadian students return home after graduation [86].

School by school
University of Cork

Programs
Students with an undergraduate degree can apply to a 4 year program. Students with an undergraduate degree who are over 23 years of age (mature students) can also apply to a 5 year program (those under 23 years of age can only apply to the 4 year program [1]).

Nationality restrictions
North American applicants are only eligible to apply to the 4 year program.

4 year program degree requirements
E.U applicants must have an upper second class honours degree in any subject. Non-E.U applicants must have an undergraduate degree in any subject.

5 year program degree requirements
Graduates from the E.U who are over 23 years of age (mature students) can apply to the 5 year program with their undergraduate qualifications; they not need to meet the secondary school (high school) requirements [1].

Admissions exam
For the 4 year program, the GAMSAT is required for all E.U applicants and the MCAT for all North American applicants. Other international applicants have not needed to write an entrance exam in the past, but should confirm with their application agency or the school directly to check their examination requirements [1]. For the 5 year program, the HPAT Ireland is required for all E.U applicants.

4 year program application documents
In the past, non-E.U, non-North American have submitted a 500 word personal statement about their experiences and why they want to study medicine at Cork.

5 year program application documents
See 4 year program application documents.

4 year program selection formula, E.U applicants
Once academic criteria are met, selection for entry is based solely on GAMSAT results. The student with the highest result is given the first position, then the second highest and so on until all of the seats are filled. There is no interview required.

4 year program selection formula, North American applicants
There is no interview [18]. The university admissions office receives copies of all the documents sent to the Atlantic Bridge Program and will make a decision based on the applicant's file. Admissions decisions are then conveyed to the student through the Atlantic Bridge Program.

4 year program selection formula, other international applicants

The selection formula depends on whether there is a recruiting agency in the applicant's country, and what their selection policy is. For applicants without a recruiting agency, selection is based on the entire application, including the personal statement.

5 year program selection formula, E.U applicants

For non-mature applicants, admission is based on high school examination results and the HPAT-Ireland examination. Applicants are given a score as described on page 387, and ranked for admission according to these scores. For mature applicants, the HPAT, educational qualifications, relevant career experience and motivation as expressed in the CAO personal statement will all be used to short list mature applicants for interview. The 2010 CAO cutoff was 725.

5 year program selection formula, other international applicants

See 4 year program, other international applicants. Applicants are not normally interviewed for this program unless the agency requires an interview [1].

Interview

For the 4 year program, only non-E.U, non-North American applicants are interviewed. For the 5 year program, mature applicants and non-E.U, non-North American applicants may be interviewed.

Cost of studies 2011-2012

EU student fees = €12,780 per year. Non-E.U student fees = €39,200 per year

4 year program statistics

In 2010, There were also approximately 20 places available for North American students [18]. There were a total of 20 places available for E.U students in the 4-year program in 2009.

5 year program statistics

There were a total of approximately 85 positions available for E.U students in the 5-year program in 2009, with 3-4 places for mature applicants.

Contact

Rm 2.59, Brookfield Health Sciences Complex, College Road, Cork, Ireland
Tel: +353 21 4901575
medschool@ucc.ie

Ref: 189. *University College Cork*. Available from: http://www.ucc.ie/.

University College Dublin

Programs

Students with an undergraduate degree can apply to a 4 year or a 6 year program. Students who are eligible to apply for the 4 year program are expected to apply to this program rather than the 6 year program, but graduates who do not qualify for the 4 year program should apply to the 6 year program [1]. Approximately 20 students each year in previous years have completed the 6 year program in 5 years. Students offered a place in the 5-year program are generally mature students, students with an appropriate undergraduate degree, or students who have performed very well in chemistry [1].

Nationality restrictions

North American applicants are not eligible to complete the 6 year program in 5 years.

4 year program academic requirements

E.U applicants must have an upper second class honours degree in any subject. Non-E.U applicants must have an undergraduate degree in any subject.

6 year program A-level requirements

In previous years, non-mature E.U applicants needed 2 subjects at grade C or above at A-level, with another 4 at grade C or above in GCSE or higher level. Students needed English, another language, math, a laboratory science subject and 2 other subjects from the list of recognized courses available from: www.nui.ie/college/docs/

gCE_GCSE.pdf The minimum points for admission vary from year to year.

6 year program IB requirements

Non-mature E.U applicants have needed 2 HL subjects with minimum grades of 4, and 4 SL subjects at minimum grades of 4. Note that those who completed IB in French or Spanish have required 25 points. English with 4 at HL (or 5 at HL if IB done in a language other than English) was also required. Equivalents to the requirement are usually accepted. In addition, students have needed another language, math, a laboratory science subject and 2 other subjects. Math studies is not acceptable for the math requirement. A minimum of 480 CAO points from IB levels was required in order to apply in 2010.

6 year program other qualifications

Requirements and conversions for E.U countries are available from: https://myucd.ucd.ie/programme_info/eu_app.ezc Requirements and conversions for many non-E.U countries are available from: https://myucd.ucd.ie/programme_info/overseas.ezc

Admissions exam

For the 4 year program, the GAMSAT is required for all E.U applicants, and North Americans need to write the MCAT.

Admissions exam (Cont'd)

For the 6 year program, the HPAT Ireland is required for all E.U applicants. For all others, there are no exam requirements unless listed at https://myucd.ucd.ie/programme_info/overseas.ezc

4 year program selection formula, E.U applicants

Once academic criteria are met, selection for entry is based solely on GAMSAT results. The student with the highest result is given the first position, then the second highest and so on until the seats are filled. The GAMSAT cutoff in 2009 was 60. There is no interview in the admissions process.

4 year program selection formula, North American applicants

There is no interview. Selection for admission is based on the full application including the personal statement and reference letters [18].

4 year program selection formula, other international applicants

Other applicants may be required to attend an interview before admission.

6 year program selection formula, E.U applicants

For non-mature and mature applicants, admission is based on high school examination results and the HPAT-Ireland examination. Applicants are given a score based on these, and ranked for admission. In 2010 the CAO cutoff was 725.

6 year program selection formula, North American

See 4 year program selection formula, North American applicants.

6 year program selection formula, other international applicants

See 4 year program selection formula, other international applicants.

Interview

Interviews are only held for mature E.U applicants at the discretion of the admissions committee, and for non-E.U applicants if their agency requires an interview. North American applicants are not normally interviewed.

Cost of studies 2011-2012

For the 4 year program, E.U student fees = €13,915 per annum, and non-E.U student fees = €39,200 per year. For the 6 year program, E.U student fees = €8,862 and non-E.U student fees = €31,000.

4 year program statistics

In the 2011-2012 application cycle, there were approximately 75 places in the 4 year program, of which roughly 30 places were available for non-E.U applicants [1].

6 year program statistics

In the 2010-2011 application cycle, there were approximately 122 E.U students accepted to the 6 year program, with approximately 10 positions available for North American students [1].

Contact

UCD School of Medicine & Medical Science
Room C310, Health Sciences Centre
University College Dublin
Belfield, Dublin 4, Ireland.
Tel: + 353 1 716 6655
healthscience@ucd.ie

Refs: 190.   *University College Dublin, 4-year program.* Available from: https://myucd.ucd.ie/admission/med_graduate.ezc.
191.   *University College Dublin, 5 and 6-year programs.* Available from: https://myucd.ucd.ie/program.do?programID=18.

National University of Ireland, Galway

Programs
Students with undergraduate degrees can apply to a 5 year and a 6 year program. Note that for E.U students, admission to the program is based on secondary school results, not the undergraduate degree.

Nationality restrictions
None.

5 year program academic requirements
North Americans must hold an undergraduate degree in any discipline, but students are strongly advised to have completed courses in chemistry, biology and physics in order to be considered. In previous years, E.U applicants applied for entry to the 6-year program and then once admitted, asked if they could join the 5-year program. Usually, the school allows applicants to complete the program in 5 years if they have the equivalent of A-level biology and chemistry [1]. Criteria are similar for non-E.U, non-North American applicants, but may differ if they apply through an agency in their country.

6 year program academic requirements
In 2011, E.U students were expected to have the equivalent of Irish HC3 (usually a grade of C at A-level) in two subjects and four other higher or standard level courses. The exact conversions are not published on their website, and students are advised to contact the admissions office to see if their qualifications are eligible. Subjects generally must include English and a laboratory subject.

Admissions exam
Graduates from the E.U must write the HPAT Ireland. There is no examination required for non-E.U applicants.

Selection formula, E.U applicants
Admission is based on high school examination results and the HPAT-Ireland examination. Applicants are given a score as described on page 387, and ranked for admission according to these scores. In 2010, the minimum entry cutoff for the CAO application was 719.

Selection formula, North American applicants
There is no interview [18]. The Atlantic Bridge program forwards all application materials to the school admissions committee. Admission is based on the entire application including personal statement and reference letters.

Selection formula, other international applicants
There is usually no interview required for other non-E.U applicants [1]. Applicants with an agency should apply through the agency, and all other applicants apply directly to the school.

Cost of studies 2011-2012

E.U student fees = €9,297 per year. Non-E.U student fees = €31,000 per year.

Statistics

In the 2011-2012 application cycle, there were approximately 60 places available in the 6 year program and 80 available in the 5 year program [1]. Roughly 100 of these places were for E.U applicants and the rest for non-E.U applicants. There is some variation in the number of places for both categories awarded each year [1].

Contact

Department of Medicine, Clinical Science Institute
National University of Ireland, Galway, University Road, Galway, Ireland.
Tel: +353 91 544 475
medschool@nuigalway.ie

Ref: 192. *National University Ireland, Galway.* Available from: http://www.nuigalway.ie/courses/undergraduate-courses/surgery-obstetrics.html.

University of Limerick

Programs
Students with an undergraduate degree are eligible to apply to the 4 year program.

Nationality restrictions
None.

Academic requirements
E.U applicants must have an upper second class honours degree in any subject. Non-E.U, non-North American applicants are expected to have the equivalent of an upper second class honours in their degree as well [1]. North American applicants must have an undergraduate degree in any subject.

Admissions Exam
The GAMSAT is required for all E.U applicants and the MCAT required for all North American applicants. Other international applicants have had the choice of writing the GAMSAT or the MCAT in previous years [1].

Application documents
The application form for non-E.U, non-North American applicants includes a personal statement and the contact information of two people the university can contact for a reference.

Selection formula, E.U applicants
Once academic criteria are met, selection for entry is based solely on GAMSAT results. The student with the highest result is given the first position, then the second highest and so on until all of the seats are filled. There is no interview in the admissions process. The GAMSAT cutoff was 55 for entry in 2008 and 56 for entry in 2009. The cutoffs have ranged between 55 and 60 [1].

Selection formula, North American applicants
Applicants are required to attend an interview. Applicants' entire files are taken into account, including the personal statements, reference letters and interviews to select students for admission [18].

Selection formula, other international applicants
Initial screening is based on having the equivalent of an upper second class honours degree and the GAMSAT or MCAT score. Whether or not an interview is required for admission depends on the country of origin and which agency the applicant applies through, if an agency is available [1].

Interview

Interviews are generally held for North American applicants and sometimes other non-E.U applicants, but not E.U applicants. For North Americans, interviews are normally held at a few Canadian universities each year and consist of 2 parts. First, applicants are broken into groups of approximately 8 students. These students are given a task and are observed by members of the admissions committee who evaluate their interaction in the team environment. The second part of the interview is a panel interview with 2-3 members of the admissions committee. It lasts approximately 20-30 minutes [1].

Cost of studies 2010-2011

E.U student fees = €12,780 per year, and non-E.U student fees = €38,500 per year.

Statistics

In the 2011-2012 application cycle, there were 80-90 positions available, approximately 50 for E.U applicants and the other 30 or 40 positions for non-E.U applicants [1].

Contact

Admissions Office
University of Limerick
Limerick, Ireland
Tel: +353 61 202015
International office: +353-61-202414
medicalschool@ul.ie

Ref: 193. *University of Limerick, medical school website.* Available from: http://www2.ul.ie/web/WWW/Faculties/Education_%26_Health_Sciences/Departments/Graduate_Medical_School.

Royal College of Surgeons in Ireland (RCSI)

Programs
Students with an undergraduate degree can apply to a 4 year, 5 year and a 6 year program. E.U applicants to the 5 and 6 year programs are considered based on their secondary school results.

Nationality restrictions
None.

4 year program degree requirements
E.U applicants must have an upper second class honours degree in any subject. Non-E.U applicants must have an undergraduate degree in any subject, but are expected to have taken basic science courses [18, 81].

5 year program A-level requirements
To be competitive, E.U applicants should have at least one A-level at grade A and two A-levels at grade B [1]. In the past, to receive credit for the foundation year, applicants needed at least 6 GCSEs with English, math and a second language at minimum grade C. Three of physics, chemistry, biology and math were needed to enter the 5-year program as well. Otherwise, applicants did not receive credit for the foundation year and were admitted to the 6-year program. Note that the committee reviews the courses and grades achieved on a case by case basis to determine who is granted exemption from the foundation year [1].

5 year program IB requirements
E.U applicants needed 34 points in the IB program to be competitive in recent years [1]. To be considered for the 5 year program, students have needed courses similar to the A-level courses listed above. The admissions committee reviews courses and grades on a case by case basis to determine who is granted exemption from the foundation year [1].

5 year program, other qualifications
Requirements for non-EU students are available from www.rcsi.ie/index.jsp?p=112&n=202&a=748 under "entry requirements for non-EU applicants."

6 year program A-level requirements
See 5 year program A-level requirements.

6 year program IB requirements
Applicants needed 30 points in the IB program to be competitive in previous years [1], as well as 3 HL and 3 SL subjects. Subject requirements included English, Math and at least one science subject.

6 year program, other qualifications
See 5 year program, other qualifications

Admissions exam
For the 4 year program, the GAMSAT is required for all E.U applicants and the MCAT required for all North American applicants.

Admissions exam (cont'd)

Other international applicants must write either the GAMSAT or the MCAT. The MCAT average for entry in 2009 was 29, and the GAMSAT cutoff for entry in 2010 was 63. For the 5 and 6 year programs, E.U applicants must write the HPAT Ireland. Other applicants may be expected to write an exam if listed at www.rcsi.ie/index.jsp? p=112&n=202&a=748 under "entry requirements for non-EU applicants." For example, US applicants are strongly encouraged to have taken an AP, IB, SAT, SAT II or ACT exam, while this is not necessarily expected of Canadian students.

4 year program selection formula, E.U applicants

Once academic criteria are met, selection for entry is based solely on GAMSAT results. The student with the highest result is given the first position, then the second highest and so on until all seats are filled. There is no interview in the admissions process.

4 year program selection formula, North American applicants

Students are required to attend an interview. Selection for admission is based on the full application including the personal statement, reference letters and interview performance [18].

4 year program selection formula, other international applicants

An interview is usually required for admission. Most applicants will be required to submit a personal statement and reference letter as well which will be evaluated for admission.

5 and 6 year program selection formulas, E.U applicants

For applicants under 23 years of age, admission is based on high school examination results and the HPAT-Ireland examination. Applicants are given a score as described on page 387, and ranked for admission according to these scores. A-level scores are converted to LCE scores at RCSI as shown in table 53. The CAO cutoff score in 2010 was 721. Note that recent A-level graduates have different grade conversions according to a new system incorporating A* grades [1]. For mature applicants, students are first ranked based on their HPAT scores, and those who are short-listed are invited to submit a CV and a personal statement, and will also be invited for an interview.

5 and 6 year program selection formulas, North American applicants

Selection for interview is based on the full application including the personal statement and reference letters. Students who have earned a degree but are applying to the 5 or 6 year programs will have their academic performance evaluated according to their high school grades (as well as SAT scores for US students) [1].

5 and 6 year program selection formulas, other international applicants

See 4 year program selection formula, other international applicants.

Interview

Interviews are only held for non-E.U applicants, and mature E.U applicants. For mature applicants, the interviews last approximately 30 minutes with 2 interviewers, of whom one or both are usually academics or lecturers from the university [1]. For North Americans, interviews are usually held in New York and Toronto. The interviews last year were approximately 20-30 minutes and were conducted by a panel of 3 interviewers from the RCSI admissions committee. For other international applicants, interviews are held at several locations including Kuala Lumpur, Bahrain and London each year. Additional interviews are occasionally held in Singapore, Hong Kong, Australia, Trinidad and Jordan.

Cost of studies 2011-2012

For the 4 year program, E.U students fees = €25,780 per year, however, the Higher Education Authority contributes €11,000 per year towards the fee. Students thus pay the remaining €13,080 per year. Non-E.U student fees = approximately €47,500 per year. For the 5 and 6 year programs, E.U students fees = €7,767 per year, and non-E.U students fees = approximately €46,000 per year.

Additional information

The 4-year program forms a separate class for the classroom years (the first two years) and will be joined by the 5 and 6-year program students in their clinical rotations. Note that North Americans applicants with undergraduate degrees have been allowed to apply to the 4 and 5-year programs simultaneously in previous years, however, this may be changing in the coming years [1]. North Americans applying to the 4-year program have not been eligible to apply to the 6-year program simultaneously in recent years. E.U applicants who want to apply to the 5 and/or 6 year medical program cannot choose whether they apply to the 5-year or 6-year program. They apply to the 5/6-year program and the admissions committee will choose which program they are eligible for. The 6-year program students do a foundation year which includes human biology, medical physics, biochemistry and some other core subjects. They then join the entering 5 year program students in the second year of study.

4 year program statistics

In the 2011-2012 application cycle, there are approximately 60 places available, with approximately 30 for E.U applicants and 30 for non-E.U applicants.

5 year program statistics
In the 2011-2012 application cycle, there were slightly less than 150 places available in the 5 year program [1], with roughly 15 places available for North American applicants and a few places for other non-E.U applicants. Note that the number of seats allocated to E.U and non-E.U applicants may change significantly from year to year [1]. In 2011, there was a quota of 49 E.U students admitted to the 5 and 6 year programs combined, with the rest of the places allocated to non-E.U applicants [1].

6 year program statistics
In the 2011-2012 application cycle, there are approximately 150 places available in the 5/6 year program [1], with 30 places available for North American applicants and a few places for other non-E.U applicants. Note that the number of seats allocated to E.U and non-E.U applicants may change significantly from year to year [1].

Contact
Admissions Office
Royal College of Surgeons in Ireland
Coláiste Ríoga na Máinleá in Éirinn
123 St Stephen's Green,
Dublin 2, Ireland.
Tel: +353 1 402 2100
admissions@rcsi.ie

A-level grade		Points awarded
	A	150
	B	130
A2 level	C	105
	D	80
	E	40
	A	75
	B	65
AS level	C	55
	D	40
	E	20

Table 53. Number of points awarded based on A-level grades at RCSI

Trinity College Dublin

Programs

Students with an undergraduate degree are eligible to apply to the 5 year program.

Nationality restrictions

None.

Degree requirement

E.U applicants must have completed secondary school. North American applicants must have completed an undergraduate degree.

A-level requirements

Students must have grades of B and C in two of physics, chemistry, biology or agricultural science. Students who do not have physics qualification may need a minimum grade of C or above in GCSE math.

IB requirements

Students wishing to use IB qualification must have at least two of physics, chemistry and biology at higher level [1]. Points for entry are calculated as follows: (Total points less bonus points) / 42 * 600. Thus, a total score less bonus points of 34 would translates to 486 CAO points. More details on IB grade conversions at Trinity College Dublin are available from: www.tcd.ie/Admissions/undergraduate/requirements/matriculation/other/

Other qualifications

Other equivalencies including EB and Cambridge pre-University are available from: www.tcd.ie/Admissions/undergraduate/requirements/matriculation/gcse/ and www.tcd.ie/Admissions/undergraduate/requirements/matriculation/other/

Admissions Exam

The HPAT Ireland is required for all E.U applicants. There has previously been no admissions exam required for non-E.U applicants [1].

Application documents

For mature E.U applicants, in addition to filling in the CAO of Ireland undergraduate medicine application, students are required to fill in a supplemental mature student application form available from: www.tcd.ie/Admissions/undergraduate/apply/forms/index.php#mature-student. This application form includes information about post-secondary education, employment, volunteer work, hobbies and interests, the applicant's interest in the course, the relevance of their life experience to the course and any additional information they wish to share.

Application documents (cont'd)

Non-E.U, non-North American applicants submit an international application form that includes education and personal comments in support of their application. References are not required initially for non-E.U, non-North American applicants but may be requested at a later stage in the application process.

Selection formula, E.U applicants

Only mature applicants are required to attend an interview. The university takes the full application into account including the interview and the HPAT to select candidates for admission [1].

Selection formula, North American applicants

There is no interview. Selection for admission is based on the full application including the personal statement and reference letters [18].

Selection formula, other international applicants

Students applying through agencies are sometimes required to attend interviews with their agencies, but those applying to the school directly are typically not required to attend an interview, and are selected for admission based on the content of their application forms and reference letters, if reference letters are requested by the school.

66

Interview

There is a mandatory interview held at the university for mature E.U applicants [1].

Cost of studies 2011-2012

E.U student fees = €6,371 per year, and non-E.U student fees = €31,000 per year.

Additional Information

Both E.U and non-E.U applicants with degrees in dentistry may be eligible to enter directly into the 3rd year of the program [1].

Statistics

In the 2011-2012 application cycle, there were approximately 134 seats available with approximately 94 places for E.U applicants and roughly 40 places for non-E.U applicants. The number of non-E.U applicants who will be admitted in future years may change significantly [1]. Of these roughly 94 places available for E.U students, 15% were allocated to students from non-traditional backgrounds, which included mature students as well as socio-economically disadvantaged students and students with disabilities.

Contact

Tel: +353 1 896 1039/3664
International office: +353 1 896 4444
admissons@tcd.ie

Ref: 194. *Trinity College Dublin*. Available from: http://medicine.tcd.ie/education/undergraduate/admissions/.

Poland
Medical programs in English

1. Medical Academy of Bialystok, 4 year and 6 year programs
2. Medical University in Bydgoszcz, Faculty II, 6 year program
3. Medical Academy of Gdansk, 6 year program
4. Medical University of Lodz, 4 year program (6 year program not for students with a degree)
5. Medical University of Lublin, 4 year and 6 year programs
6. Jagiellonian University Medical College, 4 year and 6 year programs
7. Pomeranian Academy of Medicine, 6 year program
8. Poznan School of Medicine, 4 year and 6 year programs
9. Medical University of Silesia, 4 year and 6 year programs
10. Medical University of Warsaw, 4 year and 6 year programs
11. Wroclaw Medical University, 6 year medical program

University Rankings

The QS World University Rankings have ranked two of the ten universities in Poland offering medical programs in English. The Polish universities ranking in the top 640 according to this source are:

> 304. Jagiellonian University
> 364. Warsaw University

The other Polish universities offering programs in English were not ranked that year. The Shanghai Consultancy also ranked both these universities in 2010 as 301st overall. The other universities in Poland were not ranked in the top 500 according to this source, and none were ranked in the top medical schools worldwide by either agency. More details on these rankings are available on page 118.

School by school

Medical Academy of Bialystok

Programs
Students with an undergraduate degree can apply to a 4 year and a 6 year program.

Nationality restrictions
Only students from North America can apply to the 4-year program [1]. The university currently has a 6 year program that is mostly for Scandinavian students, but is planning to introduce a 6 year program for North Americans in 2012 [1].

Academic requirements
Applicants to the 6 year program need strong secondary school grades in physics, chemistry and biology. Applicants to the 4 year program should have a good background in the sciences necessary to apply to medicine in Canada or the US [1].

Admission Exam
Students must write the MCAT to apply to the 4 year program. Students usually need scores of 23 or 24 to gain admission, depending on the year [1]. For the North American 6 year program, students may be required to take the SAT [1]. No admission exam is required for the European 6 year program.

Selection formula
Applicants to the 4 year program are interviewed. The entire application including extracurricular activities and dedication to medicine are considered when selecting students [1]. For the 6 year program, students are selected primarily on their secondary school or university grades. Good grades in biology, chemistry and physics are expected as there is no entrance examination.

Application documents
The application form includes basic demographic information and a 1 page personal statement.

Interview
There is a mandatory interview for students applying to the 4 year program.

Cost of studies 2011-2012
For the 4 year program and American 6 year program, approximately USD40,000 per year. Students may need to pay more if they want to complete their clinical studies in the US (something the university hopes to offer in the future) [1]. For the European 6 year program, approximately €9500 for the 1st year and €9000 per year for years 2-6.

Statistics

In the 2011-2012 application cycle, there were up to 17 places available in the 4 year program and up to 50 places available in the 6 year program. There were approximately 4 applicants for each place in the 6 year program [1]. A maximum of 34 students will be accepted to the North American 6 year program in 2012 [1].

Contact

Medical University of Bialystok
Kilińskiego 1 street, 15-089 Bialystok
Tel: +48 85 748 55 01
ed@umwb.edu.pl

Ref: 195. *Medical Academy of Bialystok, English Division.* Available from: http://ed.umb.edu.pl/.

Medical University in Bydgoszcz, Faculty II

Programs

Students with an undergraduate degree are eligible to apply to a 6 year program.

Nationality restrictions

This program will be open to all nationalities starting in the 2012-2013 application cycle [1].

Academic requirements

In previous years, the school has required students to have completed at least 2 of biology, chemistry and physics at secondary school level. The requirements for the 2012-2013 admission cycle will be available by April or May, 2012 [1].

Admission Exam

There will be an admissions exam in the 2012-2013 application cycle [1].

Selection formula

Students are required to attend an interview for admission.

Application documents

The application form may differ for European and non-European students in 2012 [1], but has included summaries of awards, employment and extracurricular activities as well as a personal statement up to 1 page in length in the past.

Interview

Students may be required to attend an interview.

Cost of studies

Approximately USD13,500 or €9,500 per year.

Contact

Faculty of Medicine - Dean's Office
Full-time Studies in English for Foreigners
Medical Program
Jagiellońska street, 13-15
Building A, room 04, 85-067
Bydgoszcz, Poland
Tel: +48 52 – 5853890
studiesinenglish@cm.umk.pl

Ref: 196. *Medical University in Bydgoszcz.* Available from: http://www.amb.bydgoszcz.pl/

Medical Academy of Gdansk

Programs

Students with an undergraduate degree are eligible to apply to a 6 year program.

Academic requirements

Students must have a secondary school diploma with courses in biology and chemistry.

Admission Exam

All applicants except those from Poland who have passed the matura are required to write an entrance exam [1]. The exam consists of secondary school chemistry and biology. Students usually write the exam in May or mid July each year, either at the university or in their home country if their local agency organizes an examination [1].

Application documents

Basic application form.

Selection formula

All aspects of the application are taken into consideration in the admissions decision including the admission exam, the personal statement and the interview for those who are required to attend an interview.

Interview

Only those students who did not perform well on the exam or in high school (or both)

but who are still being considered by the admissions committee will be invited for interview. The interview focuses mainly on questions from biology and chemistry.

Cost of studies 2011-2012

Approximately PLN44,000 per year, equal to roughly €15,500 per year.

Statistics

There are roughly 350 applicants for the 150 places available each year [1].

Contact

Medical University of Gdańsk
University Admission Office
Al. Zwycięstwa 41-42
80-210 Gdansk, Poland
Tel: +4858 349 13 90
admission@gumed.edu.pl
Regional contacts for several countries are available from: www.admission.mug.edu.pl/1447.html

---

Ref: 197. *Medical University of Gdansk, MD Programme admissions.* Available from: http://www.admission.mug.edu.pl/1447.html.

Medical University of Lodz

Programs

Students completing an undergraduate degree can apply to a 4 year program. Note that a 6 year program is available, but applicants who have completed a degree cannot apply [1]. Applicants with degrees who do not have the prerequisite courses are encouraged to complete the prerequisite requirements and apply to the 4 year program the following year [1].

Academic requirements

Applicants must hold an undergraduate degree and must have completed a full year of the following prerequisites at undergraduate level: general chemistry, organic chemistry, biology and physics Students who majored in chemistry, biology and physics will be given an advantage.

Admission exam

Students with MCAT scores above 24 are exempt from the entrance exam. Students who have not achieved this score or who have not taken the MCAT are given an interview examination on skype.

Selection formula

Selection is based on all aspects of the application including interview performance.

Application documents

Application form with financial information, summaries of awards, employment and extra curricular activities. Reference letters and records from past health experience can be submitted as well if the applicant chooses.

Interview

The skype interview tests 1st year university level biology and chemistry as well as secondary school (high school) physics.

Cost of studies

Approximately €12,500 per year.

Statistics

Most students admitted to the 4 year program are North Americans [1]. There are currently around 400 students enrolled in the 4 and 6 year programs combined [1].

Contact

Administration Center for Studies in English
Plac Hallera 1, 90 - 647
Lodz, Poland
Tel: +48 42 639 33 13
admission@umed.lodz.pl

69 198.   *Medical University of Lodz*. Available from: http://www.umed.lodz.pl/eng/.

Medical University of Lublin

Programs
Students completing an undergraduate degree can apply to a 4 year and a 6 year program.

4 year program academic requirements
Applicants need to hold an undergraduate degree and must have completed one full year at university level in the following prerequisite subjects: general chemistry, organic chemistry and biology. A semester in physics and either math or calculus is also required. In some circumstances, the university may consider well qualified students with 3 years of undergraduate study (minimum 90 credits) that have not completed their degree.

6 year program academic requirements
A secondary school diploma is required for admission. As a general rule, the secondary school education or equivalent should allow the student to apply to higher education institutions in their own country.

Admission Exam
North American students must write the MCAT for the 4-year program. SAT scores and PCAT scores can also be submitted.

Selection formula
All aspects of the application are taken into consideration in the admissions decision including the essay, the work experience, the motivation letter for those who are required to submit one and the interview for those who are required to attend one.

Application documents
North Americans submit an application form which includes financial information, extracurriculars, languages, and publications. An essay is also required on "why I want to become a physician". European and Asian applicants submit a different application form which includes a summary of work experience and other activities. A motivation letter is also required.

Interview
There is a mandatory interview for some applicants, depending on their country of origin.

Cost of studies 2010-2011
Approximately USD10,950 per year, or between €8,500 - 9,000.

Additional information
Note that just like other schools in Europe, the University of Lublin splits students into groups of 10 for a significant part of their education.

Statistics

In 2010, there were approximately 80 North American applicants, of which 90% were accepted to the program. Those who were not admitted were rejected because of not meeting the minimum degree requirements [1]. There were also 60 E.U applicants admitted and roughly 80 Asian applicants to the two programs [1].

School contact

Dean's Office for English Language Students
Collegium Novum, Al. Racławickie 1
20-950 Lublin, Poland
Tel: +48 81 528 8818

North American program contact

Hope Medical Institute:
Tel: +1 757-873-3333
gethope@hmi-edu.net.

European Program contact

Henning Tollefsen:
Tel: +47 91119423
henning@akuttmed.no
or Tommy Naess
Tel: +48 505818392 or
+47 90753500 (July and August)
tommy@akuttmed.no

Asian program contact

Jimmy Lin
Tel: +886932264755
jimmy@liemg.com

Ref: 199. *Medical University of Lublin.* Available from: http://www.umlub.pl/index2.html.

Jagiellonian University Medical College

Programs

Students completing an undergraduate degree can apply to a 4 year and a 6 year program.

4 year program academic requirements

Applicants need to hold an undergraduate degree and must have completed the following prerequisites: 1 semester of general chemistry, 1 semester of organic chemistry, 2 semesters of biology, 2 semesters of physics, 2 semesters of humanities or social sciences and 2 semesters of math. An alternative to 2 semesters of math is 1 semester of calculus. For Quebec students, a CEGEP degree with a minimum 70% average is sufficient.

6 year program academic requirements

Students must have secondary school courses in chemistry and biology. Courses in physics and math are recommended but not required. Students from Scandinavia should contact Ellen Bergene, +47 95 24 29 90 for subject requirements.

Admission Exam

For the 4 year program, the MCAT or GAMSAT is required for admission. The minimum MCAT score for the 2010-2011 application cycle was 21 [1]. For the 6 year program, a multiple choice entrance exam in biology and chemistry is held each year in Krakow, Poland and other locations such as Chicago, USA and Kuala Lumpur, Malaysia

in the past. A guide to help prepare for the exam is sent upon receipt of the application and registration fee.

4 year program selection formula

The most important factor in gaining admission is the MCAT score [1]. In the 2011-2012 application cycle, those with scores below 28 minimum were not interviewed. After the interview, applicants are given a score out of 5 for their GPA, 10 for their MCAT/GAMSAT results, and 10 for their interview. The GPA, MCAT and GAMSAT scoring is shown in table 54.

6 year program selection formula

Students are selected based on their ranking in the admissions exam [1].

Application documents

Students submit a brief application form which includes a one page personal statement on the applicant's reasons for choosing medicine. Applicants to the 4 year program must also submit 1-3 letters of recommendation, and a C.V.

Interview

For the 4 year program, there is a mandatory interview held in Toronto, Canada or Chicago, US.

Interview (cont'd)

Interviews in New York and Los Angeles, US, and Krakow, Poland can be arranged as well, or alternatively, applicants can be interviewed by phone at the discretion of the admissions committee. The interview is conducted by two people and covers the applicant's motivation, experience in humanitarian organizations, interpersonal and communication skills, and interests.

Cost of studies 2011-2012

Approximately €12,000 per year

4 year program statistics

In the 2011-2012 application cycle, there were approximately 90 applicants for the roughly 30 places available. Almost all students in the program are North American [1].

6 year program statistics

In the 2011-2012 application cycle, there were roughly 200 applicants for the 70 places available. Most students in the program come from outside North America [1].

Additional information

Prospective students from North America and Europe can contact previous graduates who have secured residencies. Contact information for Canadian, US, UK and other international graduates from the 4 year and 6 year programs is available from www.medschool.cm-uj.krakow.pl/zawartosc.php?grupy_kod=2

Contact

School of Medicine in English, School Office
ul. Sw. Anny 12, room 4,
31-008 Kraków Poland
Tel: +4812 422-80-42
smeoffice@cm-uj.krakow.pl

71

GPA	MCAT	GAMSAT
Points = $4 \times \dfrac{(cGPA - min)}{(max - min)} + 1$ cGPA = Average cumulative GPA Max = highest grade on scale Min = lowest grade on scale For example, a 3.0 GPA on a 4.0 scale would give: $4 \times \dfrac{(3.0 - 0.0)}{(4.0 - 0.0)} + 1 = 4$ points	34 and up = 10 points 33 = 9 points 32 = 8 points 31 = 7 points 30 = 6 points 29 = 5 points 28 = 4 points 27 = 3 points 26 = 2 points 24 - 25 = 1 point	77 and up = 10 points 74 - 76 = 9 points 71 - 73 = 8 points 68 - 70 = 7 points 65 - 67 = 6 points 62 - 64 = 5 points 59 - 61 = 4 points 56 - 58 = 3 points 53 - 55 = 2 points 50 - 52 = 1 point

Table 54. Number of points awarded based on GPA, MCAT and GAMSAT scores at Jagiellonian University Medical College

Ref: 200. *Jagiellonian University Medical College*. Available from: https://www.erk.uj.edu.pl/en/studia/katalog.

Pomeranian Academy of Medicine

Programs
Students with an undergraduate degree are eligible to apply to a 6 year program.

Academic requirements
Students must have completed courses in chemistry, as well as either biology or physics. Having both biology and physics will give students an advantage.

Admission Exam
There is currently no entrance exam, but the university may begin requiring an entrance examination in the future [1].

Selection formula
There is currently no interview or admissions exam, but all other aspects of the file are considered including awards, extra-curricular activities and academics. Academics are the most important part of the application [1].

Application documents
Application form with financial information, summaries of awards, employment and extra curricular activities. Documents proving medicine-related experience can be submitted as well.

Cost of studies 2011-2012
Approximately €9500-9800 per year

Statistics
In the 2010-2011 application cycle, there were approximately 500 applicants for the roughly 90 places available. In total there are approximately 5 or 6 North American students studying in all years of the program [1].

Contact
Pomeranian Medical University,
English Program
1 Rybacka Street
70-204 Szczecin
Poland
Tel: +4891 4800810
ep@sci.pam.szczecin.pl

Ref: 201. *Pomeranian Academy of Medicine.* Available from: http://www.ams.edu.pl/english/english-program.

Poznan School of Medicine

Programs
Students completing an undergraduate degree can apply to a 4 year and a 6 year program.

Nationality restrictions
Polish citizens are not eligible. Dual citizens and ethnically Polish people who are not Polish citizens are eligible to apply.

4 year program academic requirements
Applicants must hold an undergraduate degree from an accredited institution and must have completed a year in each of the following prerequisite subjects: general chemistry, organic chemistry, biology, physics and English. Students from all majors are eligible to apply.

6 year program academic requirements
Applicants must have strong grades in physics, chemistry and biology.

Admission Exam
For the 4 year program, all North American students must submit MCAT scores no more than three years old. There is no admissions exam required for the 6 year program.

Selection formula
All aspects of the application are taken into consideration in the admissions decision including the work experience, the letters of recommendation and the interview.

4 year program application documents
The application form includes summaries of awards, employment and extra curricular activities. Students must also submit 2 letters of recommendation from science faculty. Applicants can submit additional letters if they wish.

6 year program application documents
The application form includes summaries of awards, employment and extra curricular activities. Students must also submit 2 reference letters, one from a science teacher and one from their guidance office.

Interview
There is a mandatory interview for both programs currently held at Mercy College in New York, and at PUMS in Poznan. Interviews are held 4 times per year. There are no telephone interviews. Students from outside North America who have not taken the MCAT are interviewed in Poznan to test their knowledge in biology, chemistry and physics.

Cost of studies 2011-2012
Approximately USD15,000 per year for the 4 year program, and approximately USD12,107 per year for the 6 year program.

Additional Information

Preliminary interviews are available where the school can advise an applicant on what they can do to strengthen their application, including courses they can take and activities they can engage in.

Statistics

At Poznan University, most students come from North America, but there are also many Taiwanese students. There are also students from the E.U and other non-E.U countries. In 2009, there were approximately 350 North American students enrolled in the 4 year program and 300 in the six year program.

Contact

Poznan School of Medicine
41 Jackowskiego Street
Poznan, 60-812 Poland
Tel: +48 61 847 74 89
Contacts for several countries are available from: ump.edu.pl/eng/? strona=3_162_1050412646&am=235,244

Ref: 202. *Poznan University School of Medicine, MD program.* Available from: http://ump.edu.pl/eng.

Medical University of Silesia

Programs
Students completing an undergraduate degree can apply to a 4 year and a 6 year program. Student's undergraduate course curricula are compared with the medical school courses to determine how much credit toward their medical studies will be awarded.

4 year program academic requirements
Applicants need to hold an undergraduate degree or have some pre-medical experience.

6 year program academic requirements
Applicants must a secondary school degree.

Admission Exam
For the 4 year program, all North Americans and Indian students must submit MCAT scores no more than three years old. There is no admissions exam required for the 6 year program. Students from other countries may have admissions exams through their recruitment agencies as well [1].

Selection formula
All aspects of the application are considered including the essay (when applicable), work experience and the interview.

Application documents
The application for North Americans and applicants from India includes financial information, extracurricular activities, languages, and publications. An essay is also required on "why I want to become a physician". Taiwanese and Israeli citizens submit their applications to outside agencies listed on the school's website. Other nationals submit a basic application form.

Interview
North Americans and applicants from India are interviewed through Hope Medical Foundation. Other applicants are often interviewed at the school before enrolling [1].

Cost of studies
Approximately €10,000 per year for the first 4 years, then roughly €100-270 per week for clinical rotations starting in year 5 depending on where the rotations are completed.

Statistics
There are currently 404 students studying in the English medical program, as well as 1213 students in the Polish medical program.

Contact
Tel: +48 (32) 2088 689
smk@sum.edu.pl

Ref: 203. *Medical University of Silesia.* Available from: http://www.smk.sum.edu.pl/.

Medical University of Warsaw

Programs
Students completing an undergraduate degree can apply to a 4 year and a 6 year program.

4 year program academic requirements
Applicants must have 1200 hours of premedical coursework and either a Bachelor of Arts or a Bachelor of Science (or equivalent). To prove this, they are asked to have their university fill out a form outlining the number of hours they have completed [1].

6 year program academic requirements
Applicants must have passed chemistry, biology and physics at standard or advanced secondary school level [1].

Admissions Exam
There is no admissions exam for the 4 year program. For the 6 year program, students must write a multiple-choice entrance examination testing chemistry, biology and physics. In 2011 the examination was held at the end of May in Warsaw, Chicago, Kuala Lumpur and Oslo, but the locations may change in 2012 [1].

4 year program selection formula
Students are selected by the admissions committee primarily based on their university grades and prerequisite course hours [1].

6 year program selection formula
Students are selected based on their entrance examination performance [1].

Interview
None [1].

Cost of studies
Approximately €14,400 per year for the 4 year program and €11,100 per year for the 6 year program [1].

Statistics
In the 2011-2012 application cycle, there were approximately 300 applicants for the 100 places available in the 6 year program, and approximately 130 applicants for the 40 places available in 4 year program [1].

Contact
Medical University of Warsaw
2nd Faculty of Medicine, English Division
61 Żwirki i Wigury St.
02-091 Warszawa, Poland
Tel: +48 22 572 0552
natasza.rembielinska@wum.edu.pl

Ref: 204. *Medical University of Warsaw.* Available from: http://www.wum.edu.pl/english/.

Romania

Medical programs in English

1. Carol Davila University
2. Gr. T. Popa University
3. Iuliu Hatieganu University of Medicine and Pharmacy Cluj-Napoca
4. University of Oreada
5. Ovidius University of Constanta
6. University of Medicine and Pharmacy at Targu Mures
7. Victor Babeş University of medicine and pharmacy

University Rankings

In 2010, the universities in Romania with English taught medical programs were not ranked in the top 640 universities in the world according to the QS World University Rankings or the top 500 according to the Shanghai Consultancy World University Rankings.

School by school

Carol Davila University of Medicine and Pharmacy

Programs
Students with an undergraduate degree are eligible to apply to a 6 year program.

Academic requirements
Students must hold a secondary school (high school) diploma.

Admission exam
There is a mandatory English examination to obtain a place in the English program.

Selection Formula
Students submit their documentation in person (or possibly through a representative) to the rector's office. They can then receive permission to take the entrance exam, which is usually held in September. The top scoring candidates on this examination are offered admission.

Interview
Students are required to undergo an oral exam in addition to the written exam.

Cost of studies 2010-2011
E.U student fees = approximately €5,000 per year and non-E.U student fees = approximately €360 per month.

Statistics
In the 2011-2012 application cycle, there were 120 places available in the English medical program.

Contact
Tel: +40 21 318 0719

Ref: 205. *Carol Davila University of Medicine and Pharmacy.* Available from: www.univermed-cdgm.ro.

Gr. T. Popa University of Medicine and Pharmacy Iasi

Programs
Students with an undergraduate degree are eligible to apply to a 6 year program.

Academic requirements
Applicants must have a secondary school diploma.

Admission Exam
None [1].

Selection formula
There is no interview or examination required [1]. Students must have their credentials validated by the Romanian Ministry of Education or appropriate governing body. The points system used to select applicants for admission is available from www.umfiasi.ro/Pages/Default.aspx (see the second link under "Admission - 2011"). Points are given for several criteria including high grades, university study, as well as volunteer, professional, and other extracurricular activities.

Application documents
Students may gain 2 extra points in their application for submitting a letter of recommendation.

Approximately 2010-2011
Approximately €5000 per year

Additional Information
The university has held scholarship competitions for students who want to attend a Kaplan US Medical Licensing Exam Step 1 course. In previous years, the third year students scoring highest on the optional 2.5 hour multiple-choice examination were granted the scholarship.

Statistics
For entry in 2011, there are approximately 100 places available in the English medical program, as well as 100 in the Romanian medical program and 100 in the French medical program.

Contact
Gr.T.Popa University of Medicine and Pharmacy Iasi
Str. Universitatii no. 16, 700115
Iasi, Romania
Tel: +40 232 301 600
dec_med@umfiasi.ro

Ref: 206. *Gr.T.Popa University of Medicine and Pharmacy Iasi* Available from: http://www.umfiasi.ro/umf/ie2/navigation.jsp?node=2784#.

Iuliu Hatieganu University of Medicine and Pharmacy

Programs
Students with an undergraduate degree are eligible to apply to a 6 year program.

Academic requirements
Students must have a secondary school (high school) diploma.

Admission Exam
None [1].

Selection formula
There is no interview. Applications are scored based on applicants' school performance and personal achievements, and are ranked for admission based on their scores. Candidates are accepted preferentially on their fulfillment of the following:

1. International baccalaureate with at least 5 in chemistry or biology or,
2. General certificate of education with grade A+ or A who obtained at least B or B+ in biology or chemistry or,
3. Both the average of the baccalaureate marks and the average of each year's marks in biology and chemistry represent at least 70% of the maximum mark that can be obtained in the country of origin, as long as none of the individual marks is lower than 60% or,
4. Taking baccalaureate examination in biology and chemistry or,

5. Graduation from an accredited high school in the country of origin with biology and chemistry in the curriculum

The individual evaluation of the candidate also includes the following:

1. Post high school (college or university) education
2. High school type and results
3. Quality of extracurricular activities: voluntary work, professional experience in medicine-related fields, other relevant achievements
4. Letters of recommendation

Application documents
A reference letter and a copy of the applicant's CV must be submitted with the application.

Application deadline
The application deadline for last year was 29th July 2011.

Interview
None [1].

Cost of studies 2011-2012
Approximately €5,000 per year. Scholarships may be available starting in the second year of study for students who are performing well in the program.

Ref: 207. *Iuliu Hatieganu University of Medicine and Pharmacy.* Available from: http://www.umfcluj.ro/en.

Statistics
In the 2011-2012 application cycle, there will be a total of roughly 190 places available [1]. 30% of graduates to date have been from outside the country.

Contact
Universitatea de Medicina si Farmacie Iuliu Hatieganu
Cluj-Napoca, Victor Babes Street, no. 8, 400012
Tel: +40 264 406843
studentistraini@umfcluj.ro

University of Oradea

Programs
Students with an undergraduate degree are eligible to apply to a 6 year program.

Academic requirements
Applicants must have a secondary school diploma.

Admission Exam
There are two application cycles each year, each with an entrance exam. The entrance examination covers biology and chemistry. In 2011, the exams will be written in July and September.

Selection formula
European candidates are selected mainly based on the entrance examination which tests biology and chemistry. A list of topics is for the exam is available from: www.admitereuo.ro/index.php? option=com_content&view=article&id=82 &Itemid=100 All students must have their credentials approved by either CNRED (E.U applicants) or the Directorate General European Affairs and Bologna Secretariat (non-E.U applicants). There is no admissions exam for non-E.U students. No students who have been expelled from previous universities are accepted.

Application documents
Basic application form.

Cost of studies 2010-2011
Approximately €352 per month of study.

Contact
Universitatea din Oradea, Facultatea de Medicina
1 Decembrie, Nr.10
Oradea, Romania
Tel:+40 259 415 680,
medfarm@uoradea.ro
foreignstudents@uoradea.ro

Ref: 208. *University of Oradea, Faculty of Medicine admissions.* Available from: http://medfarm.uoradea.ro/eadmit.htm.

Ovidius University of Constanta

Programs
Students with an undergraduate degree are eligible to apply to a 6 year program.

Academic requirements
Students must have a secondary school diploma with grades of 50% or higher in biology, chemistry and physics.

Admission Exam
Students who come from non-English speaking countries may have to attend a test of proficiency in English Language upon arrival at the university.

Selection formula
All students submit the documents required to apply for a letter of acceptance from the Faculty of Medicine (proof of citizenship, secondary school certificate, etc.). In addition, E.U students fill in an application for recognition of their previous studies, while non-E.U students fill in an application for a letter of acceptance from the Ministry of Education. Once non-E.U students receive the letter of acceptance, they apply for a visa to study in Romania.

Interview
None.

Cost of studies
Approximately €3,600 per year.

Statistics
In the 2010-2011 application cycle, there were approximately 300 places available including the Romanian language program.

Contact
Ovidius University of Constanta
Alley No.1 University (Campus, building B)
Constanta, Romania
Tel: +40 241 605 003
C.iancu@univ-ovidius.ro

Ref: 209. *Ovidius University of Constanța*. Available from: http://www.medcon.ro/en-offer.php.

University of Medicine and Pharmacy of Targu Mures

Programs
Students with an undergraduate degree are eligible to apply to a 6 year program.

Academic requirements
Students must have a secondary school diploma.

Admission Exam
Students must write a 3 hour multiple choice examination in biology, chemistry and physics.

Selection formula
The admission exam carries approximately 80% of the weight, and secondary school grades are factored in as well.

Cost of studies
Approximately €5,000 per year.

Additional documents
E.U applicants and some other applicants may need to submit a copy of their CV with their application.

Statistics
There are approximately 70 places available in the English program.

Contact
University of Medicine and Pharmacy (UMF) Targu Mures
Str.Gh.Marinescu, Nr.38, Judetul Mures
Decanatul de Medicina - Departamentul Studenti Straini
Tel: +40-265-21 55 51

Ref: 210. *University of Medicine and Pharmacy of Targu Mures.* Available from: www.umftgm.ro/.

Victor Babeş University of Medicine and Pharmacy, Timişoara

Programs

Students with an undergraduate degree are eligible to apply to a 6 year program. The first three years of the program are in English, and the last three years are in Romanian [1]. Students who do not know Romanian may need to take courses in Romanian when they begin their studies.

Academic requirements

Students must have a secondary school diploma.

Admission Exam

There is an entrance exam with 60 biology questions and 20 organic chemistry questions.

Application documents and Selection formula

Applicants first submit their documents to the international office of the university (application form, transcripts, passport photos etc.). For E.U students, documents will be forwarded to the National Center for the Recognition and Validation of Diplomas (CNRED). E.U students may also need to have their high school diplomas validated by the Hague Apostille. For non-E.U applicants, the international office forwards the documents to the Romanian Ministry of Education, Research, Youth and Sports for approval. Once the documents are processed, students apply for a visa, submit their registration documents and enroll in the program.

Interview

None [1].

Cost of studies 2011-2012

E.U student fees = approximately €4,000 per year, and non-E.U student fees = approximately €3,200 per year.

Statistics

In 2009, there were approximately 450 places available in the Romanian and English medical programs combined. Students from several countries including E.U countries, the USA and Canada have studied in the program [1].

Contact

Victor Babeş University of Medicine and Pharmacy, International Students Office
Piata E. Murgu 2
300041 Timisoara, Romania
Tel: +40 256 220482
relint@umft.ro

Ref: 211. *Victor Babeş University of Medicine and Pharmacy.* Available from: http://www.umft.ro/newpage/en/index.htm.

Slovak Republic

Medical programs in English

1. Pavol Jozef Šafárik University in Kosice
2. Comenius University, Jessenius Faculty of Medicine in Martin
3. Comenius University, Faculty of Medicine

University Rankings

In 2010, the universities in Romania with English taught medical programs were not ranked in the top 640 universities in the world according to the QS World University Rankings or the top 500 according to the Shanghai Consultancy World University Rankings.

School by school

Comenius University in Bratislava, Faculty of Medicine in Bratislava

Programs
Students with an undergraduate degree are eligible to apply to a 6 year program.

Academic requirements
Students must have a secondary school (high school) diploma.

Admission Exam
A multiple choice entrance test in biology and chemistry is held at the university, or administered in the applicants' home country by a university representative. A revision booklet with 1000 practice questions can be purchased from the university. At the university, the tests are usually offered in late June and early July.

Selection formula
Students are ranked for admission based on their entrance examination score.

Application documents
The application form online can be submitted to a local representative, or if non exists, to the foreign student's office at the Faculty of Medicine. Students must submit a copy of their CV with the application.

Interview
None.

Cost of studies 2011-2012
Approximately €9000 per year

Statistics
There are approximately 100 places available for international students.

Contact
Tel: +4212 593 57 225
studijne.info@fmed.uniba.sk
List of international representatives:
www.fmed.uniba.sk/index.php?id=4750

Ref:212. *Comenius University in Bratislava, Faculty of Medicine in Bratislava.* Available from: www.fmed.uniba.sk/index.php?id=633.

Comenius University in Bratislava, Jessenius Faculty of Medicine in Martin

Programs

Students with an undergraduate degree are eligible to apply to a 6 year program.

Nationality restrictions

Slovak citizens are not eligible to apply.

Academic requirements

Students must have a secondary school diploma and have a background in biology, chemistry and English.

Admission Exam

Students must write a 40 question multiple choice entrance examination in biology and chemistry held at the university each year. The content of the exam is available from: eng.jfmed.uniba.sk/index.php? zobraz=ehtml&idmenu=3&iddata=79

Selection formula

The entrance examination is marked by the entrance examination board and students are informed of their results by July 31st. Students who perform well at the examination are offered a place in the program [1].

Application documents

Applicants must submit a copy of their CV with the application.

Interview

None [1].

Cost of studies 2010-2011

Approximately €8950 per year.

Statistics

There are currently approximately 300 international students studying medicine in the program, of which over 200 are from Norway. There are many students from Sweden, and also some students from other countries including the US [1].

Contact

Jessenius Faculty of Medicine, Institute for Medical Education in English Language
Mala Hora 4, 037 54
Martin, Slovakia
Tel: +421 43 423 82 99
akrajcovic@jfmed.uniba.sk

Ref: 213. *Comenius University in Bratislava, the Jessenius Faculty of Medicine in Martin.* Available from: http://eng.jfmed.uniba.sk/.

Pavol Jozef Šafárik University in Košice

Programs

Students with an undergraduate degree are eligible to apply to a 6 year program.

Academic requirements

Students must have a secondary school diploma.

Admission Exam

A multiple choice entrance examination in biology and chemistry is required.

Selection formula

Students with international representatives in their countries should first contact these representatives to apply. Although students need to meet the basic academic and language requirements, the most important part of the admissions process is the entrance examination [1].

Application documents

Applicants must submit a copy of their CV with the application.

Interview

None [1].

Cost of studies 2011-2012

Approximately €8500 per year

Statistics

In the 2011-2012 application cycle, there were approximately 100 places available for foreign students [1]. On average, there are approximately 300 applicants each year, but the number of applicants can vary significantly [1].

Contact

Pavol Jozef Šafárik University in Košice
Faculty of Medicine, Study Department
Trieda SNP 1, 040 11 Košice
The Slovak Republic
Tel: +421-55-6428 141
alena.tankosova@upjs.sk
International representatives: www.lf.upjs.sk/studium/Contact_Representative.html

---

Ref: 214. *Pavol Jozef Šafárik University in Košice.* Available from: http://www.upjs.sk/en/.

Ukraine

Medical programs in English

1. Bogomolets National Medical University
2. Bukovinian State Medical University
3. Crimea State Medical University
4. Danylo Halytsky Lviv State Medical University
5. Dnipropetrovsk State Medical Academy
6. Kharkov State Medical University
7. Lugansk State Medical University
8. I.Y. Gorbachevsky Ternopil State Medical University
9. M. Gorky Donesk National Medical University
10. Odessa State Medical University
11. Zaporozhya State Medical University

University Rankings

In 2010, the universities in Romania with English taught medical programs were not ranked in the top 640 universities in the world according to the QS World University Rankings or the top 500 according to the Shanghai Consultancy World University Rankings.

There is also a ranking of the top 200 universities in the Ukraine completed by UNESCO in 2009 based on the following criteria [87]:

1. Quality of scientific education and pedagogical training
2. Quality of education overall
3. International recognition

This ranking includes medical universities, technical universities, economics universities, etc. Four medical schools with English programs were ranked in the Ukraine's top 50 universities according this ranking:

4. Bogomolets National Medical University
14. M. Gorky Donesk National Medical University
43. Dnipropetrovsk State Medical Academy
46. Kharkov State Medical University

To the best of our knowledge, the full rankings are not available in English, but are available in Ukrainian from http://euroosvita.net/prog/data/upimages/rating2009_2.jpg. Articles discussing these rankings are available from http://mignews.com.ua/en/articles/29051.html and www.ehow.com/list_6573314_medical-universities-ukraine.html.

School by school

Bogomolets National Medical University

Programs
Students with an undergraduate degree are eligible to apply to a 6 year program.

Academic requirements
Applicants are required to have completed a secondary school (high school) diploma.

Admission Exam
None.

Selection formula
To apply, students should send an email to the medical school (amoris_pq@mail.ru), who will request the necessary documents from them (photocopies of passport, secondary school (high school) diploma, and transcripts translated into Russian or Ukrainian) [1]. Students then receive an invitation to study medicine at the school, and usually bring this to the nearest Ukrainian embassy to obtain their visa.

Application documents
Basic application form, as well as supporting documents like transcripts, birth certificate, etc. Applicants also need an open return ticket to their home country valid for the first year.

Interview
Students are interviewed by the vice-rector of education as well as other members of the admissions committee.

Cost of studies
The tuition fees are approximately USD4300 per year [1].

Statistics
Each year there are approximately 15-20 students studying in the English Medical Program [1].

Contact
O.O. Bogomolets National Medical University
Department of Foreign Students
13 Shevchenko blvd. Kyiv, Ukraine, 01601
Tel: +380 (444) 54-49-56
sasha@nmu.kiev.ua

Ref: 215. *Bogomolets National Medical University.* Available from: http://nmu.edu.ua/eng/e10.php.

Bukovinian State Medical University

Programs
Students with an undergraduate degree are eligible to apply to a 6 year program.

Academic requirements
Applicants are required to have completed a secondary school (high school) diploma and to have achieved grades above 75% in biology, chemistry and physics.

Admission Exam
There is an entrance test covering biology, chemistry and physics taken at the university prior to enrolling in the program.

Selection formula
Applicants are selected based on the interview performance.

Application documents
Indian students must obtain an eligibility certificate to study medicine abroad. Normally, this requires the 10+2 or equivalent courses in biology, physics and chemistry with minimum grades of 50%. Applicants also need an open return ticket to their home country valid for the first year.

Interview
Two faculty members visit India and other countries every year to interview applicants. All applicants are interviewed [1].

Cost of studies
The tuition fees are approximately USD3400 per year [1].

Statistics
At present more than 5,000 students are studying at BSMU and out of them nearly 800 are international students.

Contact
Bukovinian State Medical University
58002, Teatralna Square, 2,
Chernivtsy,
Tel: +380 (372) 55-37-54
Inter@bsmu.edu.ua
A list of overseas representatives is available from: www.bsmu.org.ua/index.php?option=com_content&task=view&id=3&Itemid=5

Ref: 216. *Bukovinian State Medical University.* Available from: http://www.bsmu.edu.ua/en/index.asp.

Crimea State Medical University

Programs
Students with an undergraduate degree are eligible to apply to a 6 year program.

Academic requirements
Students must have a secondary school diploma.

Admission Exam
None [126].

Selection formula
Students send an email to a university representative (either in their country or elsewhere). The company then asks for relevant documentation and sends the documents to the university. The university reviews the student's documents and sends them an invitation letter, which they bring to the closest Ukrainian embassy. After they are interviewed at the embassy, students apply for a visa and can then enroll in the program [126].

Interview
Students are interviewed by the staff at the nearest Ukrainian embassy [126].

Cost of studies
Approximately USD3500 per year.

Statistics
In 2011, there were approximately 50 students studying in the English program [126]. There are also English speaking students studying in masters programs at the medical university.

Contact
Crimea State Medical University
5/7 Boulevard Lenin,
95006-Simferopol,
Crimea, Ukraine.
Tel: +38-093-6640546
crsmu.com@gmail.com
A list of overseas representatives is available from: www.crsmu.com/representatives

---

Ref: 217. *Crimea State Medical University.* Available from: http://www.crsmu.com/.

Danylo Galician Lviv State Medical University

Programs
Students with an undergraduate degree are eligible to apply to a 6 year program.

Academic requirements
Students must have a secondary school diploma.

Admissions exam
None [127].

Selection formula
Foreigners should present all the required documents (or copies) to the university. The university will then arrange for the applicant to obtain their visa from the nearest embassy.

Application requirements
Basic application form.

Cost of studies
Approximately USD4300 per year

Interview
None [127].

Statistics
In the 2010-2011 application cycle, there were approximately 115 places available in both the Ukrainian and English medical programs. At present, over 5000 students are studying in approximately 40 departments.

There are roughly 120 students admitted to the English medical program each year [127].

Contact
Dean of foreign students
Associate professor
Eugene S. Varyvoda
79010, Lviv, Pekarska 69
+38 (032)2755927, 2757541
Varyvoda@meduniv.lviv.ua
A list of overseas representatives is available from: www.meduniv.lviv.ua/ by clicking on "prospective students" on the left, then "Officials of LNMU". Make sure the page is translated to English using google translate.

Ref: 218. *Danylo Halytsky Lviv State Medical University.* Available from: http://www.meduniv.lviv.ua/index.php?lang=en.

Dnipropetrovsk state medical academy

Programs
Students with an undergraduate degree are eligible to apply to a 6 year program.

Academic requirements
Students must have a higher secondary school certificate or 12 years of education with passes in chemistry, physics and biology.

Admissions exam
None.

Application documents
Basic application form.

Selection formula
Based solely on the forms and administrative documents submitted, the medical school may give out an invitation letter to study medicine at their university.

Application deadline
Applications are accepted from 1st March until 1st November. Classes starts from 1st September but students can join the first year class until 15th November.

Interview
None.

Contact
Tel: +380 933347754
admissions@dpsmu.com

A list of overseas representatives is available from: http://www.dpsmu.com/Overseas-representatives.php

Kharkov State Medical University

Programs
Students with an undergraduate degree are eligible to apply to a 6 year program. Students may receive credit for courses they took in their undergraduate degree, but can currently only receive up to 2 years of credit [1].

Academic requirements
Students must have a secondary school diploma.

Admission Exam
None [1].

Selection formula
Based solely on the forms and administrative documents submitted, the medical school may give out an invitation letter to study medicine at their university. Before entering the program, students attend a short interview to test their basic language and competence [1].

Interview
Students are interviewed on arrival in the Ukraine. They are given a medical textbook and are asked to answer questions on it [1].

Cost of studies
Approximately USD3500

Statistics
There are currently 21 students in the English medical program [1], and approximately 150 students in the Ukrainian medical program.

Contact
Kharkov State Medical University
Prospekt Lenina 4, Kharkov 310022
Tel: +380 57 707 51 38
interstudent@univer.kharkov.ua
ffm@univer.kharkov.ua

Ref: 219. *Kharkov State Medical University.* Available from: http://www.univer.kharkov.ua/en.

Lugansk State Medical University

Programs
Students with an undergraduate degree are eligible to apply to a 6 year program.

Academic requirements
Students must have a secondary school diploma and passing grades in chemistry, physics, and biology. If English is not the applicant's first language, a grade of pass must be obtained in English as well.

Admission Exam
None.

Selection formula
Students first send an email to the university (infolsmu.com@gmail.com) to receive the details on what they need to submit to apply (name, nationality, scanned passport photo page, etc). The school then sends the student an invitation letter, which they bring to the nearest Ukrainian embassy. Students then apply for a visa and travel to the school with their documents (notarized and translated into Ukrainian or Russian) to enroll in the program.

Interview
None.

Cost of studies
Approximately USD5900 for the first year, then USD3500 for years 2-6 [1]

Statistics
There are currently over 290 students studying medicine at the university including students from the UK, Canada, the US, Africa and Asia [1].

Contact
Lugansk State Medical University
Block 50 years, Of lugansk defence, 1.
Lugansk - 91045, Ukraine.
Tel: +38-067-6892167
infolsmu.com@gmail.com
A list of international representatives is available from: www.lsmu.com/representatives

Ref: 220. *Lugansk State Medical University* Available from: http://www.lsmu.com.

I. Y. Gorbachevsky Ternopil State Medical Academy

Programs
Students with an undergraduate degree can apply to a 6 year program.

Academic requirements
Students must have a secondary school diploma.

Admission Exam
None [1].

Selection formula
Students submit the application form available from http://www.tdmu.edu.te.ua/eng/adm_info/adm_proc.htm to the dean, along with a copy of their passport and secondary school diploma. They then receive an invitation letter which they bring to the nearest Ukrainian embassy where they will apply for a visa. Once applicants have obtained a visa, they inform the international student office of their arrival date and they are invited for an interview upon arrival. Students then gain admission after signing a contract in which they agree to pay for their first year of study.

Interview
Students are interviewed when they arrive on campus before enrolling in the program.

Cost of studies
Approximately USD3,700 per year

Statistics
There are currently approximately 3100 students studying in the faculties of medicine, pharmacy and dentistry combined. Students are split into groups of 8 during their studies [1].

Contact
I. Y. Gorbachevsky Ternopil State Medical Academy
m.Voli, 1, Ternopil, 46001
Tel: +380 352 524492
dean@tdmu.edu.te.ua
International representatives are listed at http://www.tdmu.edu.te.ua/eng/adm_info/adm_proc.htm

Ref: 221. *I. Y. Gorbachevsky Ternopil State Medical University.* Available from: http://www.tdmu.edu.te.ua/eng/general/index.php.

M. Gorky Donetsk National Medical University

Programs

Students with an undergraduate degree are eligible to apply to a 6 year program.

Academic requirements

Students must have a secondary school diploma.

Admission Exam

There is an English proficiency exam, in which a grade of proficient allows the applicant to study there, and a grade of marginal requires them to take an English class parallel to their medical training for additional cost. Those who get a grade of poor can enroll in a 1 year preparatory class in English at the university.

Selection formula

Students can submit an application online at http://donmeduni.com/apply %20online.htm if the online link is working. If it is not working, students can email the vice dean (vdeanvz@hotmail.com) who will send them a copy of the application form. They then submit this form back to the vice dean with the first page of their passport and a document confirming their completion of secondary school, and their CV if they wish [1]. Once this is done and the application fees are paid, the university sends successful applicants an invitation letter to study at the university which they bring to the local Ukrainian embassy to apply for a visa (along with other documents including photographs, an HIV/AIDS test result and official bank documents showing that they have paid half the first year's tuition). With these documents, students are guaranteed a visa. Students also need to complete an English examination on arrival in the Ukraine which determines whether they need to complete a preparation year in English language studies.

Interview

None in previous years.

Cost of studies 2010-2011

Approximately USD4,200 per year [1].

Statistics

In the 2010-2011 application cycle, there were approximately 70-80 students in the English classes. Students are separated into groups of 8 or 9 students.

Contact

Donetsk National Medical University, 16, Ilicha Avenue, Donetsk, Ukraine-83003 Tel: +380 622 955379, +380 622 955512 vdeanvz@hotmail.com

---

Ref: 222. *M. Gorky Donetsk National Medical University.* Available from: http://www.donmeduni.com/.

Odessa National Medical University

Programs
Students with an undergraduate degree are eligible to apply to a 6 year program.

Academic requirements
Students are required to have completed a secondary school (high school) diploma with minimum grades of 50% in chemistry, physics, and biology.

Admission Exam
None [1].

Application documents
There is a basic application form to fill in. Students submit their application form to the university representative in their country if one exists. If not, they submit the application to the university directly.

Selection formula
If the documents are sent to an international representative, they will pass it on to the university, who will issue an invitation letter to the student. The applicant brings this letter to the Ukrainian embassy, who will issue the student visa and allow the student to study at the university [1].

Interview
None [1].

Contact
Odessa State Medical University
Valikhovskiy lane, 2,
Odessa 65026, Ukraine
Tel : + 380 487238333
Indian representative: +91-9837029629
rector.office@odmu.edu.ua

Ref: 223. *Odessa State Medical University.* Available from: http://www.odmu.edu.ua/index.php?v=1190.

Zaporozhya state medical university

Programs
Students with an undergraduate degree are eligible to apply to a 6 year program.

Academic requirements
Students are required to have completed a secondary school (high school) diploma.

Admission Exam
None [1].

Application documents
Basic application form.

Selection formula
Once the application form and the certificates of all previous education are sent, alongside administrative requirements, an international student can be admitted. They receive an invitation given from the university authorities through the foreign agents or a firm. The whole process of being admitted can take less than 2 weeks and there are no specific grade requirements.

Interview
None [1].

Application fees
One time only fees include USD150 registration fees, USD150 admission fees, USD150 invitation fees and USD200 administrative charge. This comes to a total of USD 650 one time only fees.

Cost of studies
USD3,600 per year in tuition fees.

Contact
This list of official and authorized overseas representatives can be found here: http://www.zsmu.net/over.html and http://www.zsmu.net/indian_representative.html

Medical School Interview

The interview is your final step toward gaining admission to medical school. Like with the other steps, thorough preparation is required. We have met unsuccessful applicants who said that they did not prepare for interviews because they wanted to "be themselves". Being unprepared does not help you be more yourself. We believe that it is essential to show who you are in the interview, and that the best way to do this is to spend time beforehand thinking about yourself, what experiences you have, and doing mock interviews to make sure you communicate your messages clearly. Like with the other steps, those who prepare the best tend to do the best.

Unsuccessful applicants frequently gain admission the following year by preparing better for their interviews. For example, in Canada, the success rate for re-applicants is 7% higher than first time applicants (27.5% vs. 20.6%). In our experience, this higher acceptance rate reflects the additional preparation and experience students have the second time they go into an interview. If it is your first time interviewing, be as prepared as someone interviewing the second time around, or more prepared, and your chances will improve.

Before you start preparing, it is important to understand what the medical schools are looking for in the interviews. Here is what two medical schools say:

University of Manitoba (MMI): "The actual content of questions is not all that different from a job interview. We're interested in the same qualities in our medical students that have been identified by the medical profession as essential for physicians. Well developed oral communication skills are essential. In addition, we will explore such qualities as integrity, honesty, reliability, conscientiousness, respect, responsibility, self-assessment skills, approach to learning, and motivation."

University of Saskatchewan (MMI): "Personal attributes such as communication skills and maturity will be assessed at all MMI stations. Station scenarios may be structured to specifically judge a candidate's ethical and critical decision-making abilities, knowledge of the healthcare system, understanding of health determinants in a local or global context, commitment to helping others, nonacademic achievements, or desire for studying medicine."

<u>Cambridge University</u>: "We want to know whether you have a genuine intellectual curiosity for medical science, imagination and a breadth and flexibility of outlook, have the personal characteristics likely to make you a good doctor, and have a realistic attitude to medicine as a career."

<u>University College London</u>: "Interviewers will independently score the candidate on the following qualities: motivation for and understanding of a career in medicine, awareness of scientific and medical issues, ability to express and defend opinion, attitude and maturity of character, communication skills and individual strengths."

<u>Duke University</u>: "Interview day is, at heart, a "fit" day - a day to determine whether you and Duke make a good match. From Duke's perspective, it's a chance for us to probe more deeply the information in your application, to learn more about the depth of your intellectual curiosity, commitment to a career of service, and ethical values."

<u>Ross University, School of Medicine</u>: "The interview helps assess your overall personal and academic background, maturity, adaptability, character, aptitude, and most importantly, your motivation to become a doctor."

Although the structure of the interviews varies from one university to another, all universities are looking for some similar things in their applicants, including a good and realistic understanding of what the medical profession entails, a strong motivation and capacity to become a doctor, a maturity of character, an awareness of medical issues, communication skills as well as other personal characteristics. Certain universities like the University of Glasgow and the University of Sheffield also expect applicants to have researched their curriculum and have good reasons for wanting to attend their medical school.

Interview structures

Panel interviews

In this form of interview, the interview is in the presence of either one, two or more interviewers. The interview can be very formal with a table between the interviewee and the interviewers or it can be very much informal with chairs put together in a circle. Whether it is formal or informal, the interviewers are not there to intimidate you or ask you trick questions. Most medical school interviews are quite friendly in nature and can feel like a conversation.

Multiple Mini Interviews (MMI)

The MMI consists of a series of short, timed mini-interviews attempting to draw multiple samples of an applicant's ability to think on their feet, critically appraise information and communicate their ideas [88]. The number of stations, the types of tasks you are required to complete and the details regarding the methods of evaluation differ from one school to another. Here is what McMaster University, the pioneers of the MMI interview, says about their MMI stations:

"The stations deal with a variety of issues, which may include but are not limited to, communication, collaboration, ethics, health policy, critical thinking, awareness of society health issues in Canada and personal qualities [89]."

Here is an example of an MMI scenarios that was used in the past from the 2006 interviewer's manual of McMaster University [90].

Scenario 1:

"Dr. Blair recommends homeopathic medicines to his patients. There is no scientific evidence or widely accepted theory to suggest that homeopathic medicines work, and Dr. Blair doesn't believe them to. He recommends homeopathic medicine to people with mild and nonspecific symptoms such as fatigue, headaches, and muscle aches, because he believes that it will do no harm, but will give them reassurance. Consider the ethical problems that Dr. Blair's behavior might pose. Discuss these issues with the interviewer."

Here are the instructions the interviewers were given in assessing the candidates [88]:

1. Did the applicant express balance and sympathy for both intellectual positions?
2. Was there a clear analysis of the ethical problems paternalism raises?
3. Did the applicant suggest a course of action that is defensible and moderate?

Scenario 2:

"Your company needs both you and a coworker (Sara, a colleague from another branch of the company) to attend a critical business meeting in San Diego. You have just arrived to drive Sara to the airport. Sara is in the room."

Here are the instructions the interviewers were given in assessing the candidates [88]:

1. Did the applicant appear empathetic?
2. Did the applicant attempt to console Sara without belittling her or making light of her concerns?
3. Does the applicant help Sara considering multiple potential courses of action?

The prompt does not tell you much about Sara, and it is you as the interviewee who needs to find out what is going on. For this example, here is the background information that you can find out as you talk with Sara: "Sara is anxious regarding her safety. She had a friend who narrowly escaped being at the World Trade Center when it was destroyed. Until now, she had not experienced angst regarding air travel, but presumably there were latent feelings present, surfacing today with the immediate prospect of flying to San Diego. She had routinely travelled via air in the past, but this is the first time air travel was required since September 11th, 2001. She is gripped with fear over what might happen."

Here is a list a effective communication skills the observer will be looking for [88]:

- Listens well.
- Remains supportive.
- Avoids making light of Sara's concerns.
- Normalizes concerns, noting that these feelings of anxiety can be common.
- Confirms, without patronizing, that Sara is aware of the relative safety of air travel (e.g. better security now in place at airports, statistically tiny chance of being targeted, etc)
- Helps Sara separate the intellectual response of low danger from the emotional response of anxiety.

Some other universities like Queen's University Belfast also discuss on their websites how evaluators assess the interviewees. Here is an example of an MMI scenario from their website and the instructions to the evaluators:

Scenario: "Your mother rings you and asks you to come round and help with a major family decision. Her 70 year old father has been diagnosed with a condition that will kill him sometime in the next five years. He can have a procedure that will correct the disease and not leave him with any long term problems, but the procedure has a 10% mortality rate. He wants to have the procedure but your mother is not in favour of it. How would you help mediate this issue?"

Here are the instructions the evaluator is given to assess the candidate (the candidate does not see these criteria) [91]:

> Demonstrates sensitivity to the needs of others
> Understands the right of the patient to be fully involved in decisions about their care
> Can think of ways to help resolve a situation when emotional issues may cloud one's judgement
> Understands the limit of their own knowledge and experience

These are only a few examples, and some schools might use very different types of scenarios.

Some universities, both in Canada and the UK, have some practice MMI questions on their websites. The questions available from St. George's Medical School, the University of Saskatchewan and from the University of Calgary are available from:

1. http://www.sgul.ac.uk/undergraduate/foundation-for-medicine/interviews

2. http://www.medicine.usask.ca/education/medical/undergrad/admissions/multiple-mini-interview-mmi-information/Practice_MMI_Questions.pdf

3. http://www.ucalgary.ca/mdprogram/prospective/admissions/mmi/samples

An MMI interviewer manual is also are also available from the McMaster University website:

http://fhs.mcmaster.ca/mdprog/interviews.html under "For further details regarding the MMI and a copy of the training manual, please click here."

Some companies in the UK that prepare applicants for MMIs also have a few sample questions available, such as www.medical-interviews.co.uk.

http://www.medical-interviews.co.uk/Multi-Mini-Interviews-MMI-St-Georges.aspx

Types of questions you are asked

Questions asking for examples

1.   Describe a situation where you played an important role in a team
2.   Give us an example of when you got angry
3.   Can you remember a time when you made a mistake
4.   Describe a situation where you used your communication skills effectively
5.   Tell us about how you dealt with a conflict

You will get a question asking you for an example in almost every panel interview, and in some MMI interviews. It is very important that you have **identified examples, anecdotes and stories that you want to tell the interviewers before your interview.** It is also very important that if you are asked a question of that type, you do not talk in generalities about yourself but really think of one specific example and talk about it. For instance, with question 1, saying that you often play a crucial role on your soccer team to decide which players are going to be selected will not be as powerful as remembering one specific time the decision had to be made, and then describing in more detail what happened that time, what you thought, what you did, the result and the impact it had on the team, the game and yourself. Also, if your example involves a situation with a team, do not waste time talking about what the team did but really focus on what you did, because the panel is here to find out about you and your skills.

Last, but not least, it is essential to have a structure in your answer. We suggest:

1.   Describing the situation first (when, where, who, what was happening)
2.   What you saw/thought/felt/noticed
3.   What you did and how you did it
4.   The result of the situation and sometimes what you learned from it

This is not the only possible structure. Some books suggest that you describe the situation first, then what you did, then why and finally the result. As long as it follows logically, we do not think that there is a preferred structure. However, it is important that you have a structure that flows well and that makes your example clear to somebody who does not know you. Practice telling your stories to people that do not know you well if possible to make sure they are clear, concise and flow well.

The last important point is that preparing 5 or 10 anecdotes with lessons learned tends to serve applicants better than trying to remember 50 different stories. You will find that having 5 or 10 good anecdotes will enable you to answer almost all of the questions they ask. For example, if you have a story about leading a project and what you learned from your leadership experience, you will be able to answer many questions with this one example like "tell me about a time you led a team", "tell me about a time you have worked in a team", "tell me about a time you have handled a difficult situation", "tell me about a time you needed to communicate effectively", etc.

"Dealing with" or "coping with" questions

1. How do you handle stress
2. How do you deal with incompetent people
3. How do you handle criticism
4. How do you handle conflicts
5. How do you deal with a bad team leader

These nonspecific questions are a good opportunity to show maturity and reflection. Although they are not asking you for a specific example, it is often more effective to think of one or two examples and not talk in generalities.

Also, even if they are not specifically asking 'why do you do it that way', it is essential to explain your reasoning in your answer. Simply listing the few things you do in order to handle stress will not be as effective as explaining why and how you have developed these methods of coping with stress.

If you are not sure why you are doing something a certain way, you can try to think of why it is that you do not do it differently and that can form the basis of your reasoning. Explaining your train of thought is always going to be a better answer than simply answering with a list of things you do to cope with or deal with a situation.

Another very important point is that you need to acknowledge the problem/situation you are asked about. What we mean is that if they ask you about how you deal with stress, it is probably not a good idea to say you do not get stressed. There are many stresses that you will face as a medical student and later on as a doctor. Some examples include stress before exams, stress when making a mistake on the ward, stress when presenting to a large audience or to doctors, stress when breaking bad news or stress from not having enough time to spend with family and friends and feeling unbalanced. Even if you believe you do not get stressed, acknowledge that it may happen in certain cases and try to answer the question showing some reflection and evidence of your maturity/experience.

As with any types of questions, you need a structure to deliver your answer. Try answering questions and getting different people to listen to your answers. They will be able to tell you if your answer is difficult to follow, not well structured or if it sounds clear.

Sample answer: How do you handle stress?

1. Immediate stress: When I face a very stressful situation, I like to go to my family or a few people I have developed a good relationship with to talk and ask for advice. I find that talking and hearing someone else's perspective often helps me to not lose sight of the important matters in a stressful time.

2. Long term stress: Although hobbies and activities do not help in a specific stressful situation, I find that the fact that I take part in several activities with different peer groups every week makes me a generally more relaxed person and possibly this helps me decrease the usual stress that comes before exams.

3. Preventing stress: I also think that there are simple things I can do to help myself prepare when I know stressful situations are coming up such as exams. Making a plan, prioritising tasks, making sure I get enough sleep are all little things that together contribute to helping me cope with stressful situations.

This is certainly not a perfect answer, and there are many answers that will be stronger. However this example is here to show how an interviewee can demonstrate that they have thought about the issue, and that they have taken action to address it. Many students answer questions like this by listing how many hobbies they have and all the activities that they do but in fact, when an sudden stressful situation occurs, it is unlikely that the hobbies you do will help you adequately. In this example, the candidate give a structured answer describing how they may manage immediate stress but also the actions they take to prevent stressful situations. This answer could most certainly be improved by adding 1 or 2 specific examples of times when the applicants has done something to handle a stressful situation. Many interviewers ask this question because they have seen or heard of students who lose their balance in medical school, and perform poorly or drop out as a result. It will help your candidacy if you can show them that you take deliberate steps to keep your stress level low, and will be able to stay balanced in medical school.

Expressing an opinion, point of view, ethical questions

1. Do you think that private healthcare is better that public healthcare?
2. What do you think of doctors smoking right outside hospitals?
3. What do you think of abortion?
4. What do you think of the numbers of hours doctors work?
5. What do you think of the role of nurses in the medical team?

Just like the example related questions, these questions are very common. The panel members are not necessarily looking for somebody who agrees with their opinion but are looking for somebody who can talk about the topic from different perspectives and who can present balanced arguments in a clear, concise and structured manner. The panel also wants to know if you are knowledgeable about certain topics, for example, if you have a good idea of how the healthcare system works in the country you are applying to.

For ethical questions particularly, we strongly advise that you give the various sides of the argument before you talk about your personal point of view. When you express your own point of view, it is important that you can justify your points with solid arguments. To be able to answer a good range of ethical questions, it is a good idea to have read enough and to have reflected on the most common ethics related topics in medicine. A few books are mentioned on the University of Michigan career website which we have listed below [92]:

Books:
1. Ethical and Economic Issues Confronting Today's Practicing Physicians: A Synopsis. Charles F. Thurber, 2004
   Available from: http://www.admission-interview.com/index.html
   An ebook available for purchase for approximately 20 USD from the above website. Includes several commonly tested interview cases with analysis of both sides of the issue. We both used this book while preparing for our interviews and found it useful.
2. Classic Cases in Medical Ethics: Accounts of the Cases that have Shaped Medical Ethics, with Philosophical, Legal, and Historical Backgrounds. Gregory E. Pence, 2004
   Approximately 46 USD on amazon.com, includes analysis of ethical cases with background and historical perspective.
3. The Ethics of Health Care. Raymond S. Edge and John Randall Groves, 1999
   Approximately 31 USD on amazon.com. Introduction to healthcare ethics with exercises to help the reader practice what is taught in the book.

There are several other books available online as well.

The University of Michigan also suggested a few websites, including www.virtualmentor.org. The website has a case index exploring a variety of cases, including some that are more commonly asked about such as refusal of life-sustaining treatments, and some that are unlikely to be tested in medical school interviews but are there for medical specialists, such as ethics around Partial Androgen Insensitivity Syndrome.

In order to prepare, you may want to read about the most commonly tested topics, including cases that allow you to reflect on the ethical issues. However you choose to prepare, it is much more important to understand the recurring themes (patient's right to autonomy, requirement for beneficence and non-maleficence etc.) that apply to all cases. In reading different cases, students generally find that a few themes continue to come up again and again, and can be used in the interview. Interviewers are not looking necessarily for a "right" answer, but instead are looking to see that you can reason through both sides of an ethical decision and come to a reasonable and defensible conclusion.

Here is an example of a structure you can use to answer ethical questions. Again, it is not the only structure possible but is one example:

1. Explore ethical issue/consideration 1
2. Explore ethical issue/consideration 2 (other side of the argument)
3. Explore ethical issue/consideration 3 (third side of the argument if applicable)
4. Use of extreme examples to make your point and reconcile the different issues considered + conclude with an opinion that flows logically from your thought process
5. If asked a specific question, answer the question at this point

"What do you think of abortion?"

1. Explore ethical issue/consideration 1

On the one hand, the fetus is considered a human being by many religions, and an abortion would be taking away the life of that child.

2. Explore ethical issue/consideration 2 (other side of the argument)

On the other hand, we must also consider the autonomy that the mother should have to make decisions about her own body and health. Pregnancy and delivery does not come without its health risks to the mother.

3. Explore ethical issue/consideration 3 (third side of the argument if applicable)

There is also room for abuse. A women may be threatened by the father, her family etc. to have the abortion and lose a baby she wants to have.

4. Use of extreme examples to make your point and reconcile the different issues considered + conclude with an opinion that flows logically from your arguments

There is a wide range of scenarios that must be considered. I might think very differently about a first year law school student who was raped compared to a woman who had 3 girls, was pregnant again with another girl but wanted an abortion so that she could have a boy instead. The ethical issues to consider for each case are different because although it can be argued that both cases are about ending a life, there are other factors that need to be considered as well. Looking at these two extreme cases makes me feel like the legalisation of abortion can be very beneficial to certain people such as the raped girl, but because of the risk of abuse, strict measures should be put in place to regulate abortion.

Remember, you can conclude with a view that is opposite to the one above and still do very well. What is important is that you reflect on the different considerations, that your conclusion flows logically from your thought process and that you present your arguments before you state a conclusion.

What do they ask you about in the interview

The intention of the interview is very similar from one university to another. For the most part, they want to find out about:

1. Your motivation and interest for medicine
2. Your work experience and your volunteer experience – medically related and non-medically related.
3. Your realistic understanding and knowledge of the medical practice & the medical system

4. You strengths, weaknesses, character, attributes
5. Medical ethics and ability to communicate a balanced argument

Note that MMI interviews tend to focus much more on the last 3 areas.
We will explore answers below to questions in each of the above areas and give some insight into preparing your answers. The answers are not full answers but are bullet points to serve in helping you create your answers.

Your motivation and interest for medicine

Why do you want to be a doctor?

1. Think of when it started, what triggered it – biology classes, passion for science, science journals or magazines, doctor in the family, illness in the family, anecdote or experience from childhood, etc.
2. Think of what you like in the profession – the intellectual challenge of the science in medicine, the patient care aspects, the complexity of medical cases, the depth and breath of the material taught, the communication with patients and families, the combination of independent and team work, the teaching aspect, the research aspect, etc.
3. Make sure that your answer does not beg the question: why not a physiotherapist then?

➡These are examples of things you may want to think about but try to make sure that the answer you give could not just be given by someone else. There needs to be something about you in it that is personal.

Why not a physiotherapist/nurse/dentist?

1. Acknowledge the aspects that you are looking for in being a doctor that you could get with these professions such as patient contact, the feeling of helping people, science, etc.
2. Think of what would be missing - the depth and breath of the material taught, medicine is the broadest knowledge in healthcare, the role of leading the healthcare team in taking care of patients, etc.
3. If you have some healthcare experience, observing the role of nurses vs. doctors in the team may have given you insight into what you liked or did not like about each role. It would make your answer very interesting if your reasoning is rooted in a personal experience.

➡ Ideally your answer to " why do you want to be a doctor" should cover this question as well.

What efforts have you made to find out about medicine?

1. What experiences have you had – internships, shadowing a physician, volunteering, etc.
2. Who have you talked with – professors, doctors, family members, etc.
3. What have you read – journals, magazines, etc.

➡Talking to others and reading are important, but the efforts you have made to learn about medicine actively are the ones that carry the most weight.

Why do you want to study medicine in our program?

1. What type of university culture do you prefer - close contact with professors, problem based learning, hands on learning?
2. What parts of the curriculum appeal to you?
3. Have you had a chance to speak to anyone in their university?

➡Note that some medical schools like the University of Glasgow state specifically that the applicant's knowledge of their curriculum may be assessed in the interview. Similarly, at the University of Sheffield, knowledge of and interest in studying at Sheffield is one of the seven criteria assessed at the interview. Queens University is also known to ask this type of question.
➡Your knowledge of the program and school dynamic will reflect well at the interview.

Do you have any questions for us?

1. Some people prefer not to ask questions. This is often perfectly acceptable, depending on the interviewers and how much time they have made for questions.
2. When asking questions, it is important to ask questions that cannot easily be looked up on their website, of course.

Your work and volunteer experience

Tell me about your volunteer experience working at the hospital?

1. What aspects of medicine did you witness?
2. Maybe you understand better how a patient feels on the ward, not being able to choose when he or she eats, when he or she wakes up...how will that change the doctor you will become?
3. Maybe you observed some things you particularly admired in some doctors.
4. Maybe you understood another side of medicine, like how a medical team interacts or the role of the family in patient care.

➡ If you are asked a question like this, you should not list general things like in the list above. The list is here to help you think of elements you may want to bring up in your answer. Ideally you should try to answer referring back to an anecdote or an example from your personal volunteer experience.

What did you learn from your work that you did not know before?

1. In a question that is so specific, do not talk in generalities. Draw on what you learned from a specific example, situation or experience you had during your work or volunteer experience.
2. For example, maybe you saw one doctor being very available to the family members of a sick patient while another doctor did not have as much time to offer to them, and you really noticed how involving the family and giving them support helped guide the decision process for the patient's treatment.
3. Maybe you learned something about how patients feel on the ward by talking with them. When someone has cancer for example, their entire life revolves around the disease. When people ask them "how are you", they are often referring to their health, rather than the artist, the teacher or the cook underneath. Maybe as a volunteer you learned how to gain patients' friendship, and bring those elements of their personality out by listening to their stories and remembrances. You could talk about a specific story too if it is relevant, and how learning this as a volunteer will help you develop trusting connections with patients.
4. Maybe you understand better the interaction between the different members of the medical team. Any example is good, but be specific and draw some lessons from it that will be useful to you as a medical student or a doctor.

Tell us about a patient from your volunteer experience

Again, just like the question above, it is very important here to be specific. Maybe you remember something a patient said that touched you or surprised you. Maybe a patient impressed you with his or her courage or optimism. Maybe you were present with a patient during a very hard time and it helped you better understand some things you had not thought of before. Again, any example could be good if you are specific enough and draw some lessons from it that will be useful to you as a medical student or a doctor.

Your realistic understanding of medical practice

What in being a doctor are you looking forward to the most & least?

The question is not simply asking for the pros and cons of being a doctor but is instead asking for what aspects you are looking forward to most and least. Thus, make sure your answer is personal and not just a list of pros and cons. To help you think about your own answer, here are some pros and cons you could consider:

- Pros:
    - ‣ Opportunity to use your skills to treat patients
    - ‣ Opportunity for research – contributing to medical advancement
    - ‣ Challenging – continuous training / lifelong learning
    - ‣ Medicine is a broad field / opportunities for change within medicine
    - ‣ Varied type of work: preventive / treatment / research / teaching / public health

- Cons:
    - ‣ Can be stressful, particularly if exposed to long hours, changing work patterns, difficult patients, or having to make difficult decisions, sometimes on your own
    - ‣ Compromise on work-life balance when on call and possibly working difficult hours
    - ‣ Often dealing with uncertainty

➡ When you mention the aspects you do not look forward to, it might be a good idea to say that you have thought about those and explain why you still want to go into medicine. Remember to make your answer personal, say what you are looking forward to and most importantly explain why. It is a better idea to only choose a few points but to expand on them well.

How will you cope with the stress as a doctor?

1. You already worked toward a degree and maybe you have been employed for some time as well. Think of the methods you have used to handle stress during your first degree so you can give specific examples during your interview.

2. Even if you do not get very stressed, it is important to acknowledge that it can happen and show some maturity of thought on how you can cope with it.

3. Some things you might want to consider are sports, music, support networks of friends and/or family, religion, setting realistic goals, etc.

There is a sample answer to "How do you handle stress" on page 454.

➡ Again, a long list of methods will not give you many points in your interview. Choose a few points that correspond to you and expand on them using examples from your life.

What makes a good doctor?

1. Rather than merely giving a list of attributes that make a good doctor, it might be better to use your experience in healthcare to describe what you believe makes a good doctor. This will make your answer more personal and stronger.

2. For example, instead of saying good communication is important, maybe you have witnessed how a doctor who explained complex notions in simple terms really improved his or her relationship with his patients. You can describe your anecdote quickly and conclude with why you think good communication skills might be important.

3. Other ideas of attributes that make a good doctor are: knowledgeable, competent, confident, humble, organisational skills, caring, honest and reliable.

➡ Again, the best answer will not be the one with the most adjectives, but rather the one that is well constructed and well supported with a personal experience.

Your strengths, weaknesses, character

Why should we take you and not somebody else?

1. This is a good place to talk about your strengths which should be prepared and thought through beforehand. Your strengths might come from the way you were brought up, your educational or professional background, your experience in dealing with certain situations, etc.

2. Think of things that are unique to yourself. This can be a way of thinking, a way of reacting, your personal background and experiences, things you have achieved, etc. Try to think of examples of when these attributes of yours have come across and present those examples as part of your answer, rather than listing adjectives. It is much more powerful to describe a situation and how you contributed to creating good communication between different parties rather than just say that you have good communication skills. For example, it is less effective to say something like "I am really good at connecting with people. I have always been good at this and love working with people from all different cultures", than to ground an answer in actions you have taken: "My volunteering with patients and my work teaching children in Thailand have taught me important lessons about overcoming age and cultural barriers and connecting with people from all walks of life. I think this will be very helpful in working with a diverse patient population as a physician..."

Can you tell us your three main weaknesses and strengths

1. It is essential that you have prepared your strengths and weaknesses before you go into your interview as you will often have to talk about them in a direct or indirect way.

2. When you think of the strengths you want to present, make sure that they somewhat correspond to the attributes you believe make a good doctor as this is what you are interviewing for.

3. Just like the other questions, you need to back up your strengths with examples or anecdotes of things that you have done. Anyone can say that they are reliable but telling the panel that you volunteered weekly in a hospital for 3 years and never missed a day will make your point more powerful.

4. For your weaknesses, you need to explain what you have done to improve on them or how you are planning to work on improving them. Maybe you have difficulty stepping out of your comfort zone but have recently made particular efforts to travel on your own or try things you were not familiar with to improve in this area.

Medical ethics and scenario questions

The admissions committee wants to see if you think broad, if you think logically, if you consider several aspects of a problem. Do you try to do everything by yourself or do you get help from experienced people? Do you follow rules? Do you follow ethics? What do you do when ethics and rules clash? These types of question are common in MMI format interviews and are there to give you an opportunity to show maturity of thought.

What would you do if one of your colleagues smells like alcohol

1. I would not jump to conclusions right away. My colleague could have had a drink spilled on him or her. I would want to be tactful so as not to compromise that person's reputation and my relationship with them unnecessarily.
2. I would also want to recognise that if they had been drinking, there could be circumstances that I was unaware of such as the loss of a family member, an abusive relationship, or something else.
3. However, patient safety would be my first priority. If my colleague was drinking, I would not want them to see another patient that day and I would therefore want to talk to them right away. To protect patients' safety, if he or she had been drinking that day, I would make sure that they did not see any more patients.
4. If they left that day after we talked but the problem persisted, I would then contact our supervisor.

Should we start introducing a $10 fee for all family doctor visits?

1. On the one hand, this may reduce patient volume in the clinics and allow physicians to spend more time with patients who have greater need.
2. Implementing this policy might also generate a modest revenue to help pay for rising costs of healthcare.
3. On the other hand though, many people might delay seeing the physician as a result. For example, a patient with blood in their stool who assumed the blood was due to haemorrhoids might delay seeing the doctor for a few more months because of the cost, allowing a potential cancer to grow or spread.
4. In addition, this would disproportionately affect lower income patients, and worsen the healthcare disparities that already exist.

Should we start screening applicants for terminal diseases like Huntington's?

1. On the one hand, this policy might help ensure that more graduating medical students are able to provide many years of service to the community after graduating.

2. Also, for conditions where early treatment can improve survival (although this is not the case with Huntington's disease), we may be able to start treatment for some prospective students early and increase their life span.

3. On the other hand, many people may not want to know if they have a terminal illness, particularly if no treatment is available.

4. In addition, making this legal might cause many other professions to do the same thing. What if law firms, businesses or nursing schools started to screen the same way? It might become very difficult for someone with a terminal illness to enrol in higher education or find the job they would like.

5. Although this may allow medical schools to get more years of service to the community from their graduates, I do not think it is a good idea because it would require prospective applicants to learn information they may not want to know, and because of the potential for the policy to be taken on by many other industries.

If you the minister of health in a rural region, what would be your plan?

1. First, I would want to find out what needs exist in the community.

2. I would speak to community leaders, community members and healthcare workers. I would look at the health related data available for the region and might consider performing a survey as well.

3. In addition, I would look at the funding and human resources available.

4. In deciding where to invest these resources, I would make sure to look beyond just traditional healthcare and look at interventions that reflect the broad view of health. This could mean implementing AIDS education programs or substance abuse programs, or whatever interventions addressed the greatest needs.

5. I would also want to measure the impact of the interventions. If we were doing an STD prevention program for example, I would want to keep track of the STD statistics in the coming years to see how effective my intervention was.

➡ It is not which intervention you will pick that matters to the admission committee. Instead, it is your approach to a challenging situation.

Refer to page 456 for an example on answering a question about abortion and for a discussion of a structure you can use to answer ethical questions.

The above examples can certainly be improved, and many interviewees will give much better answers. However, the examples are here to illustrate how an applicant can express understanding of both sides, analyse the issue and come to a reasonable, defendable conclusion based on their analysis. Recall the criteria assessed by the admissions officers at McMaster University, which reflect what interviewers are generally looking for in these types of questions:

1. Did the applicant express balance and sympathy for both intellectual positions?
2. Was there a clear analysis of the ethical problems paternalism raises?
3. Did the applicant suggest a course of action that is defensible and moderate?

In many ways, the same themes tend to recur over and over for these questions. For example, potential for abuse applies to abortion, euthanasia, and performing genetic screening on prospective medical students. Not jumping to conclusions immediately and ensuring the safety of patients applies to many questions as well. By reading about medical ethics and answering several questions, a pattern will start to develop, and will allow students to analyse the issues they are given and excel in their interview.

Costs

Cost of application to medical school

The minimum cost of the application includes the MCAT, GAMSAT, BMAT and/or UKCAT registration fees, except at the relatively small number of medical schools not using any admissions tests.

The regular registration fees for the exams in the UK range between £42 and £195, without late fees or international fees. For the MCAT, the regular registration fee is approximately USD235 without late or international fees. Costs associated with preparation for the tests should also be factored in. Students might register for preparation courses or buy books to prepare. More details on these costs are available in the exam specific sections.

The fees for application range from as low as £11 (USD16) to apply to only one program on the UCAS form, to as much as CAD315 to apply to only McMaster University in Ontario (although additional schools are only CAD75 - 85 each).

Travel expenses for interviews should also be taken into account. Some schools can help with lodging to save on hotel costs when you travel for your interview.

Cost of studying medicine

Canada

The average tuition in Canadian dollars for first year Canadian students at English taught medical programs is approximately CAD15,500. The tuition for international students ranges significantly, from It ranges from approximately CAD25,000 at Dalhousie University to a high of CAD95,841 at McMaster University.

Some schools like the University of Western Ontario and Dalhousie University will provide need-based scholarships for students [93, 94]. Currently there are 29 scholarships awarded each year to medical students at the University of Western Ontario [93]. At the University of Toronto in the 2009-2010 academic year, 70% of first year students qualified for an average of

CAD5600 of grant funding for the year [95]. Some schools also have merit-based scholarships that they offer to a few selected students upon acceptance to medical school.

Some schools like the University of Manitoba have a financial incentive program to encourage students to return and practice in the school's province. At the University of Manitoba, Manitoba students can be granted CAD12,000 to CAD20,000 a year for up to 6 years during their third and fourth year as well as their residency if they agree to provide service once their training is complete [96].

At most, if not all schools in Canada, financial aid representatives work with students to ensure that no student who is offered a place in the program is unable to go to medical school for financial reasons. Several schools including the University of Toronto have this goal as their financial aid mission statement.

Alongside obtaining loans from the schools, Canadians are often eligible for very low-interest loans through the government and local banks. For example, the Canadian and provincial governments offer medical students up to CAD150,000 (or occasionally even more) of loan with no interest until 6-12 months after graduation. Students studying abroad may also be eligible for these loans. See the provincial government websites for details.

Banks such as the Royal Bank of Canada will also offer credit lines of up to CAD200,000 (or more in some cases) to eligible students. These loans will accrue interest at the prime interest rate or slightly higher in some cases. It is a good idea to meet with different bank representatives and meet with the schools' financial aid representatives once accepted to take advantage of the best loans and bursaries available.

UK

For entry in September 2012, almost all medical schools will charge new full time students from the UK/E.U up to a maximum of £9,000, based on new regulations. There will be corresponding changes in the tuition loans and funding available. For non-E.U applicants, tuition can range between approximately £13,000 to £32,000 per year.

Funding for graduate entry medicine

For most students from England and Wales entering graduate entry medicine courses lasting 4 years in the UK, the two most significant sources of funding are the NHS and the Student Loans Company (SLC). The SLC is responsible for distributing government loans throughout the UK. For the first year of the program, students need to pay for tuition themselves either by taking a tuition loan from the SLC or by finding another source of funding (savings, bank loans, etc.). The last three years' tuition fees are paid for by an NHS bursary depending on income [97].

The major details of the first year SLC tuition fee loan in the 2012-2013 academic are listed below [98, 99].

- Once students have applied and been accepted for this loan, the loan amount is given directly to the universities in most cases and will be paid directly toward the student's tuition fee.
- The maximum amount per year for tuition in the 2012-2013 academic year will be £9,000, which is adequate to cover home student tuition. This loan is only for tuition, meaning that if the tuition is £7,000, then the loan amount will be £7,000. No extra money will be made available for the student.
- The loan accrues interest during the student's study period at a rate that varies from month to month. The loan has fluctuated significantly in recent years. Due to public interest in higher education, the SLC loan interest rate was set at 0% from September 1st, 2009 to August 31st, 2010. The loan will accrue interest at inflation + 3% while studying, then between 0 and 3% more than inflation after graduation depending on income.
- No payments of any sort need to be made while the student is still in university.
- Once the student begins earning over £21,000 per year, the payments will automatically be deducted from their salaries.
- Once earning over the £21,000 threshold, the repayment amount is calculated at 9% of the difference between the student's gross taxable income and the £21,000 threshold. Thus, a student earning the average salary in foundation year 1 of approximately £30,200 [100] would pay approximately £69 a month, or £833 a year toward their loan from their salary. A foundation year 2 student earning on average £37,500 [100] would pay approximately £191 a month, or £2,297 a year toward their loan until the loan is paid. Note that these salaries can vary significantly depending on the hospital.

The SLC tuition loan is the main source of funding for most first year students. In addition, there are NHS bursaries available throughout medical school including the first year. These bursaries can be either income assessed (eligibility criteria include household income) or non-income assessed (eligibility is independent of household income). More details on these bursaries are available at http://www.nhsbsa.nhs.uk/students, and a bursary calculator is available from www.ppa.org.uk/StudentBursariesCalculator/reset.do

Furthermore, if students qualify for an income assessed loan through the NHS, they are eligible for an additional loan through the SLC called a maintenance loan, intended to help pay for living expenses, books etc. Students who only qualify for non-income assessed bursaries through the NHS are usually not eligible for these additional loans.

The last category of financial support from the SLC is targeted support. These grants are specifically for students with dependents, students who are parents or students with disabilities. There is also a grant for students at UK institutions who have large travel costs for their studies or clinical rotations. See http://www.slc.co.uk for details on the different types of loans and grants available.

A table showing the funding available in England based on income for the 2012-2013 academic year is available from the UK Government Department for Business Innovation and Skills, which is included below [101]. These maintenance loans in this table are for students living away from home outside London. The maintenance loan decreases by approximately £1,125 if living at home, and increases by approximately £2,175 if living away from home in London [102]. There will also be a £150 million national scholarship programme introduced in 2012 to help students from lower income households.

Residual income*	Amount of tuition fee loan available	Amount of maintenance grant available	Amount of maintenance loan available for those studying outside London and away from home
Up to £25,000	£9,000	£3,250	£3,875
£30,000	£9,000	£2,341	£4,330
£35,000	£9,000	£1,432	£4,784
£40,000	£9,000	£523	£5,239
£45,000	£9,000	Nil	£5,288
£50,000	£9,000	Nil	£4,788
£55,000	£9,000	Nil	£4,288
£60,000	£9,000	Nil	£3,788
Over £62,500	£9,000	Nil	£3,575

Table 55. Funding available in England based on income for the 2012-2013 academic year

*Household residual income is your household's gross income minus a few allowances, including roughly £1,100 for each dependent child, and allowances for pension schemes and superannuation payments eligible for tax relief. If a student is dependent on their parents, their parents' income is taken into account, minus the allowances. If not, their spouse or partner's income is taken into account minus allowances. Student earnings are generally excluded from household residual earnings [103, 104].

A student loan calculator estimating tuition, maintenance, and other loans and grants is available from www.studentfinance.direct.gov.uk at: www.studentfinance.direct.gov.uk/portal/page?_pageid=153,4680136&_dad=portal&_schema=PORTAL

In addition to the NHS and SLC websites, another good website is www.money4medstudents.org, established by the British Medical Association. Many students also choose to meet or speak with the financial aid advisors at universities that accepted them to determine which scholarships they may be eligible for.

Some of these loans and bursaries are not available for students from Scotland and Northern Ireland. There is a specific student finance website for England, Wales, Northern Ireland, Scotland and another website for students from other E.U countries. Students wishing to study in the UK can access information on what funding sources are available and apply for some of this government funding directly through the websites. Each of these links are listed below.

England	www.direct.gov.uk/StudentFinance
Wales	www.studentfinancewales.co.uk/
Northern Ireland	www.studentfinanceni.co.uk
Scotland	www.saas.gov.uk
E.U students from outside the UK planning to study in England, Wales or Northern Ireland	www.direct.gov.uk/studentfinance-eu

Table 56. Sources of information on government funding for different E.U countries

Funding for 5 and 6 year programs

For 5 and 6 year programs, the funding options are somewhat similar except for two changes. First, only the fifth and sixth years of medical school are eligible for NHS bursaries for students from England and Wales, rather than the second, third and fourth year as is the case for graduate entry programs. Thus, applicants usually secure funding through other sources for the first four years. Second, graduate applicants are not eligible for the tuition fee loans mentioned at the beginning of the previous section for the 5 and 6 year programs, however, they are eligible for the maintenance loans if they qualify and need more money for tuition or living expenses.

USA

For in-state students, the average first-year medical school fees in the 2010-2011 year were USD40,775 for private medical schools and USD21,248 for public medical schools. For non-residents, the average fees were approximately USD42,301 at private medical schools and USD42,210 at public medical schools. The tuition fees for first-year students at a few private and public US medical schools in the 2010-2011 year are listed below [105]:

Private Medical Schools	Tuition for all students	
Columbia University College of Physicians and Surgeons	$46,212	
Cornell University Medical College	$45,543	
Creighton University School of Medicine	$46,752	
Dartmouth Medical School	$45,075	
George Washington University School of Medicine	$48,687	
Georgetown University School of Medicine	$43,616	
Harvard Medical School	$45,050	
Johns Hopkins University School of Medicine	$41,200	

Public Medical Schools	Out-of-State/ International	In-State
University of Hawaii, John A. Burns School of Medicine	$27,000	$56,184
University of Kentucky College of Medicine	$28,144	$53,282
University of Minnesota Medical School - Minneapolis	$32,049	$41,139

Table 57. Tuition for first-year students in the 2010-2011 academic year [105]

The estimated costs of rent, food and other living expenses is usually between USD15,000 and USD22,000 per year. Health insurance usually costs between USD1,500 and USD2,500 per year. The most up-to-date figures on tuition fees, living expenses and health insurance costs at each school are available from the AAMC at http://services.aamc.org/tsfreports/

The average indebtedness of US medical school graduates in 2009 was USD141,00 [106]. It is estimated that this figure has increased and will continue to increase at approximately 6-7% per year [107]. The average graduating debt for each university is given in the MSAR book every year.

Most students use a combination of subsidized loans (loans through the government or through the school with no interest cost to students during school, during the grace period and during any deferment periods) and unsubsidized loans. Note, however, that most government loans are only available to U.S citizens and permanent residents. Federal and military loans are listed in MSAR and there are several other loans available through schools and private lenders. Most medical schools also give a presentation on their tuition and financial aid on the day of the interview.

For international students, some US schools will ask students to prove that they can pay the tuition for the first year of medical school before they enroll. This usually involves taking a loan or converting money a few months in advance. A few schools like Johns Hopkins will ask students to establish a separate bank account prior to enrolling with funds sufficient to pay for the full cost of the four years of their education. In 2008, this amount was approximately USD252,000 [108]. Several US schools give financial aid regardless of international status. Examples include Dartmouth, Harvard, and Yale Medical Schools.

At most schools, students are required to submit details on their own income and savings as well as the income and savings of their spouses, their children and their parents. This is done using the Free Application for Federal Student Aid (FAFSA) and additional school specific financial aid forms. The financial aid offices use the information submitted to calculate the expected contribution of the student and their family. They then award financial aid accordingly based on the difference between this expected contribution and the remaining costs, as well as the funds available to the school. Students whose parents and family are not able to contribute as much as the expected contribution can usually access additional corporate loans offered through the school or other loans from the government and private lenders.

At most schools, if a student is accepted or wait-listed at a U.S medical school and is eligible for financial aid at that school, the applicant can submit the financial aid forms early and have the financial aid office at that school calculate the amount of financial aid they are eligible for. This information can be helpful for students who are accepted at more than one school and are deciding which school to attend.

Australia

The cost of studies in Australia is generally comparable to tuition in the US for out of state students. The tuition ranges from approximately AUD43,300 to AUD60,000 per year. Some schools including the Australian National University and the University of Queensland offer a few scholarships for international students to help cover the costs of tuition. North American and European students usually have the same options for federal loan funding available to students studying at home.

Caribbean

The cost of studies are also generally cheaper in the Caribbean than they are in the US. The costs of studies at the four most widely accredited schools in the Caribbean are listed below. Note that since applicants can start at 3 different times during the year in most cases and can thus accelerate or lengthen the program based on the amount of vacation they wish to take, these costs may differ. The average costs per year below are determined assuming the applicant will finish their studies in 48 months as they would at most schools in the US or Canada.

University	Total Cost of all semesters (USD)	Average Annual Tuition assuming completion in 48 months (USD)
American University of the Caribbean [115]	$162,000	$40,500
Ross School of Medicine [122]	$165,000	$41,250
SABA School of Medicine [123]	$98,500	$24,625
St. George's University [118]	$205,000	$51,250

Table 58. Tuition for first-year students at Caribbean medical schools in the 2010-2011 academic year

Some Caribbean schools provide scholarships for students who demonstrate financial need and/ or academic excellence. Schools providing these scholarships include the Ross University School of Medicine and St. George's University School of Medicine [109, 110].

Croatia

Tuition fees at the University of Split and the University of Zagreb in Croatia are much cheaper than in the above countries. Students paid approximately €7,000 per year in tuition in the 2011-2012 academic year.

Czech Republic

The cost of studies in the Czech republic is slightly more expensive than in Croatia, but still significantly cheaper than in Western countries and in Ireland. Tuition ranges from approximately €9,000 to per year to €13,000 per year. At Charles University, Second Faculty of Medicine, students performing in the top 10% of the class are given a tuition fee reduction from €11,600 per year to €10,000 per year.

Hungary

The cost of studies in Hungary ranges from roughly USD10,000 to USD16,400 per year. At Simmelweis University, students performing very well are eligible for a 10-15% tuition fee reduction.

Ireland

The tuition fees for Irish medical schools are shown in the table below.

	University	European Union Students	International Students [85]
	The Royal College of Surgeons in Ireland	€13,080 in 2011	€47,500 in 2011

Four-year programs	University College Cork	€12,780 in 2011	€39,200 in 2011
	University College Dublin	€13,915 in 2011	€39,200 in 2011
	The University of Limerick	€12,780 in 2010	€38,500 in 2010
Five-year programs	National University of Ireland, Galway	€9,297 in 2011	€31,000 in 2011
	The Royal College of Surgeons in Ireland	€7,767 in 2011	€46,000 in 2011
	Trinity College Dublin	€6,371 in 2010	€31,000 in 2011
	University College Cork	€13,915 in 2011	€39,200 in 2011
	University College Dublin	€8,862 in 2011	€31,000 in 2011
Six-year programs*=	National University of Ireland, Galway	€9,297 in 2011	€31,000 in 2011
	University College Dublin	€8,862 in 2011	€31,000 in 2011
	The Royal College of Surgeons in Ireland	€7,767 in 2011	€46,000 in 2011

Table 59. Tuition for first-year students at Irish medical schools

Note that the figures in table 59 do not include living expenses. In general, living expenses come to approximately USD15,000 per year, or £10,000. Scholarships are not available for US and Canadian applicants through the Irish schools [18], however, Canadian students are eligible for most of the government and bank loans available to students studying locally, including bank credit lines of up to CAD200,000 at prime interest rates or slightly higher. Some of these credit lines offer payment deferral until 12 months after completion of the MD program [18]. US students studying in Ireland are also eligible for most federal loans that are available to US students studying at home.

E.U residents are often eligible for some of the funding outlined on page 469.

Poland

The cost of studies in Poland is similar to that of other Eastern European countries, with tuition ranging from approximately €9,000 per year to €15,500 per year. The 4 year program and the American 6 year program at the Medical University of Bialystok are exceptions to this rule, charging approximately $40,000 per year. The University of Warsaw charges more for its 4 year program than its 6 year program (€14,400 per year for the 4 year program, €11,100 per year for the 6 year program).

Romania

Romanian schools charge relatively little compared to most other countries considered in this guide. International students studying in all Romanian schools pay tuition fees of between €3,200 - €5,000 per year.

Slovak Republic

The three schools in the Slovak Republic offering medical programs in English charge between €8,500 - 9,000 per year.

Ukraine

Ukrainian schools have the lowest tuition fees of any schools considered in this guide, with tuition fees ranging from approximately USD3,400 to USD4,300 pear year.

Bibliography

1.   *Obtained from speaking with the Admission office.*

2.   Guadian.co.uk. *Tuition fees 2012: what are the universities charging?* ; Available from: www.guardian.co.uk/news/datablog/2011/mar/25/higher-education-universityfunding.

3.   *University of Calgary, Medical School webpage.* Available from: http:// medicine.ucalgary.ca/.

4.   *McMaster University Medical school Admission webage.* Available from: http:// fhs.mcmaster.ca/mdprog/admissions.html.

5.   *Canadian medical education statistics.* Available from: www.afmc.ca/publications-statistics-e.php, 2010. **32**.

6.   *Queens University - medical school admissions.* Available from: http://meds.queensu.ca/ undergraduate/prospective_students/method_of_selection.

7.   *University of Toronto, Medical School webpage.* Available from: http:// www.facmed.utoronto.ca/site4.aspx.

8.   *University of Ottawa, school of Medicine webpage.* Available from: http:// www.medicine.uottawa.ca/eng/.

9.   *Northern Ontario School of Medicine webpage.* Available from: http://www.normed.ca/ education/ume/default.aspx?id=352&ekmensel=c580fa7b_96_0_352_1#.

10.   *Université de Montréal, Faculté de Medecine webpage.* Available from: http:// www.med.umontreal.ca/.

11.   *Université de Sherbrooke, Faculté de Medecine webpage.* Available from: http:// www.usherbrooke.ca/medecine/.

12.   *Université Laval, Faculté de Medecine webpage.* Available from: http:// w3.fmed.ulaval.ca/site_fac/.

13.   *University of Saskatchewan, College of Medicine webpage.* Available from: http:// www.medicine.usask.ca/.

14.   *The AAMC - Applicants and Matriculants Data.* Available from: https://www.aamc.org/ data/facts/applicantmatriculant/, 2010.

15.   Zanten, M.V. and J.R. Boulet, *Medical Education in the Caribbean: A Longitudinal Study of United States Medical Licensing Examination Performance, 2000 –2009* Academic Medicine, 2009. **86**(2).

16.   *Charles University, 2nd Faculty of Medicine.* Available from: http://www.lf2.cuni.cz/ Studium/pr/eindex.htm.

17.   *Atlantic Bridge FAQ.* Available from: http://www.atlanticbridge.com/med/faqs/ fqindex.htm.

18. *Call with the Atlantic Bridge Program Office.*
19. Jones, R., *The effect of commercial coaching courses on performance on the MCAT.* Academic Medicine, 1986. **61**(4).
20. center, C.I.i., *IMG specific programs.* Available from: http://www.img-canada.ca/en/resources/img_programs.htm.
21. *Medical Council of Canada website.* Available from: http://www.mcc.ca/en/.
22. CaRMS, *Operational Reports.* Available from: www.carms.ca/eng/operations_R1reports_10_e.shtml, 2010.
23. (ECFMG), E.C.f.F.M.G., *2010 information booklet.* Available from: http://www.ecfmg.org/2010ib/index.html, 2010.
24. *University of British Columbia, Faculty of Medicine admissions statistics.* Available from: http://www.med.ubc.ca/education/md_ugrad/MD_Undergraduate_Admissions/MD_Undergraduate_Admissions_Statistics.htm
25. *OMSAS instruction booklet.* Under 'instruction booklet']. Available from: http://www.ouac.on.ca/omsas/
26. *MD-PhD handout from Yale,* Yale university.
27. *UBC MD/Ph.D program overview.* Available from: http://www.med.ubc.ca/education/md_ugrad/mdphd/overview.htm.
28. *University of Alberta, MD/Ph/D FAQ.* Available from: http://www.med.ualberta.ca/Home/Education/MScPhD/mdphd-faq.cfm.
29. *McGill MD/MBA requirements.* 2011; Available from: http://www.mcgill.ca/desautels/mdmba/.
30. *University of Calgary, Haskayne school of business combined degree programs.* Available from: http://haskayne.ucalgary.ca/grad/mba/haskayne/combineddegrees/#md.
31. *Medical School Admission Requirements (MSAR).* 2009-2010: AAMC.
32. *University of Alberta - Medical school Admission webpage.* Available from: http://ume.med.ualberta.ca/ProspectiveLearners/MDAdmissions/Pages/default.aspx.
33. *FAQ from Dalhousie medical school website.* Available from: http://admissions.medicine.dal.ca/faqs.htm#fq07
34. *University of Saskatchewan, admissions timeline.* Available from: http://www.medicine.usask.ca/education/admissions/calendar-for-applicants.
35. *University of British Columbia, MD undergraduate Webpage.* Available from: http://www.med.ubc.ca/education/md_ugrad.htm.
36. *University of Calgary Applicant's Manual.* 2008-2009; Available from: http://medicine.ucalgary.ca/med/files/med/Applicants%20Manual%2020072008Updated111308.pdf.

37. *University of Toronto - Non-academic qualifications.* Available from: www.md.utoronto.ca/admissions/information/requirements/Non-Academic.htm.

38. *University of Toronto - Application tips.* Available from: www.md.utoronto.ca/quick-info/Top10.htm.

39. *Memorial University - Faculty of medicine - FAQ.* Available from: http://www.med.mun.ca/Admissions/FAQ-s.aspx.

40. Council, B., *Learning infosheets: Medicine.* Available from: www.britishcouncil.org/learning-infosheets-medicine.pdf, 2006.

41. *Routes into medicine.* Available from: www.wanttobeadoctor.co.uk/main.php?page=15.

42. *University of Aberdeen.* Available from: http://www.abdn.ac.uk/medicine/prospective/.

43. *Importance of early application.* Available from: http://www.medschoolready.com/app/earlyearlyapplication.asp.

44. *Yale University - applying to medical school book.* 2008-2009; Information on the early decision program, the MCAT, the AMCAS, essays, letters of recommendation, joint MD-PHD programs, financing medical shool and more]. Available from: www.yale.edu/career/students/gradprof/media/redbook.pdf.

45. *University of Texas Medical School at Southwestern 2008 entering class profile.* Available from: http://www.utsouthwestern.edu/utsw/cda/dept20676/files/397484.html#profile

46. AAMC, *Medical School Application Requirements 2012-2013 online guide.* 2011.

47. *AMCAS 2009 Instructional manual.* 2009: AAMC.

48. *The AMCAS 2008 Application worksheet.* 2008; Available from: www.aamc.org/students/amcas/2008applicationworksheet.pdf.

49. *AAMC Update for Experienced Admissions Advisors.* Powerpoint presented March 2011.

50. *AMCAS Application Tips.* 2008; Available from: http://www.aamc.org/students/amcas/2008tips.pdf.

51. *University of Chicago - MSTP - FAQ.* Available from: http://pritzker.uchicago.edu/jointdegrees/mstp/faq.shtml.

52. *Standford University - MSTP - Admission webpage.* Available from: http://mstp.stanford.edu/admissions.html.

53. *The AAMC website - Combined degrees page.* Available from: http://services.aamc.org/currdir/section3/degree2.cfm.

54. *Boston University school of Medicine Admission webpage.* Available from: http://www.bumc.bu.edu/admissions/.

55. *Tufts University MD/MPH programs.* Available from: http://www.tufts.edu/med/education/phpd/mph/pathways/mdmph/index.html.

56.   *Vanderbilt Law School Joint degree programs.* Available from: http://law.vanderbilt.edu/prospective-students/joint-degree-programs/index.aspx

57.   *University of Pennsylvania School of Medicine, Joint Degree Programs.* Available from: http://www.med.upenn.edu/educ_combdeg/mdjd.shtml

58.   *Association of MD/MBA programs.* Available from: http://mdmbaprograms.com/5.html.

59.   *Harvard Medical School Admission webpage.*

60.   *Columbia Medical school Admission webpage.*

61.   *John Hopkins medical school website* Available from: http://www.hopkinsmedicine.org/ADMISSIONS/intstudents.html.

62.   *Penn State Hershey, requirements for admission.* Available from: http://pennstatehershey.org/web/md/admissions/overview/requirements.

63.   *Harvard Medical School Admissions FAQ.* Available from: http://hms.harvard.edu/admissions/default.asp?page=admissions

64.   *University of Nebraska College of Medicine admissions information.* Available from: http://www.unmc.edu/dept/com/index.cfm?CONREF=3.

65.   *Loma Linda Medical School Admissions FAQ.* Available from: http://www.llu.edu/medicine/admissions/faqs.page.

66.   *Johns Hopkins School of Medicine, admissions requirements.* Available from: http://www.hopkinsmedicine.org/admissions/apps.html

67.   *Weill Cornell School of Medicine admissions requirements.* Available from: http://www.med.cornell.edu/education/admissions/app_req.html

68.   *Student doctor forum.* Available from: www.studentdoctor.net.

69.   *Boston University Medical College application information.* Available from: http://www.bumc.bu.edu/admissions/applicationprocess/.

70.   *Creighton University, School of Medicine application information.* Available from: http://medschool.creighton.edu/medicine/oma/app/index.php

71.   *Harvard Medical School Letters of Evaluation FAQ.* Available from: http://hms.harvard.edu/admissions/default.asp?page=researchapply.

72.   *Florida International University College of Medicine admissions.* Available from: http://medicine.fiu.edu/admissions.php?ss=attc.

73.   *University of Washington Medical School Admission webpage.* Available from: http://uwmedicine.washington.edu/Education/MDProgram/Admissions/ApplicationProcedure.htm.

74.   *AMCAS transcript FAQ.*

75.   *AMCAS 2011 Instructional manual.* 2010: AAMC.

76. *AMCAS FAQ.* Available from: https://www.aamc.org/students/applying/amcas/ 63174/faqs/.

77. *CAO Graduate Entry Medicine Application handbook.* link under 'Graduate Entry Medicine']. Available from: http://www.cao.ie/index.php

78. *CAO Undergraduate Entry Medicine application handbook.* link under ' Undergraduate Entry Medicine']. Available from: http://www.cao.ie/index.php

79. *HPAT Ireland Brochure.* Available from: http://www.hpat-ireland.acer.edu.au/ index.php?option=com_content&view=article&id=56%3Ainformation-booklet&catid=11%3Adownload-booklet&Itemid=5.

80. *HPAT Ireland wepage.* Available from: http://www.hpat-ireland.acer.edu.au/ index.php?option=com_content&view=frontpage&Itemid=1.

81. *RCSI FAQ.* Available from: http://www.rcsi.ie/index.jsp? 1nID=93&pID=99&nID=1438.

82. *CAO application handbook.* Available from: http://www.cao.ie/index.php? page=downloads

83. *Royal College of Surgeons Ireland, graduate entry medicine.* Available from: http:// www.rcsi.ie/index.jsp?1nID=93&pID=99&nID=1438.

84. *Trinity College Dublin undergraduate prospectus.* Available from: http://www.tcd.ie/ Admissions/undergraduate/.

85. *Atlantic Bridge website.* Available from: http://www.atlanticbridge.com/.

86. *Royal College of Surgeons Ireland, FAQ.* Available from: http://www.rcsi.ie/index.jsp? 1nID=93&pID=99&nID=1438.

87. Lenovytska, O., *"Top 200 Ukraine" in 2009.* Available from http://dt.ua/projects/ top200/articles/60393 through google translate, 2010.

88. *Manual for interviewers 2006, McMaster University.* Available from: http:// www.acupunctureprogram.com/articles/Manual_for_Interviewers_2006.pdf.

89. *McMaster University - Undergraduate MD program admission page.* Available from: http://65.39.131.180/ContentPage.aspx?name=Admissions_Interviews.

90. *McMaster University, Faculty of Medicine interview information.* Available from: http:// fhs.mcmaster.ca/mdprog/interviews.html.

91. *Queen's University Belfast MMI interview examples.* Available from: www.qub.ac.uk/ schools/mdbs/medicine/Prospectivestudents/MultipleMiniInterviews/.

92. *University of Michigan career services, medical school interview preparation.* Available from: http://www.careercenter.umich.edu/students/med/mainterviews.html under "2. Peruse resources to familiarize yourself with current issues in medical education and practice [PDF].".

93. *The University of Western Ontario - Medicine admission webpage.* Available from: http://www.schulich.uwo.ca/education/admissions/medicine/.

94. *Dalhousie University Medical School webpage.* Available from: http://dlm.cal.dal.ca/_MEDI.htm#3.

95. *University of Toronto, Faculty of Medicine financial aid.* Available from: http://www.md.utoronto.ca/students/finance/financialaid/.

96. *University of Manitoba, faculty of medicine, admission webpage.* Under 'Applicant Information Bulletin']. Available from: http://www.umanitoba.ca/faculties/medicine/admissions/index.html.

97. *Medical and dental student bursary eligibility.* NHS Business Services Authority; Available from: www.nhsbsa.nhs.uk/Students/3262.aspx.

98. *Student Loan Company website.* Available from: http://www.slc.co.uk/.

99. *Obtained from a call with Student Loan Company.*

100. *NHS career website.* Available from: http://www.nhscareers.nhs.uk/details/Default.aspx?Id=553.

101. *Thinking of Going to Uni in 2012.* UK Department for Business Innovation and Skills; Available from: www.bis.gov.uk/assets/biscore/higher-education/docs/t/11-789-thinking-of-uni-2012-financial-support.pdf.

102. *Student loans.* Direct.gov; Available from: www.direct.gov.uk/en/EducationAndLearning/UniversityAndHigherEducation/StudentFinance/Applyingforthefirsttime/DG_171539.

103. *University of Manchester, funding information.* Available from: http://www.manchester.ac.uk/undergraduate/funding/home/residualincome/.

104. *Student Loan Company 2010 Statistics report.*

105. AAMC, *Tuition and Student Fees, First-Year Medical School Students 2010-2011.* Available from: services.aamc.org/tsfreports/select.cfm?year_of_study=2011, 2011.

106. Hopkins, K., *10 Medical Schols That Lead to Most Debt.* Available from: www.usnews.com/education/best-graduate-schools/articles/2011/04/14/10-medical-schools-that-lead-to-most-debt, 2011.

107. *AAMC reporter : With debt on the rise, students and schools face an uphil battle.* january 2008; Available from: http://www.aamc.org/newsroom/reporter/jan08/debt.htm.

108. *Johns Hopkins School of Medicine international student admissions.* Available from: http://www.hopkinsmedicine.org/admissions/intstudents.html.

109. *St George's University - School of Medicine webpage.* Available from: http://www.sgu.edu/som/index.html?opendocument&.

110. *Roos University - Medical School webpage.* Available from: http://www.rossu.edu/medical-school/.

111. *Creighton Medical School, 2008 class profile.* Available from: http://medschool.creighton.edu/medicine/oma/profiles/2008classprofile/index.php.
112. *George Washington School of Medicine admissions handbook.* Available from: http://www.gwumc.edu/edu/admis/
113. *University of Hawaii, John A. Burns School of Medicine admissions.* Available from: http://jabsom.hawaii.edu/JABSOM/admissions/mdprogram.php?l1=mdp&l2=proS
114. *University of Kentucky, College of Medicine admissions FAQ.* Available from: http://www.mc.uky.edu/meded/admissions/faq.asp
115. *American University of the Caribbean - Tuition and fees.* Available from: http://www.aucmed.edu/prospective/tuition-fees.html.
116. *University of Pennsylvania 2008 entering class profile.* Available from: http://www.med.upenn.edu/admiss/2006_class.html
117. *Jefferson Medical College admissions FAQ.* Available from: http://www.jefferson.edu/jmc/admissions/faq.cfm.
118. *St. George's University School of Medicine - tuition and fees.* Available from: http://www.sgu.edu/financial-services/som-tuition.html
119. *University of Bristol - medicine 5 year program.* Available from: http://www.medici.bris.ac.uk/general/Undergraduate/.
120. *Dartmouth Medical School Admissions.* Available from: http://dms.dartmouth.edu/admissions/admission/.
121. *Univerity of Minnesota Medical School pre-med admissions requirements overview* under 'overview (PDF)]. Available from: http://www.meded.umn.edu/admissions/premedday/.
122. *Ross School of Medicine, tuition and fees.* Available from: http://www.rossu.edu/medical-school/files/MedRatesBSClinical0809final.pdf.
123. *SABA School of Medicine - financial aid.* Available from: http://www.saba.edu/admissions_financial.php.
124. *University of Alberta.* Available from: http://www.med.ualberta.ca/education/ugme/admissions/dofm.cfm.
125. *University of Waterloo pre medical website.* Available from: www.uwpremed.uwaterloo.ca/downloads/Ontarian_Medical_Schools.doc
126. *Obtained from speaking with university representative Global Career Makers Delhi,* gcmdelhi@gmail.com, +91 99100 726 05.
127. Kumar, R., *Obtained from speaking with university representative Ace Edvisors, Delhi,* contact@aceedvisors.com, +91 96 79 36 6893.
128. *University of Calgary Admissions.* Available from: www.ucalgary.ca/mdprogram/prospective/admissions.

129.   *University of Manitoba.* Available from: http://www.umanitoba.ca/faculties/medicine/.

130.   *University of Saskatchewan, Medical School Admissions.* available from: http://www.medicine.usask.ca/education/admissions/.

131.   *OMSAS Information.* Available from: http://www.ouac.on.ca/omsas/omsas-answers.html

132.   *McMaster University, Medical School Admissions.* Available from: http://fhs.mcmaster.ca/mdprog/admissions.html.

133.   *Medical School Admissions Requirements, Online Database.* Available from: https://services.aamc.org/30/msar/.

134.   *Queen's University, Medical School Admission.* Available from: http://meds.queensu.ca/undergraduate/prospective_students.

135.   *University of Toronto Handout from OMSAS 2009.* Available from: www.ouac.on.ca/omsas/pdf/toronto.pdf

136.   *McGill University Admission webpage.* Available from: http://www.mcgill.ca/medicine/admissions/criteria/selection/evaluations/.

137.   *Memorial University, medical school admission webpage.* Available from: http://www.med.mun.ca/Admissions/Home.aspx

138.   *University of Cambridge.* Available from: http://www.cam.ac.uk/admissions/undergraduate/courses/medicine/.

139.   *University of East Anglia.* Available from: http://www.uea.ac.uk/med/course/mbbs.

140.   *Barts and the London School of Medicine and Dentistry, Queen Mary, University of London.* Available from: http://www.smd.qmul.ac.uk/admissions/medicine/index.html.

141.   *King's College London - Medicine Graduate Entry Programme.* Available from: http://www.kcl.ac.uk/ugp09/programme/649.

142.   *King's College London - Medicine 5 year course.* Available from: http://www.kcl.ac.uk/ugp09/programme/85.

143.   *Imperial College London, 4-year program.* Available from: http://www1.imperial.ac.uk/medicine/teaching/undergraduate/ge/.

144.   *Imperial College London, 6-year program.* Available from: http://www1.imperial.ac.uk/medicine/teaching/undergraduate/medicine/.

145.   *St George's Hospital Medical School - Graduate Stream entry requirements.* Available from: http://www.sgul.ac.uk/students/undergraduate/medicine/mbbs-gep.cfm.

146.   *University College London.* Available from: http://www.ucl.ac.uk/medicalschool/index.shtml.

147.   *University of Birmingham, 4-year program.* Available from: http://www.medicine.bham.ac.uk/ug/gec/guidance.shtml.

148. *University of Birmingham, 5-year program.* available from: http://www.medicine.bham.ac.uk/ug/mbchb/.

149. *Keele University, applicant brochure.* Available from: http://www.keelemedicalschool.org.uk/keele_medical_school/resources/MedSch_Brochure.pdf.

150. *Keele University - Medical School - Admissions and Entry Criteria.* Available from: http://www.keele.ac.uk/depts/ms/undergrad/courseinfo/entryrequirements.htm.

151. *University of Leicester - Graduate Entry Program.* Available from: http://www.le.ac.uk/ugprospectus/courses/medicine/main.html.

152. *University of Nottingham - Graduate Entry Medicine webpage.* Available from: http://www.nottingham.ac.uk/mhs/gem/students/index.php.

153. *University of Nottingham - Facutly of medicine and health science webpage.* Available from: http://www.nottingham.ac.uk/mhs/.

154. *University of Warwick - Graduate Entry Medicine.* Available from: http://www2.warwick.ac.uk/fac/med/study/ugr/.

155. *Hull York Medical School.* Available from: http://www.hyms.ac.uk/.

156. *University of Leeds, School of Medicine.* Available from: http://www.leeds.ac.uk/medicine/mbchb/.

157. *Newcastle University, medicine admissions brochure.* Available from: http://mbbs.ncl.ac.uk/public/admissions/.

158. *Newcastle University, 5-year program.* Available from: http://www.ncl.ac.uk/undergraduate/course/A100/Medicine_and_Surgery.

159. *University of Sheffield.* Available from: www.shef.ac.uk/medicine/prospective_ug/applying.

160. *University of Liverpool, 4 year program.* Available from: http://www.liv.ac.uk/study/undergraduate/courses/A101.htm.

161. *University of Manchester School of Medicine.* Available from: http://www.medicine.manchester.ac.uk/.

162. *Brighton and Sussex medical school.* Available from: http://www.bsms.ac.uk/undergraduate/index.php.

163. *Oxford University, 4-year program.* available from: http://www.medsci.ox.ac.uk/study/medicine/courses/accelerated.

164. *University of Oxford - Graduate Entry Medicine - prospectus.* Available from: http://www.medsci.ox.ac.uk/study/medicine/courses/prospectus.pdf/at_download/file.

165. *Oxford University, 6 year program.* Available from: http://www.medsci.ox.ac.uk/study/medicine/courses/preclin.

166. *University of Southampton.* Available from: http://www.som.soton.ac.uk/undergrad/course/.

167. *University of Southampton - School of Medicine Brochure.* Available from: http://www.som.soton.ac.uk/undergraduates/pdf/BM-programmes.pdf.

168. *University of Bristol School of Medicine.* Available from: http://www.bris.ac.uk/medical-school/.

169. *University of Bristol, 2011 prospectus.* Available from: http://www.bristol.ac.uk/prospectus/undergraduate/2011/sections/MDYF/dept_intro.

170. *Peninsula medical School - Admissions.* Available from: http://wdbdev.pcmd.ac.uk/pms/undergraduate/apply.php.

171. *University of Dundee, medicine admissions.* Available from: http://www.dundee.ac.uk/medschool/undergraduate/admissions.

172. *University of Edinburgh, medical school admissions.* Available from: http://www.ed.ac.uk/schools-departments/medicine-vet-medicine/undergraduate/medicine/applying/how-to-apply.

173. *University of Glasgow.* Available from: www.gla.ac.uk/faculties/medicine/undergraduatestudy/medicine/mbchbdegreeprogramme.

174. *University of St. Andrews.* Available from: http://medicine.st-andrews.ac.uk/prospectus/index.aspx.

175. *Cardiff University.* Available from: http://medicine.cf.ac.uk/en/degree-programmes/undergraduate/.

176. *Cardiff University, 2011 undergraduate prospectus.* Available from: http://www.cardiff.ac.uk/for/prospective/ug/prospectus/.

177. *University of Wales, Swansea.* Available from: http://www.swansea.ac.uk/medicine/GraduateEntryMedicineProgramme/.

178. *Queen's University Belfast.* Available from: http://www.qub.ac.uk/schools/mdbs/ProspectiveStudents/.

179. *University of Split.* Available from: http://www.mefst.hr/default.aspx?id=47.

180. *University of Zagreb.* Available from: http://mse.mef.hr/.

181. *Charles University in Prague, Faculty of Medicine in Pilsen.* Available from: http://web.lfp.cuni.cz/studies/studies and http://www.lfp.cuni.cz/study_english.aspx.

182. *Charles University in Prague, First Faculty of Medicine.* Available from: http://www.lf1.cuni.cz/en.

183. *Charles University, 3rd Faculty of Medicine.* Available from: http://old.lf3.cuni.cz/english/.

184. *Masaryk University.* Available from: http://www.med.muni.cz/index.php?id=9.

185. *Palacky University*. Available from: http://www.upol.cz/en/faculties/faculty-of-medicine-and-dentistry.

186. *University of Pécs*. Available from: http://www.pote.hu/index.php?&nyelv=eng.

187. *Semmelweis University*. Available from: http://english.sote.hu/.

188. *University of Szeged, Albert Szent-Györgyi Medical University*. Available from: http://www.szote.u-szeged.hu/AOK/eng/.

189. *University College Cork*. Available from: http://www.ucc.ie/.

190. *University College Dublin, 4-year program*. Available from: https://myucd.ucd.ie/admission/med_graduate.ezc.

191. *University College Dublin, 5 and 6-year programs*. Available from: https://myucd.ucd.ie/program.do?programID=18.

192. *National University Ireland, Galway*. Available from: http://www.nuigalway.ie/courses/undergraduate-courses/surgery-obstetrics.html.

193. *University of Limerick, medical school website*. Available from: http://www2.ul.ie/web/WWW/Faculties/Education_%26_Health_Sciences/Departments/Graduate_Medical_School.

194. *Trinity College Dublin*. Available from: http://medicine.tcd.ie/education/undergraduate/admissions/.

195. *Medical Academy of Bialystok, English Division*. Available from: http://ed.umb.edu.pl/.

196. *Medical University in Bydgoszcz*. Available from: http://www.amb.bydgoszcz.pl/

197. *Medical University of Gdansk, MD Programme admissions*. Available from: http://www.admission.mug.edu.pl/1447.html.

198. *Medical University of Lodz*. Available from: http://www.umed.lodz.pl/eng/.

199. *Medical University of Lublin*. Available from: http://www.umlub.pl/index2.html.

200. *Jagiellonian University Medical College*. Available from: https://www.erk.uj.edu.pl/en/studia/katalog.

201. *Pomeranian Academy of Medicine*. Available from: http://www.ams.edu.pl/english/english-program.

202. *Poznan University School of Medicine, MD program*. Available from: http://ump.edu.pl/eng.

203. *Medical University of Silesia*. Available from: http://www.smk.sum.edu.pl/.

204. *Medical University of Warsaw*. Available from: http://www.wum.edu.pl/english/.

205. *Carol Davila University of Medicine and Pharmacy*. Available from: www.univermed-cdgm.ro.

206. *Gr.T.Popa University of Medicine and Pharmacy Iasi* Available from: http://www.umfiasi.ro/umf/ie2/navigation.jsp?node=2784#.

207. *Iuliu Hatieganu University of Medicine and Pharmacy.* Available from: http://www.umfcluj.ro/en.

208. *University of Oradea, Faculty of Medicine admissions.* Available from: http://medfarm.uoradea.ro/eadmit.htm.

209. *Ovidius University of Constanta.* Available from: http://www.medcon.ro/en-offer.php.

210. *University of Medicine and Pharmacy of Targu Mures.* Available from: www.umftgm.ro/.

211. *Victor Babeş University of Medicine and Pharmacy.* Available from: http://www.umft.ro/newpage/en/index.htm.

212. *Comenius University in Bratislava, Faculty of Medicine in Bratislava.* Available from: www.fmed.uniba.sk/index.php?id=633.

213. *Comenius University in Bratislava, the Jessenius Faculty of Medicine in Martin.* Available from: http://eng.jfmed.uniba.sk/.

214. *Pavol Jozef Šafárik University in Košice.* Available from: http://www.upjs.sk/en/.

215. *Bogomolets National Medical University.* Available from: http://nmu.edu.ua/eng/e10.php.

216. *Bukovinian State Medical University.* Available from: http://www.bsmu.edu.ua/en/index.asp.

217. *Crimea State Medical University.* Available from: http://www.crsmu.com/.

218. *Danylo Halytsky Lviv State Medical University.* Available from: http://www.meduniv.lviv.ua/index.php?lang=en.

219. *Kharkov State Medical University.* Available from: http://www.univer.kharkov.ua/en.

220. *Lugansk State Medical University* Available from: http://www.lsmu.com.

221. *I. Y. Gorbachevsky Ternopil State Medical University.* Available from: http://www.tdmu.edu.te.ua/eng/general/index.php.

222. *M. Gorky Donetsk National Medical University.* Available from: http://www.donmeduni.com/.

223. *Odessa State Medical University.* Available from: http://www.odmu.edu.ua/index.php?v=1190.

224. *MCAT essentials.*